NORTHEAST COMMUNITY COLLEGE LIBRARY

WITHDRAWN

D1569475

RUMEN MICROBIOLOGY

Rumen Microbiology

Burk A. Dehority

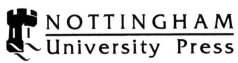
NOTTINGHAM
University Press

Nottingham University Press
Manor Farm, Main Street
Thrumpton, Nottingham, NG11 0AX, UK

NOTTINGHAM

First published 2003
© BA Dehority

All rights reserved. No part of this publication
may be reproduced in any material form
(including photocopying or storing in any
medium by electronic means and whether or not
transiently or incidentally to some other use of
this publication) without the written permission
of the copyright holder except in accordance with
the provisions of the Copyright, Designs and
Patents Act 1988. Applications for the copyright
holder's written permission to reproduce any part
of this publication should be addressed to the publishers.

British Library Cataloguing in Publication Data
A catalogue record for this book is available from the British Library

ISBN 1-897676-99-9

Disclaimer

Every reasonable effort has been made to ensure that the material in this book is true, correct, complete and appropriate at the time of writing. Nevertheless the publishers, the editors and the authors do not accept responsibility for any omission or error, or for any injury, damage, loss or financial consequences arising from the use of the book.

Typeset by Nottingham University Press, Nottingham
Printed and bound by Biddles Ltd, Guildford, Surrey

PREFACE

The motivation for writing this book actually began in 1969, when the decision was made to offer a graduate course in Rumen Microbiology in the Department of Animal Science. Other than Hungate's book "The Rumen and Its Microbes", published in 1966, there were no books available to serve as possible textbooks. In addition, a considerable amount of new information had been reported in the literature since Hungate's book had been published. Thus, information was gathered from various sources, including the most recent Journal publications and a series of lectures was prepared. Each succeeding time the course was taught, an attempt was made to incorporate the new information available in the literature. Eventually these notes evolved into the present book.

The primary objective of teaching a course in rumen microbiology was not to train future rumen microbiologists, but rather to give students an insight into the "black box" of the rumen. Specific questions which I believed needed to be addressed were: (1) What is the anatomy of the gastrointestinal tract of ruminants and other herbivores and how do they differ from non ruminants? (2) What organisms are present in the rumen which convert feed materials, particularly the structural carbohydrates of forage plants, to energy sources which can be utilized by the host animal? (3) What factors effect the rate and extent of microbial digestion? (4) How do the different types of organisms interact with each other? Obviously, the second question was the major one to be addressed, which would involve enumeration, description, activity and factors controlling the concentration of anaerobic protozoa, bacteria and the more recently discovered fungi. Most of the descriptive information on the rumen organisms is based on classical methods of microbiology. However, introduction of the newer techniques of molecular biology should provide the information needed for more precise genotypic classification rather than the phenotypic criteria used previously.

Because the "hands-on" approach is such a powerful learning tool, it was decided that a laboratory section should be included as part of the course. Although at least an undergraduate course in microbiology would be desirable as a prerequisite, the anaerobic techniques needed for culture of the rumen organisms essentially required starting from the beginning with all students. In general, most investigators would suggest that the bacteria are the most important organisms in the rumen fermentation and should be dealt with first. However, I have chosen to present the protozoa first, primarily because it was more appropriate to begin laboratory work with the protozoa. Collection of rumen contents, sampling, and microscopic counting are easier for students to accomplish and allows them a good introduction into lab work.

A working outline of the experiments developed over the years for this course are presented in the Appendix. With appropriate laboratory equipment and facilities, it is hoped that these experiments would be useful to both students and instructors.

CONTENTS

Preface		v
1	Herbivores: animals adapted through microbial fermentation in the gastrointestinal tract to feed solely on plant materials	1
2	Gross anatomy, physiology and environment of the ruminant stomach	19
3	Classification and morphology of rumen protozoa	43
4	Establishment, numbers and diurnal changes in the concentration of rumen protozoa	73
5	Metabolism, nutrition and growth of rumen protozoa	101
6	Distribution, specificity and role of the rumen protozoa	129
7	Rumen bacteria - history, methods of *in vitro* culivation, and discussion of mixed culture fermentations	157
8	Cellulose digesting rumen bacteria	177
9	Species of rumen bacteria active in the fermentation of hemicelluose	209
10	Pectin-fermenting species of rumen bacteria	229
11	Starch digesters, other less numerous species and facultative anaeorbes in the rumen	243
12	Numbers, factors affecting the population and distribution of rumen bacteria	265
13	Rumen fungi	267
14	Additional metabolic activities and interactions among rumen microoganisms	321
Appendix		347
Index		365

CHAPTER 1

HERBIVORES: ANIMALS ADAPTED THROUGH MICROBIAL FERMENTATION IN THE GASTROINTESTINAL TRACT TO FEED SOLELY ON PLANT MATERIALS

In the evolution of the herbivores, there was a failure to develop enzymes capable of attacking cellulose and other complex plant polysaccharides (Moir, 1965; Bauchop, 1977; Dehority, 1986). Cellulose, potentially the most abundant energy source in the world for animals, consists of glucose units joined together by ß 1-4 glycosidic linkages. Hemicellulose primarily consists of xylose units linked together by ß 1-4 xylosidic linkages, with lesser amounts of arabinose, glucose, galactose, rhamnose and glucuronic acids. Pectin, the other major carbohydrate in plants is a rather heterogenous molecule, containing α 1-4 linked polymers of galacturonic acid plus small amounts of galactose, glucose, arabinose and glucuronic acids (Whistler and Smart, 1953).

As a means of obtaining energy from these plant polysaccharides, the herbivores have developed a symbiotic relationship with anaerobic microorganisms (bacteria, protozoa and fungi). Two major types of herbivores have evolved, the ruminant and ruminant-like animals, which have a pre-gastric microbial fermentation of plant material, and another group of animals in which fermentation occurs in the hindgut (Moir, 1965; Hungate, 1966; Bauchop, 1977). Evolution and anatomy of the digestive tract of herbivores has been reviewed by Hume and Warner (1980) and Dehority (1986).

Herbivore types

HINDGUT FERMENTATION

An excellent review of hindgut fermentation in mammals has been published by Hume (1997), in which he compares movement of fluid and particulate material through the hindgut (large and small intestine) to chemical reactors. Chemical reactors are defined on the basis of whether the input is continuous or intermittent, and whether or not the reactants are mixed prior to entering the reactor. The different types of chemical reactors are diagrammatically illustrated in Figure 1.1. The small intestine is similar to a plug-flow reactor, with a continuous flow through a tubular reaction chamber where material mixes radially but not along the flow axis. There is thus a continuous decrease in reactant concentration and an increase in end product concentration from the inlet to outlet. Continuous flow stirred-tank reactors are characterized by the continuous flow of material through a spherical reaction vessel of small volume. The concentration of the reactants is immediately reduced as it enters the vessel. Composition tends to be uniform throughout

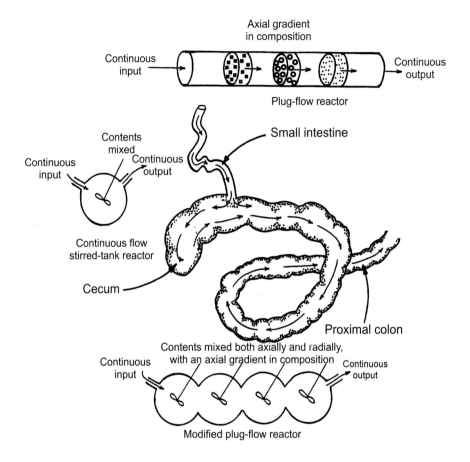

Figure 1.1. Three different types of chemical reactors and their relationship to movement of particulate matter through the hindgut (redrawn with modifications from Hume, 1997).

the reactor, not changing with time. Flow of digesta through diverticula such as the cecum would best fit the stirred-tank model. If several stirred-tank reactors were connected in sequence, flow characteristics would be intermediate between the plug-flow and stirred-tank reactor. Hume (1989) refers to this as a "modified plug-flow reactor." In this system, incoming reactants are mixed both radially and axially, i.e., within each vessel-like section and along the axis. The antiperistaltic and the peristaltic contraction in the proximal colon results in digesta movement similar to a modified plug-flow reactor. Obviously, these models are oversimplifications of the more complex systems which actually occur biologically; however, they do provide insight about composition and flow of digesta through the hindgut.

Insects

Insects which feed on living, dead or decomposing plant material have developed an enlarged pouch in the hindgut in which plant structural carbohydrates can be degraded by microbial activity (Kane, 1997). Figure 1.2 compares a typical insect digestive tract with that of a wood-eating termite. The paunch region in the wood-eating termite has a pH which ranges from 6 to 7.5 and a redox potential between -50 to -270 mV, conditions which are favorable for an anaerobic fermentation. Apparently flagellate protozoa hydrolyze wood polysaccharides and ferment liberated glucosyl units to acetate, H_2 and CO_2. The termite is able to use acetate as a source of carbon and energy and acetogenic bacteria convert most of the H_2 and CO_2 to acetate; however, some CH_4 is also produced.

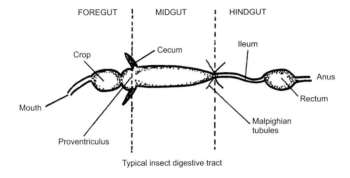

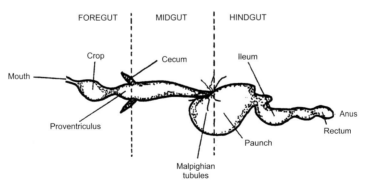

Figure 1.2. Comparison of a typical insect digestive tract with that of the wood-eating termite, *Reticulitermes flavipes* (redrawn from from Kane, 1997).

In some species of termites which are devoid of hindgut protozoa, there is evidence which suggests that the termites themselves may produce cellulase (Slaytor, 1992); however, other gut microorganisms are apparently required to utilize the resulting oligosaccharides. All attempts to isolate cellulolytic bacteria from the hindgut of termites have failed (Varma et al., 1994); however, Schäfer et al. (1996) recently were able to isolate a number of hemicellulose-degrading bacteria and yeasts from the paunch of termites.

One genus of cockroach, *Cryptocercus*, feeds strictly on wood and harbors cellulolytic protozoa in its hindgut. Many other species of insects feed on plants, but the more refractile components like lignocellulose are excreted unchanged (Kane, 1997).

Fish and reptiles

Although anaerobic microorganisms are present in the posterior intestine of herbivorous fish and reptiles, their ability to digest lignocellulosic materials appears to be extremely limited. Hindgut chambers, present in some species, are well separated from the rest of the gut (Clements, 1997; Bjorndal, 1997).

Birds

Microorganisms have been found throughout the entire length of the avian digestive tract; however, there is little evidence that any appreciable amount of cellulose digestion occurs in most species of birds (Vispo and Karasov, 1997). Several exceptions to this would be found in the hoatzin, the ratites (ostriches, emus and rheas) and geese. The hoatzin (*Opisthocomus hoazin*), a leaf-eating bird from northern South America, has an enlarged foregut (crop), where an extensive amount of microbial cellulose digestion occurs (Grajal et al., 1989).

Two species of ratites, the ostrich and rhea, have enlarged ceca which harbors a large microbial population capable of digesting dietary cellulose. Concentrations of obligately anaerobic bacteria between 10^{10} and 10^{11}/g of wet weight have been reported to occur in cecal contents (Mead, 1989). Colon fermentation also occurs in the ostrich, where microbial numbers surpassed those in the cecum and were similar to concentrations in the rumen (Swart et al., 1993b). However, concentrations of cellulolytic bacteria were much lower. Figure 1.3 presents diagrammatic sketches of the hindgut anatomy in the ostrich, rhea and emu. Ostriches and rheas are herbivorous, i.e., adaptable grazers/browsers, eating mainly grasses, leaves and new shoots from shrubs and trees. The emu however is an opportunistic feeder, feeding primarily on fruits, seeds, flowers, insects and young forages (Angel, 1996). The enlarged ceca in the ostrich and rhea obviously slow down rate of passage which in turn allows adequate time for microbial activity. Digesta retention time in the ostrich has been estimated at 48 h (Swart et al., 1987; 1993a), compared to 5.5 h in the emu (Herd and Dawson, 1984). Capacity of the cecum and colon in the ostrich hindgut is approximately 40%, as compared to 6 and 10 % in the emu and rhea, respectively (Cho et al., 1984; Skadhauge et al., 1984).

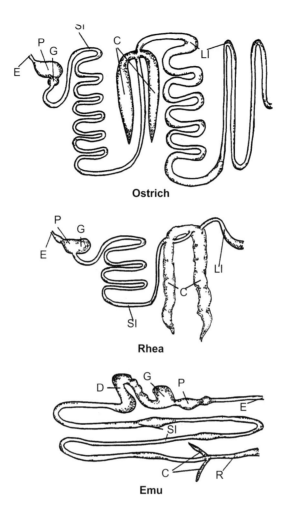

Figure 1.3. Diagrammatic sketches of the gastrointestinal tracts of the ostrich, rhea and emu. C - ceca; E - esophagus; G - gizzard; LI - large intestine; P - proventriculus; R - rectum; SI - small intestine (redrawn from Cho *et al.*, 1984; Skadhauge *et al.*, 1984; Swart *et al.*, 1987).

Cellulose digestibilities ranging from 18 to 45% have been reported to occur in the hindgut of Canada geese as well as barnacle and snow geese (Buschbaum et al., 1986; Prop and Vulink, 1992; Sedinger *et al.*, 1995).

In general, cellulolytic bacteria have been reported to occur in a wide number of other avian species (chickens, ducks, geese, turkeys and grouse); however, as pointed out by Vispo and Karasov (1997), the isolation of cellulolytic bacteria does not prove that digestion of cellulose is of importance to the host. The concentration of cellulose and overall composition of the ingesta entering the ceca and hindgut, as well as the rate of short-chain fatty acid production by these organisms, may severely limit their nutritional contribution.

6 *Rumen microbiology*

Mammals

There are two major types of hindgut fermenting mammals, i.e., cecum fermentors and colon fermentors (Hume and Warner, 1980). In the cecum fermentation model, an enlarged cecum retains solutes and small particles for fermentation. The less digestible fibrous particles pass rapidly on through the large intestine, allowing utilization of a high fiber diet without the encumbrance of a large hindgut. This is an advantage for smaller animals because of the relationship between body size and food requirements. The rabbit, guinea pig, capybara, tapir and warthog are the most common cecum fermentors. Larger herbivores such as the horse, ass, zebra, rhinoceros and elephant, are the colon fermenting type, where contents of the cecum and colon mix freely and act as one large fermentation vat. These differences are illustrated in Fig. 1.4, which compares the hindgut anatomy of the rabbit (cecum fermentation), horse (cecum-colon fermentation) and sheep (foregut fermentation). Relative capacity of the different compartments as a percent of the total digestive tract are also shown (Parra, 1978, Argenzio, 1984).

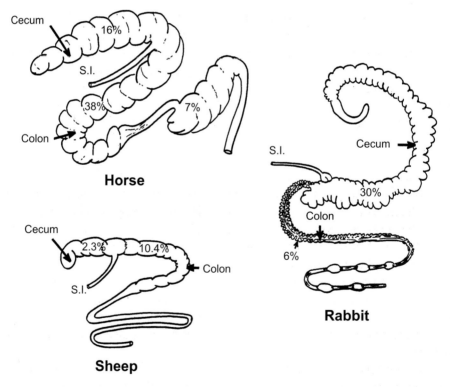

Figure 1.4. Hindgut anatomy of the rabbit (cecum fermentation), horse (cecum and colon fermentation) and sheep (foregut fermentation). S.I. - small intestine. Figures redrawn with modifications from Van Soest (1982). Capacities of the individual organs, as a percent of the total gastrointestinal tract, are shown. Note that the colon of the horse is divided into two well separated segments by the pelvic flexure (the ventral or proximal colon and the dorsal or distal colon).

Cellulolytic bacteria, isolated in pure culture from cecal contents of both the guinea pig and rabbit, have been identified as atypical species of ruminococcus (Hall, 1952; Dehority, 1977). Davies (1964) isolated several cultures of cellulolytic bacteria from the hindgut of the horse in 1964; however, the species were not identified. In a more recent study, bacterial concentrations were determined in various segments of the gastrointestinal tract of 11 horses by Mackie and Wilkens (1988). Mean concentrations in the small intestine were 1.96, 8.07 and 25.50 x 10^6 per g of contents in the duodenum, jejunum and ileum, respectively. Much higher concentrations were found in the cecum and colon, 21.20 and 12.70 x 10^8 per g of contents. Total and functional groups of bacteria were also determined in cecum and colon contents of a single horse and white rhinoceros. Total culturable counts per g of ingesta in the cecum and colon, respectively, were 6.0 and 3.5 x 10^8 in the horse and 15.8 and 1.4 x 10^8 in the white rhino. In both organs, cellulolytic and hemicellulolytic numbers were higher in the horse than the white rhino. The horse was fed on natural mixed grass pasture, while the rhino was shot in the wild. Whether the differences between the two species is real or based on diet remains to be determined.

Moore and Dehority (1993) determined total and cellulolytic bacterial concentrations in cecum and colon contents of six ponies, both when they were faunated and subsequently defaunated. Total bacterial concentrations in the cecum and colon when faunated were 9.17 and 32.4 x 10^8 per g of contents, respectively. When defaunated, mean concentrations were 11.4 and 15.1 X 10^8, respectively. These values are fairly similar to those reported from the horse by Mackie and Wilkens (1988). The mean percentage cellulolytic bacteria in faunated animals at both sites was 1.4% compared to 5.8% in the defaunated animals.

The microflora in the gastrointestinal tract of two species of wild monkeys, vervet and samango, in the family Cercopithecidae was studied by Bruorton *et al.* (1991). In contrast to monkeys in the family Colobinae, which have four compartments in their stomach and carry out a pre-gastric fermentation, the Cercopithecidae have a simple stomach with an enlarged, sacculated cecum and colon. Since their diet contains leaves and other foliar material, it seemed likely that a microbial fermentation might occur somewhere in the hindgut. Culturable counts in the cecum and colon ranged from 0.78 to 4.47 x 10^{10} per g of contents, which is considerably greater than the concentrations previously reported from the hindgut of the horse. A fairly high percentage of bacterial isolates, particularly from the cecum and colon of the samango monkey, were able to digest carboxymethyl cellulose, which is indicative of their possible ability to digest insoluble cellulose.

Low numbers of ciliate protozoa have been observed in the cecum of the guinea pig, while quite high concentrations have been found in the capybara and other larger herbivores. However, species of hindgut protozoa differ markedly from those of the rumen and the majority are classified within separate families (Hungate, 1966; Dehority, 1986).

In the case of the rabbit and other rodents, soft feces are excreted, which are immediately reingested (coprophagy). The soft feces differ from the rest of the fecal output, which is not consumed (McBee, 1977). By this procedure, the deficiencies of the hindgut fermentation such as limited absorption and loss of synthesized microbial protein are overcome. Limited coprophagy has also been observed with horses, particularly with foals. Inoculation of the gut of the young animal appears to take place by ingestion of feces from its mother (McBee, 1977; Hörnicke and Björnhag, 1980).

Although probably not of major importance, a definite hindgut fermentation occurs in ruminants. Partially digested materials may undergo further digestion in the hindgut and contribute to the overall efficiency of digestion in ruminants (McBee, 1977; Hume and Warner, 1980). DM digestibilities, ranging from 10.7 to 23.4%, were measured in the hindgut of sheep by Lewis and Dehority (1985). The highest amount of digestion occurred when an all-hay diet was fed. It has generally been assumed, though not known with any degree of certainty, that the rumen and cecal fermentation are somewhat similar. This idea would be supported by the fact that bacteria isolated from cecal contents of both ruminants and non-ruminants are similar to the predominant ruminal species (Hall, 1952; Davies, 1964; Mann and Ørskov, 1973; Ulyatt *et al.*, 1975; Dehority, 1977; Lewis and Dehority, 1985).

FOREGUT FERMENTATION

With the evolutionary development of multi-chambered stomachs, pre-gastric microbial fermentations became established (Dehority, 1997). In general, these additional chambers are non-glandular and are thought to have been derived from the esophagus or cardiac region of the stomach. Food materials in these chambers are separated from the acid conditions in the pyloric region of the stomach, thus allowing microbial growth. The Hamster rat probably has the simplest multi-chambered stomach, essentially consisting of two chambers connected by a narrow orifice (Moir, 1965). The langur monkey, and other Old World monkeys of the subfamily Colobinae, possess multi-chambered stomachs (Hill, 1952; Kuhn, 1964; Bauchop, 1977). The langur monkey's stomach contains four compartments, the first two of which harbor an extensive microbial fermentation. However, rumination has not been observed (Bauchop, 1977). The two-toed and three-toed tree sloths are both polygastric, possessing stomachs with three separate chambers (Bauchop, 1977). It is of interest that ciliate protozoa have not been observed in the stomachs of any of the above described ruminant-like species.

Various stages of foregut evolution can be found in the suborder Suina. Stomach anatomy ranges from that of the simple stomach in the pig to the development of small blindsacs or pouches in the peccary and finally to the large complex stomach of the hippopotamus (Figure 1.5). No microbial fermentation occurs in the highly acid single compartment of the pig's stomach. A limited bacterial fermentation occurs in the first three compartments of the peccaries' stomach (anterior and upper blindsacs and the gastric pouch). The pH in these compartments is around 6.0, compared to much lower values in the glandular stomach. Protozoa were not observed in any of the compartments (Dehority, 1997). The hippopotamus stomach contains four chambers (Moir, 1965; Bauchop, 1977). Food passing from the esophagus enters into a small chamber, which has openings into two large chambers or diverticula and the tubular body of the stomach. The large tubular chamber has an esophageal groove along its lesser curvature that leads to the pyloric portion which is well separated from the fermentative section. A large population of both bacteria and ciliate protozoa are present. Although the protozoa are fairly unique, they do belong to the same family as the protozoa occurring in the hindgut of the horse rather than those commonly found in the rumen (Thurston and Grain, 1971; Thurston and Noirot-Timothée, 1973; van Hoven, 1974).

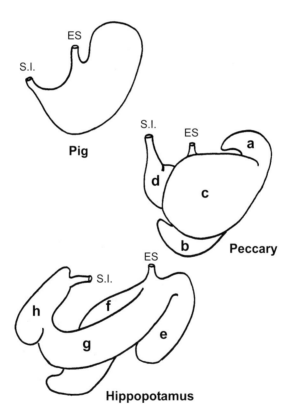

Figure 1.5. Forestomach anatomy in the suborder Suina. Key: ES - esophagus; S.I. - small intestine Peccary: (a) anterior blindsac; (b) upper blindsac; (c) gastric pouch; (d) glandular stomach (redrawn from Bauchop, 1977). Hippopotamus: (e) left diverticulum; (f) right diverticulum; (g) anterior stomach; (h) posterior stomach, pyloric section (redrawn from Langer, 1976).

10 *Rumen microbiology*

The foregut of the macropod marsupials (quokka, wallaby, kangaroo) is anatomically quite different. Four separate regions, not externally visible, can be observed internally and appear to correspond to functionally distinct areas (Bauchop, 1977). Fig. 1.6 illustrates the type of stomach which occurs in the kangaroo. The sacciform forestomach, sometimes called the anterior blindsac or gastric cecum is anterior to the entrance of the esophagus, followed by an elongated portion called the tubiform forestomach, which is heavily sacculated on the outer curvatures. Stomach contents range in pH from 4.6 to 8 and an extensive microbial fermentation takes place in the sacculated region. The inner or lesser curvature has an esophageal groove which bypasses the fermentation area. Relatively high concentrations of both bacteria and protozoa are present in the stomach ingesta (Bauchop, 1977; Dehority, 1996).

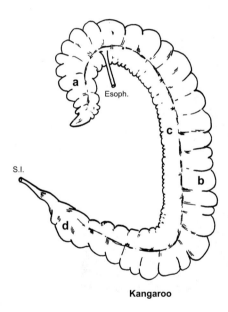

Figure 1.6. Diagrammatic sketch of the kangaroo stomach. ESOPH. - esophagus; S.I. - small intestine; (a) sacciform forestomach; (b) tubiform forestomach (lined with an epithelium of mucous secreting cardiac glands); (c) esophageal groove area (lined with smooth stratified epithelium); (d) pyloric region (redrawn from Van Soest, 1982)

Pseudoruminants

Old World camels and the related camelids in the New World (llama, alpaca, vicuña and guanaco) are classified in a separate family from ruminants, and sometimes referred to as pseudoruminants. Although they do ruminate, distinct morphological differences in their multi-chambered stomach separates them from true ruminants (Figure 1.7). The camel stomach contains three compartments: the first compartment is quite large, containing about 83% of the total gastric volume. A smaller second chamber and an elongated third compartment, which contains a small, well separated pyloric region at its terminal end, contain 6% and 11% of the total gastric volume, respectively (Bauchop, 1977; Moir, 1968; Vallenas *et al.*, 1971). An esophageal groove is present which terminates at the opening to the third compartment. The first compartment in the camel stomach is lined with smooth stratified epithelium, except in the bottom portion where recessed glandular saccules are present. The smooth stratified epithelial lining extends into the second compartment; however, most of the surface is lined with papillated glandular mucosa. Although the exact function of the secretory cells is unknown, evidence suggests that they probably secrete both mucous and buffers. Glands similar to those in the first two compartments are found in the initial four-fifths of the elongated third compartment, with gastric and pyloric glands in the final one-fifth. The camelid stomach contains a large bacterial and ciliate protozoal population, quite similar to that of ruminants (Dogiel, 1926 and 1928; Lubinsky, 1964; Selim *et al.*, 1996; Kubesy and Dehority, 2002).

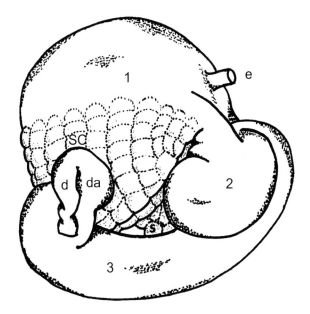

Figure 1.7. Diagrammatic sketch of the llama stomach. (1) first compartment; (2) second compartment; (3) third compartment; (d) duodenum; (da) duodenal ampulla; (e) esophagus; (s) sacculated area in cranial sac; (sc) sacculated area in caudal sac. Redrawn from Vallenas et al. (1971). From Dehority (1997).

The fatty acid composition of depot fats in both the hippopotamus and camel are similar to those of the ruminant animal, containing a high percentage of stearic acid and odd-numbered n-fatty acids. Supposedly these arise through the microbial hydrogenation of dietary unsaturated C_{18} fatty acids and by intestinal digestion of microbial structural

12 Rumen microbiology

lipids. Moir (1965) and Bauchop (1977) have used the composition of depot fats as one criteria for the existence of a pre-gastric fermentation.

Preruminants

The chevrotains, sometimes called preruminants, are similar to the pseudoruminants in that they also have three stomach compartments. However, in contrast, the first two compartments are entirely lined with stratified squamous epithelium. They are differentiated from true ruminants in that they lack an omasum and are classified in a separate family, Tragulidae. There are two genera: *Hyemoschus,* which contains a single species, *aquaticus,* is called the water chevrotain and is found in Africa; the second genera, *Tragulus,* contains six species, which occur in India and southeast Asia, and are commonly known as mouse deer (Church, 1976; Dehority, 1997). Mouse deer are about half the size of the water chevrotain, weighing between 2.5 and 4.0 kg with an overall length of about 0.5 m (Walker, 1964). A diagrammatic sketch of the chevrotain stomach is shown in Figure 1.8.

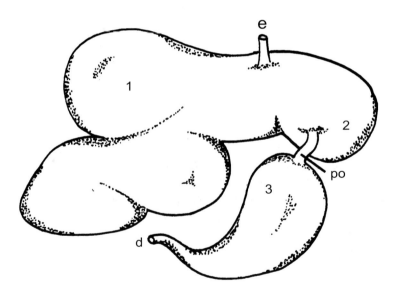

Figure 1.8. Diagrammatic sketch of the chevrotain stomach. (1) rumen; (2) reticulum; (3) abomasum; (d) duodenum; (e) esophagus; (po) preomasum. Redrawn from Moir (1968). From Dehority (1997).

Conclusions

Animals with a pre-gastric fermentation derive three important nutritional advantages from the presence and activities of the microorganisms. First, cellulose and other plant polysaccharides not normally hydrolyzed by the constitutive enzymes of the animal are brought into solution and become available as energy sources. Thus, the volume of dry matter passing onto the post-rumen portion of the gut is markedly reduced. Second, the microbial population can utilize non-protein nitrogen for growth, converting it into microbial protein which is in turn available to the animals dietary amino-acid pool. Third, vitamin synthesis by the microbial population makes the animal virtually independent of dietary sources of all vitamins, except A and D.

The majority of herbivores in the world are ruminants, i.e., their stomach has four distinct compartments (rumen, reticulum, omasum and abomasum) and they ruminate or regurgitate and rechew their food. (Hungate, 1966; Church, 1969, 1976; Hofmann, 1988). Anatomy, physiology and environment of the ruminant stomach are presented in detail in Chapter 2.

References

Angel, C. R. (1996) A review of ratite nutrition. *Animal Feed Science and Technology*, **60,** 241-246.

Argenzio, R. A. (1984) Introduction to gastrointestinal function. In: Dukes' *Physiology of Domestic Animals*. Edited by M. J. Swenson. Cornell University Press, Ithaca, NY. USA. pp. 262.

Bauchop, T. (1977) Foregut fermentation. In: *Microbial Ecology of the Gut*. Edited by R. T. J. Clarke and T. Bauchop. Academic Press, New York, NY. USA. pp. 223-250.

Bjorndal, K. A. (1997) Fermentation in reptiles and amphibians. In: *Gastrointestinal Microbiology – Vol. 1*. Edited by R. I. Mackie and B. A. White. Chapman & Hall, New York, NY. USA. pp. 199-230.

Bruorton, M. R., C. L. Davis and M. R. Perrin. (1991) Gut microflora of vervet and samango monkeys in relation to diet. *Applied and Environmental Microbiology*, **57,** 573-578.

Buchsbaum, R., J. Wilson and I. Valiela. (1986) Digestibility of plant constituents by Canada geese and Atlantic brant. *Ecology*, **67,** 386-393.

Cho, P., R. Brown and M. Anderson. (1984) Comparative gross anatomy of ratites. *Zoo Biology*, **3,** 133-144.

Church, D. C. (1969) *Digestive Physiology and Nutrition of Ruminants*. Vol. 1. O.S.U. Book Stores Inc., Corvallis, OR. USA.

Church, D. C. (1976) *Digestive Physiology and Nutrition of Ruminants*. Vol. 1. Second Edition. O.S.U. Book Stores, Inc., Corvallis, OR. USA.

Clements, K. D. (1997) Fermentation and gastrointestinal microorganisms in fishes. In: *Gastrointestinal Microbiology – Vol 1*. Edited by R. I. Mackie and B. A. White. Chapman & Hall, New York, NY. USA. pp. 156-198.

Davies, M. E. (1964) Cellulolytic bacteria isolated from the large intestine of the horse. *Journal of Applied Bacteriology*, **27**, 373-378.
Dehority, B. A. (1977) Cellulolytic cocci isolated from the cecum of guinea pigs (*Cavia porcellus*). *Applied and Environmental Microbiology*, **33**, 1278-1283.
Dehority, B. A. (1986) Protozoa of the digestive tract of herbivorous mammals. *Insect Science and its Application*, **7**, 279-296.
Dehority, B. A. (1996) A new family of entodiniomorph protozoa from the marsupial forestomach, with descriptions of a new genus and five new species. *Journal of Eukaryotic Microbiology*, **43**, 285-295.
Dehority, B. A. (1997) Foregut fermentation. In: *Gastrointestinal Microbiology - Vol. 1*. Edited by R. I. Mackie and B. A. White. Chapman & Hall, New York, NY. USA. pp. 39-83.
Dogiel, V. A. (1926) Sur quelques infusoires nouveaux habitant l'estomac du dromadaire (*Camelus dromadarius*). *Annales de Parasitologie*, **4**, 241-271.
Dogiel, V. A. (1928) La faune d'infusoires habitant l'estomac du buffle et du dromadaire. *Annales de Parasitologie*, **6**, 328-338.
Grajal, A., S. D. Strahl, R. Parra, M. G. Dominguez and A. Neher. (1989) Foregut fermentation in the hoatzin, a neotropical leaf-eating bird. *Science* **245**, 1236-1238.
Hall, E. R. (1952) Investigations on the microbiology of cellulose utilization in domestic rabbits. *Journal of General Microbiology*, **7**, 350-357.
Herd, R. M. And T. J. Dawson. (1984) Fiber digestion in the emu, *Dromaius novaehollandiae*, a large bird with a simple gut and high rates of passage. *Physiological Zoology*, **57**, 70-84.
Hill, W. C. O. (1952) The external and visceral anatomy of the olive colobus monkey (*Procolobus verus*). *Proceedings of the Zoological Society of London*, **122**, 127-186.
Hofmann, R. R. (1988) Anatomy of the gastrointestinal tract. In: *The Ruminant Animal, Digestive Physiology and Nutrition*. Edited by D. C. Church. Prentice Hall, Englewood Cliffs, NJ. USA. pp. 14-43.
Hörnicke, H. and G. Björnhag. (1980) Coprophagy and related strategies for digesta utilization. In: *Digestive Physiology and Metabolism in Ruminants*. Edited by Y. Ruckebusch and P. Thivend. MTP Press, Lancaster, UK. pp. 707-730.
Hume, I. D. (1989) Optimal digestive strategies in mammalian herbivores. *Physiological Zoology*, **62**, 1145-1163.
Hume, I. D. (1997) Fermentation in the hindgut of mammals. In: *Gastrointestinal Microbiology - Vol. 1*. Edited by R. I. Mackie and B. A. White. Chapman & Hall, New York, NY. USA. pp. 84-115.
Hume, I. D. and A. C. I. Warner. (1980) Evolution of microbial digestion in mammals. In: *Digestive Physiology and Metabolism in Ruminants*. Edited by Y. Ruckebusch and P. Thivend. MTP Press, Lancaster, UK. pp. 665-684.
Hungate, R. E. (1966) *The Rumen and Its Microbes*. Academic Press, New York, NY. USA.

Kane, M. D. (1997) Microbial fermentation in insect guts. In: *Gastrointestinal Microbiology - Vol. 1*. Edited by R. I. Mackie and B. A. White. Chapman & Hall, New York, NY. USA. pp. 231-265.

Kubesy, A.A. and B.A. Dehority. (2002) Forestomach ciliate protozoa in Egyptian dromedary camels (*Camelus Dromedarius*). *Zootaxa*, **51,** 1-12.

Kuhn, H.-J. (1964) Zur Kenntnis von bau und funktion des Magens der Schlankaffen (Colobinae). *Folia Primatologica,* **2,** 193-221.

Langer, P. (1976) Functional anatomy of the stomach of *Hippopotamus amphibius* L.1758. *South African Journal of Science,* **72,** 12-16.

Lewis, S. M. and B. A. Dehority. (1985) Microbiology and ration digestibility in the hindgut of the ovine. *Applied and Environmental Microbiology.* **50,** 356-363.

Lubinsky, G. (1964) Ophryoscolecidae of a guanaco from the Winnipeg Zoo. *Canadian Journal of Zoology,* **42,** 159.

McBee, R. H. (1977) Fermentation in the hindgut. In: *Microbial Ecology of the Gut*. Edited by R. T. J. Clarke and T. Bauchop. Academic Press, New York, NY. USA. pp. 185-222.

Mann, S. O. and E. R. Ørskov. (1973) The effect of rumen and post-rumen feeding of carbohydrates on the cecal microflora of sheep. *Journal of Applied Bacteriology,* **36,** 475-484.

Mackie, R. I. and C. A. Wilkens. (1988) Enumeration of anaerobic bacterial microflora of the equine gastrointestinal tract. *Applied and Environmental Microbiology*, **54,** 2155-2160.

Mead, G. C. (1989) Microbes of the avian cecum: types present and substrates utilized. *Journal of Experimental Zoology*, **3(suppl),** 48-54.

Moir, R. J. (1965) The comparative physiology of ruminant-like animals. In: *Physiology of Digestion in the Ruminant*. Edited by R. W. Dougherty. Butterworth, Inc., Washington, DC. USA. pp. 1-14.

Moir, R. J. (1968) Ruminant digestion and evolution. In: *Handbook of Physiology*. Edited by C. F. Code. Sect. 6, Vol. 5. American Physiological Society, Washington, D.C. USA. pp. 2673-2694.

Moore, B. E. and B. A. Dehority. (1993) Effects of diet and hindgut defaunation on diet digestibiltiy and microbial concentrations in the cecum and colon of the horse. *Journal of Animal Science*, **71,** 3350-3358.

Parra, R. (1978) Comparison of foregut and hindgut fermentation in herbivores. In: *The Ecology of Arboreal Folivores*. Edited by G. G. Montgomery. Smithsonian Institution Press, Washington, D.C. USA. pp. 205-229.

Prop, J. And T. Vulink. (1992) Digestion by barnacle geese in the annual cycle: the interplay between retention time and food quality. *Functional Ecology*, **6,** 180-189.

Schäfer, A., R. Konrad, T. Kuhnigk, P. Kämpfer, H. Hertel and H. König. (1996) Hemicellulose-degrading bacteria and yeasts from the termite gut. *Journal of Applied Bacteriology*, **80,** 471-478.

Sedinger, J. S., R. G. White and J. Hupp. (1995) Metabolizability and partitioning of energy and protein in green plants by yearling lesser snow geese. *Condor*, **97**, 116-122.

Selim, H. M., S. Imai, O. Yamato, E. Miyagawa and Y. Maede. (1996) Ciliate protozoa in the forestomach of the dromedary camel (*Camelus dromedarius*), in Egypt, with description of a new species. *Journal of Veterinary Medical Science*, 58, 833-837.

Skadhauge, E., C. N. Warui, J.M.Z. Kamau and G.M.O. Maloiy. (1984) Functions of the lower intestine and osmoregulation in the ostrich: preliminary anatomical and physiological observations. *Quarterly Journal of Experimental Physiology*, **69**, 809-818.

Slaytor, M. (1992) Cellulose digestion in termites and cockroaches: what role do symbionts play? *Comparative Biochemistry and Physiology,* **103B,** 775-784.

Swart, D., R. I. Mackie and J. P. Hayes. (1987) For feathers and leathers. *Nuclear Active, International Journal of the Atomic Energy Corporation. No. 36,* **36,** 2-9.

Swart, D., R. I. Mackie and J. P. Hayes. (1993a) Influence of live mass, rate of passage and site of digestion on energy metabolism and fibre digestion in the ostrich. *South African Journal of Animal Science,* **23,** 119-126.

Swart, D., R. I. Mackie and J. P. Hayes. (1993b) Fermentative digestion in the ostrich. (*Struthio camelus* var. *domesticus*). *South African Journal of Animal Science*, **23,** 127-135.

Thurston, J. P. and J. Grain. (1971) Holotrich ciliates from the stomach of *Hippopotamus amphibius* with descriptions of two new genera and four new species. *Journal of Protozoology,* **18,** 133-141.

Thurston, J. P. and C. Noirot-Timothée. (1973) Entodiniomorph ciliates from the stomach of *Hippopotamus amphibius* with descriptions of two new genera and three new species. *Journal of Protozoology,* **20,** 562-565.

Ulyatt, M. J., D. W. Dellow, C. S. W. Reid and T. Bauchop. (1975) Structure and function of the large intestine of ruminants. In: *Digestion and Metabolism in the Ruminant.* Edited by I. W. McDonald and A. C. I. Warner. University of New England Publishing Unit, Armidale, Australia. pp. 119-133.

Vallenas, A., J. F. Cummings and J. F. Munnell. (1971) A gross study of the compartmentalized stomach of two new-world camelids, the llama and guanaco. *Journal of Morphology*, **134,** 399-424.

van Hoven, W. (1974) Ciliate protozoa and aspects of the nutrition of the hippopotamus in the Kruger National Park. *South African Journal of Animal Science,* **70,** 107-109.

Van Soest, P. J. (1982) *Nutritional Ecology of the Ruminant.* O & B Books, Inc. Corvallis, OR. USA.

Varma, A., B. K. Kolli, J. Paul, S. Saxena and H. König. (1994) Lignocellulose degradation by microorganisms from termite hills and termite guts: A survey on the present state of art. *FEMS Microbiology Reviews,* **15,** 9-28.

Vispo, C. And W. H. Karasov. (1997) The interaction of avian gut microbes and their host: an elusive symbiosis. In: *Gastrointestinal Microbiology – Vol 1.* Edited by R. I. Mackie and B. A. White. Chapman & Hall, New York, NY. USA. pp. 116-155.

Walker, E. P. (1964) *Mammals of the World.* Vols. I and II. Johns Hopkins University Press, Baltimore, MD. USA.

Whistler, R. L. and C. L. Smart. (1953) *Polysaccharide Chemistry.* Academic Press, New York, NY. USA.

CHAPTER 2

GROSS ANATOMY, PHYSIOLOGY AND ENVIRONMENT OF THE RUMINANT STOMACH

Rumen-reticulum

The ruminant stomach lies on the left side of the abdominal cavity, occupying about 3/4 of the total space (Church, 1969, 1976; Hofmann, 1988). The gross anatomy is shown in Figure 2.1.

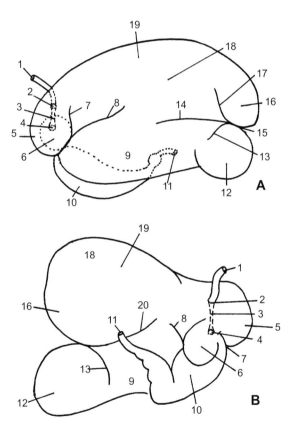

Figure 2.1. Diagrammatic sketch of the ruminant stomach; A - left side, B - right side. Key: (1) esophagus; (2) cardia or esophageal opening; (3) esophageal groove; (4) reticulo-omasal opening; (5) reticulum; (6) omasum; (7) rumino-reticular fold; (8) cranial groove; (9) ventral sac; (10) abomasum; (11) duodenum; (12) caudo-ventral blind sac; (13) ventral coronary groove; (14) left longitudinal groove; (15) caudal groove; (16) caudo-dorsal blind sac; (17) dorsal coronary groove; (18) dorsal sac; (19) rumen; (20) right longitudinal groove. Drawn from photographs and illustrations in Church (1969, 1976) and Hoffman (1988).

The interior of the rumen itself is divided into sacs by the reticulo-ruminal fold and various pillars, which are marked by shallow grooves on the external surface. These pillars aid in the contraction of the various sacs and thus circulate and mix the ingesta. The epithelial lining of the reticulum is raised into folds forming a honeycomb structure, while the rumen itself is lined with papillae of varying size and shape. Papillae are most dense in the ventral parts of the cranial and ventral sacs, presumably where the most absorption occurs. When food is eaten by the animal, it enters into the reticulum from the esophagus and passes back into the rumen area. Orderly and synchronized contractions occur in the rumen-reticulum, which aid in mixing newly ingested food, regurgitation, eructation of gas and movement of food on into the omasum.

In young nursing animals, the milk flows down the reticular or esophageal groove and passes directly into the omasum. Lips or folds of tissue on each side of the groove come together forming a closed tunnel which leads directly from the end of the esophagus (cardia) to the reticulo-omasal orifice. Closure of the groove, the esophageal groove reflex, primarily occurs in the young animal and is thought to be stimulated by suckling (Ruckebusch, 1988). Ørskov and Benzie (1969), studying the esophageal groove reflex in young lambs accustomed to sucking from a teat before weaning, found that any liquid suspension sucked from a bottle passed entirely into the abomasum. This was demonstrated using $BaSO_4$ in protein suspensions and taking radiographs of the animals. The response could be demonstrated in sheep up to 12 months of age. In a further study, it was found that reflex closure of the groove could be maintained in lambs weaned from their mother and trained to drink small meals from a trough (Ørskov et al., 1970). The lambs clearly distinguished between the liquid suspension brought to them in a trough at feeding time and the drinking water always present in an identical trough. The former they consumed with eager excitement, the latter they quietly sipped from time to time. The authors concluded that the trough feed, like a teat-bottle feed was accepted as a substitute for suckling and not associated with the relief of thirst. Thus, they believe the reflex closure of the groove can be conditioned by the feeding procedure adopted at weaning so that it no longer depends on the stimuli associated with sucking and swallowing.

Abe et al. (1979) were able to maintain reflex closure of the groove in calves up till 16 weeks of age by feeding a warm liquid milk substitute either from a nipple-pail or open bucket. After training with the milk-substitute up to 4 weeks of age, closure could be effected by drinking warm water from the bucket. The *ad lib* feeding of solid food (roughage and concentrate) or giving of cold water did not disturb reflex closure of the groove up to 16 weeks of age. Experimentally this technique could be of use in studies where it is desirable for the nutrients to bypass fermentation in the rumen, i.e. evaluation of various protein sources (Potter et al., 1972).

OMASUM

The interior of the omasum is partially filled by longitudinal folds or leaves, which are diagrammatically illustrated in Figure 2.2. The spaces between the leaves are generally packed very tightly with finely divided ingesta. A groove extends along the lower side of the omasum, from the reticulo-omasal opening to the omaso-abomasal opening. Small particles of ingesta and fluids can either pass directly down this groove into the abomasum or move up between the leaves. The surface area of the omasal leaves has been estimated to equal to about 1/3 of the total forestomach in the bovine (Church, 1969, 1976).

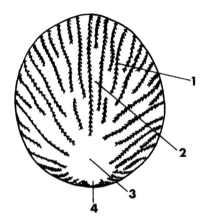

Figure 2.2. Diagrammatic sketch of omasal cross section. Key: (1) omasal leaves or laminae; (2) interlaminar recesses; (3) omasal canal; (4) omasal groove (redrawn after Hofmann, 1988).

ABOMASUM

Ingesta passes from the omasum into the abomasum or "so-called" true stomach, which connects the omasum with the small intestine. A constriction divides the interior of the abomasum into the fundus and pyloric regions. In contrast to the other portions of the multi-chambered stomach, which are lined with non-glandular epithelia, the fundus is lined with a true mucosa containing specialized secretory or glandular cells which produce pepsin and hydrochloric acid. Fewer glandular cells are present in the pyloric region; however, these are the cells which are believed to produce mucin. The pyloric sphincter is located at the posterior end of the abomasum, regulating the passage of digesta into the small intestine (Church, 1969, 1976; Hofmann, 1988).

From the abomasum on, the digestive tract of the ruminant is quite similar to that of the non-ruminant. Thus, the unique aspects of the ruminant stomach which set it apart from other mammalian orders lie in the first three stomach compartments, i.e., the rumen, reticulum and omasum.

FISTULATION OF THE RUMINANT STOMACH

One of the most useful techniques in studying the physiology of the ruminant stomach has been through the use of fistulas, or surgical openings into the various stomach compartments. Fistulation of the rumen is a relatively simple operation which is generally performed in two stages (Johnson, 1966). First an incision is made in the body wall on the left side, behind the ribs and below the lumbar area. This is followed by blunt dissection through the muscle layers to the surface of the rumen. The muscle layers are sutured back by stitches through the body wall, peritoneum and surface of the rumen, taking care not to puncture the rumen. The wall of the rumen is scarified and the body wall is sewn up and allowed to heal for a week to 10 days during which time the rumen wall adheres to the body wall. In essence, a hernia has been formed at that spot. The second stage involves a small surgical opening through this area into the rumen and insertion of a cannula. The wound then heals and a permanent opening into the rumen is obtained.

Omasal, abomasal and duodenal fistulas are also used, but surgical techniques are a bit more complex and the fistulas tend to be useful for shorter periods of time.

Ingestion and passage of feed through the rumen

INGESTION AND RUMINATION

Ingested feed is usually chewed only enough to mix the food with saliva and form a bolus of a suitable size and consistency to swallow easily. The bolus is projected into the stomach with considerable force and is deposited in the anterior portion of the rumen, in the area of the reticulo-ruminal fold. Although not thoroughly understood at present, animals will consume a large amount of feed quickly and then spend a fairly long time in the process of rumination. This involves a series of steps, i.e., regurgitation of the ingesta from the reticulo-rumen, swallowing of regurgitated liquids, re-chewing of solids accompanied by further salivary secretion and finally re-swallowing of the bolus (Hungate, 1966; Church, 1969, 1976; Ruckebusch, 1988). Several theories have been developed to explain why animals ruminate: (1) the predator theory, that is after eating in the open the animal retreats to a safe place to rest and rechew the food; (2) addition of oxygen to the ingesta, stimulating the growth of facultative anaerobes; (3) increases passage rate into the omasum; and (4) decreases forage particle size. The arguments for and against these theories are discussed in detail by Gordon (1968) and Dehority (1997). Whether one or a combination of the reasons listed, or some other as yet unknown reason is responsible for rumination, this process has enabled a large group of herbivores to survive and multiply in environments where only poor-quality forages were available.

Saliva plays an important role in the ruminant animal, both in the original ingestion of feed and subsequent rumination. With the exception of feeding on lush pasture, feed is often dry and may even be of a powdery nature that would be extremely difficult to swallow if not for the moistening effect of saliva. Fairly high concentrations of both sodium and potassium bicarbonate and phosphate are found in saliva, which help buffer the acids produced during fermentation in the rumen. In addition, nitrogen, primarily as urea, mucin, phosphorus, magnesium and chlorine are also present in fairly high concentration, and undoubtedly serve as a readily available supply of nutrients to the microorganisms. Recycling of nitrogen in the saliva can be very important in instances of low dietary nitrogen intake. The quantity of saliva produced per day, depends on the type and quantity of feed, ranging from about 5-15 liters for sheep and 75-190 liters for cattle (Hungate, 1966; Church, 1969, 1976, 1988).

The amount of time an animal spends ruminating is thought to be controlled by the particle size of the ingesta. For example, feeding only grain or finely ground roughage results in cessation of rumination. If an animal is fed hay through a fistula rather than by mouth, rumination time is increased. An excellent series of studies on rumination in sheep have been published by Welch and Smith (1968, 1969a, b, 1970) and Welch *et al.*, (1970). Briefly they found that marked diurnal patterns occurred in rumination time, the peak activity taking place during the night. Fasting caused a rapid decline in normal rumination activity, which ceased entirely after 36 hours. Rumination was initiated soon after the first meal following a fast. During an average 24 hour period, their animals spent approximately 6 hours eating (chopped forage fed twice a day at 15% excess), 9 hours ruminating and 9 hours idle. Poor quality roughage with high fiber content caused an increase in rumination time. Rumination time increased with increased size of single meals and was higher than for an equal weight of hay fed continuously. In subsequent studies with cattle, decreasing forage quality increased rumination time, and a difference in rumination time was observed between four breeds of dairy cattle fed an identical ration.

PASSAGE OF INGESTA FROM THE RUMEN-RETICULUM

Level of intake, particle size, specific gravity, and concentration of solids all appear to be factors which can influence the rate of ingesta movement through the reticulo-rumen (Hungate, 1966; Church, 1969, 1976; Owens and Goetsch, 1988). Rumen solids turnover times in cattle have been observed to range from 1.3 to 3.7 days, with most values averaging about 2.1 to 2.7 days or 50-60 hours. Turnover times are somewhat less in sheep, ranging from 0.8 to 2.2 days with the majority of values being slightly over one day.

Rumen volumes and fluid turnover rates were measured in the same sheep fed either 100% hay or 60% corn-40% hay at equal dry matter intakes (Grubb and Dehority, 1975). Rumen volume decreased in two of the three sheep when the concentrate ration was fed; however, no significant differences were observed in fluid turnover rate (Tables 2.1 and 2.2). In contrast, dry matter turnover time was significantly longer when the concentrate diet was fed (Table 2.3). However, dry matter digestion was also significantly higher with the concentrate diets. This apparent discrepancy is explained on the basis that when feed consumption is constant the rumen can contain undigested residues from a greater amount of highly digested feed, i.e., more daily ration allotments than when feed digestibility is low. Thus, when turnover rate is based on an indigestible component, such as lignin in this case, the solids turnover time for concentrate feed may actually be longer. It is suggested that under these circumstances fluid turnover rate may be a better index of rumen function (Hungate, 1966).

Table 2.1. EFFECT ON RUMEN VOLUME OF FEEDING AN EQUAL WEIGHT (800 g) OF EITHER ORCHARDGRASS HAY OR 60% CRACKED CORN-40% ORCHARDGRASS HAY TO THE SAME SHEEP[a]

Diet	Sheep no.	Rumen volume (liters)[b]		
		1	2	3
Orchardgrass hay		6.45 ± 0.47^x	5.96 ± 0.35	5.13 ± 0.17^x
60% cracked corn-40% orchardgrass hay		4.78 ± 0.10^y	5.72 ± 0.25	4.54 ± 0.14^y

[a]Data from Grubb and Dehority (1975).
[b]Mean and standard error of the mean.
[x,y]Means within a column followed by different superscripts are significantly different at $P<0.05$.

Table 2.2. EFFECT ON RUMEN FLUID TURNOVER RATE OF FEEDING AN EQUAL WEIGHT (800 g) OF EITHER ORCHARDGRASS HAY OR 60% CRACKED CORN-40% ORCHARDGRASS HAY TO THE SAME SHEEP[a]

Diet	Sheep no.	Fluid turnovers per day[b]		
		1	2	3
Orchardgrass hay		1.62 ± 0.08	1.43 ± 0.06	1.77 ± 0.10
60% cracked corn-40% orchardgrass hay		1.57 ± 0.07	1.18 ± 0.04	1.63 ± 0.10

[a]Data from Grubb and Dehority (1975).
[b]Mean and standard error of the mean.

Table 2.3. EFFECT ON DIGESTION AND RUMEN DRY-MATTER TURNOVER TIME OF FEEDING AN EQUAL WEIGHT (800 g) OF EITHER ORCHARDGRASS HAY OR 60% CRACKED CORN-40% ORCHARDGRASS HAY TO THE SAME SHEEP[a]

Diet	Digestion in the rumen (%)	Turnover time (days)
Orchardgrass hay	52.5 ± 3.5^x	1.80 ± 0.07^x
60% cracked corn-40% orchardgrass hay	68.4 ± 1.6^y	2.38 ± 0.18^z

[a]Data from Grubb and Dehority (1975).
[x,y]Means within a column followed by different superscripts are significantly different at $P<0.01$.
[x,z]Means within a column followed by different superscripts are significantly different at $P<0.05$.

To evaluate effects of intake level and forage type on ruminal turnover rates, Varga and Prigge (1982) fed alfalfa and orchardgrass to lambs at two levels of intake, 90% of voluntary consumption and 60% of that intake for both forages. Liquid turnover rate was twice as fast at the higher level of intake, i.e., 1.73 vs 0.79. Although solids turnover rates tended to be faster at the higher intake level, the difference was not significant. A similar increase in liquid passage from the rumen of cattle was observed by Haaland and Tyrrell (1982) when intake was increased from maintenance to two times maintenance.

Intake of forages by ruminants is generally considered to be limited by the amount of forage present in the rumen, which in turn reflects the length of time that forage particles are retained in the rumen. Retention of solid particles in the rumen appears to be a function of size, which is primarily reduced by chewing during eating and rumination (Balch and Campling, 1962; Smith *et al.*, 1983; Ulyatt *et al.*, 1986). Little material passes out of the rumen when particle size exceeds 1.0 to 2.0 mm in sheep and between 2.0 to 4.0 mm in cattle. This size does not appear to vary much over a wide range of diets (Ulyatt *et al.*, 1986). These authors concluded that chewing, both during eating and rumination, was the most important process in particle size reduction, and of the two, chewing during rumination played the largest role. They also suggested that particle size reduction may not be the rate limiting step in rumen clearance, but rather the amount of material that passes per contraction of the rumen.

McLeod and Minson (1988) determined the proportions of large forage particles which were broken down to small insoluble particles by primary mastication (eating), rumination, and digestion plus detrition (rubbing). Large particles were defined as those retained during wet sieving on a screen with an aperture of 1.18 mm. Primary mastication was determined by obtaining samples of masticated feed through an esophageal fistula. Breakdown by secondary mastication or rumination was measured by collection of regurgitated digesta after chewing. The quantity of forage broken down by digestion, plus detrition was estimated as the difference between the amount of large particles eaten and the quantity broken down by primary mastication and rumination and the quantity of large particles excreted in the feces, corrected for loss by digestion using the lignin ratio in feed and feces. Based on measurements from four forages fed to steers (separate leaf and stem fractions from rye grass and alfalfa) the mean values for the percentage breakdown of large particles was as follows:

Primary mastication	-	25.5%
Rumination	-	50.1%
Digestion and detrition	-	16.7%
Excreted in feces	-	7.7%

The overall proportion of large particle breakdown was similar for all four forages and did not appear to be related to voluntary intake. These data would clearly support the previous conclusions of Ulyatt *et al.* (1986) on the importance of chewing.

Shaver et al. (1988), studied the effects of feed intake, forage physical form and forage fiber contents on passage of particulate matter. They found that feeding long or chopped hay at low or high feed intake had little influence on particle size in the rumen. They also found that nearly 60% of the ventral rumen and reticulum DM and 40% of the dorsal rumen DM for both long and chopped hay could theoretically pass through the reticulo-omasal orifice. Since chewing time was essentially the same for both the long and chopped hay, they questioned whether particle size is really the rate limiting step in particulate passage from the rumen. The authors concluded that the rate of escape of small particles from the rumen is an important factor in rumen retention time, and may be closely associated with particle specific gravity. The larger, low-density particles may also contribute to mat formation, which could serve to trap the smaller particles.

Further support for the theories on particle passage were reported by Prigge et al. (1990). These authors found that neither passage rate of digesta from the rumen, voluntary intake or diet digestibility were related to particle size of the rumen digesta. Their data also suggested that the threshold size for ruminal passage of particles in cattle was probably between 3 and 5 mm. This would agree with the 2 to 4 mm proposed earlier by Ulyatt et al. (1986). They speculated that intake and digestibility of forage diets may be influenced more by specific gravity, rate of hydration and possibly rate of digestion than by particle size.

Gerson et al. (1988) found that the number of attached bacterial cells per m^2 was much larger for the large particles, although the ml of gas produced per bacterial cell was the same for all particle sizes. This results in a faster rate of fermentation for the larger particles, which would agree with the previously reported results of Ehle et al. (1982), who found particle size reduction to be greatest *in situ* for large particles, decreasing as particle size decreases.

Another factor which influences the passage of particles from the rumen is functional specific gravity (Hooper and Welch, 1985a, b). Functional specific gravity differs from specific gravity in that air- and gas-filled voids or pockets in the particle are not eliminated in the measurement. Specific gravity of particles in the rumen is obviously influenced by entrapped air and gas, and when particle size is reduced the entrapped gasses are released. The functional specific gravity of small particles is thus greater than larger particles and appears to increase at a faster rate in legumes than in grasses. At zero time, about 80% of approximately $200\mu^3$ mixed hay and mature alfalfa particles had a functional specific gravity of less than 0.9; however, this figure was reduced to 28% after 1 h in the rumen and 5.5% after 2 h. After 4 h in the rumen, 50% or more of the feed particles had attained a functional specific gravity exceeding 1.10 which should allow fairly rapid passage out of the rumen. Similar results were obtained in more recent studies by Siciliano-Jones and Murphy (1991) and Wattiaux et al. (1991, 1992).

Using synthetic spheres (polypropylene, lucite and teflon) of different size (.32, .64 and 1.27 cm) and density (.91, 1.34 and 2.30 g/ml), Ehle and Stern (1986) measured the effects of these two factors upon passage rate. In general, both parameters influenced passage rate; however, density appeared to be more important than particle size.

A symposium paper by Welch (1986), "Physical parameters of fiber affecting passage from the rumen," provides an excellent summary of the available information in these areas. Particle size and functional specific gravity appear to be the critical factors affecting passage of particulate matter from the rumen. In general, particles of 0.2 mm or less with a functional specific gravity of about 1.2 appear to have the maximum rate of passage. Particles with functional specific gravities of 1.17 and below (.90 and .96) were the most heavily ruminated. Passage was greatest for particles with functional specific gravities of 1.17 and above (1.42, 1.77 and 2.15). Passage was slightly less for particles with 2.15 specific gravity, which agrees with the results of Ehle and Stern (1986). Apparently specific gravity can be too light or too heavy for particles to pass from the rumen at so-called normal rates. Not only is the composition of rumen fluid a factor in functional specific gravity, but surface chemistry of the particle and water-holding capacity properties of the various fiber components are probably also involved.

Microbial fermentation in the rumen is the primary factor altering the physical form of ingested feed so that particle size and specific gravity are favorable for passage on down the tract. In addition, and equally important, the microflora can convert the otherwise unavailable energy sources in the feed (cellulose, hemicellulose, etc.) to forms which the animal can use.

The rumen environment

The rumen-reticulum has been likened to a large fermentation vat, varying in size from 3-15 liters for sheep and from 35-100 liters for cattle (Church, 1969, 1976; Hofmann, 1988). Through a number of different physiological mechanisms, the host animal maintains a rather constant environment within the rumen; however, the microbial fermentation within the rumen can almost be considered "outside" of the host animal itself. In other words, the animal simply provides a suitable site and feed for the microorganisms. The microbes in turn then provide a pre-gastric digestion service, which in the case of roughage feeds, could not be carried out by the host; an excellent example of symbiosis between the animal and microorganisms. The steady supply of food and continuous removal of microbial fermentation products (VFA, CO_2 and CH_4) and food residues provides ideal conditions for the development and growth of an extremely dense microbial population, which consists of anaerobic bacteria, ciliated protozoa and lower numbers of fungi. The primary factors which influence the growth and activity of the rumen microbial population are temperature, pH, buffering capacity, osmotic pressure, dry matter content and oxidation-reduction potential.

TEMPERATURE

In general, the temperature in the rumen is relatively constant, ranging between 38 and

40°C in normally fed animals (Church, 1969, 1976; Clarke, 1977). The homeothermic maintenance of this relatively high temperature accounts for the rapid fermentation which occurs in the rumen. Immediately after feeding when an active fermentation is occurring, the temperature may rise as high as 41°C, but is usually between 39 and 40.5°C. The only marked change in rumen temperature appears to result from the ingestion of large quantities of cold water or frozen forage. In this case, rumen temperatures can fall from 5-10°C and as long as 1-2 h may be required for the temperature to return to normal; however, this appears to exert little effect on overall food utilization. It should also be noted that the rumen protozoa do not survive temperatures much above 40°C, especially if held at that temperature for an extended period (Hungate, 1966).

pH

Rumen pH is probably one of the most variable factors in the fermentation environment (Hungate, 1966; Church, 1969, 1976; Clarke, 1977). Fluctuations occur with time after feeding, nature of the feed and frequency of feeding. Actually the pH reflects the amount of acids produced by the microflora, as mediated by absorption and buffering capacity of the saliva that is produced. The normal range of pH is approximately between 5.5 and 7.0 with animals fed a so-called "normal" ration. Outer limits on ruminal pH lie between 4.5 and 7.5. With once a day feeding, the minimum pH is generally attained about 2-6 h after feeding, which in turn corresponds to maximum acid production. Ruminal pH, measured just prior to 0800, was found to be higher ($P < 0.01$) in sheep fed once daily at 0800, as compared to sheep fed the same total amount of feed 6 times or 24 times per day (Dehority and Tirabasso, 2001). Some typical pH curves are shown in Fig. 2.3 for two sheep fed once or twice per day. The animals were fed a 35% concentrate diet. Note the variation in response to feeding, both between sheep and between days.

Figure 2.4 is a graph showing the mean rumen pH values from four sheep fed diets ranging in composition from all corn (0% hay) to 100% orchardgrass hay. Measurements were taken on days 14 and 21 after changing diets. The pH curves decrease fairly linearly as the percent corn in the diet increases, except for the 0% and 20% diets. Diets high in soluble carbohydrates which are readily fermentable can reach minimum values of pH 5.0 or lower. The rumen ciliates are more sensitive to pH changes than the bacteria and disappear if pH rises above 7.8 or falls to about 5.0 (Clarke, 1977).

Although most investigators measure pH on fresh rumen contents, work has shown that loss of CO_2 can give pH readings higher than that which exists in the rumen itself. The most accurate method for measurement of rumen pH is probably by the use of a recording pH meter with electrodes inserted into the rumen. Kovacik *et al.* (1986) continuously recorded rumen pH in sheep given ad libitum access once daily for 1.5 h to a 50% hay-50% concentrate diet. Results were calculated as the percentage of time per day that rumen pH was below 6.6, 6.2, 5.8, 5.4 and 5.0. Rumen pH was 5.8 or below

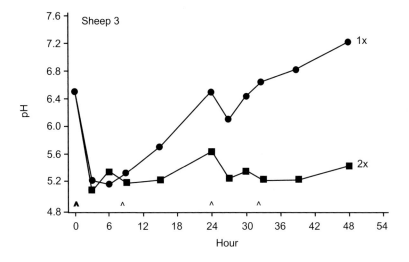

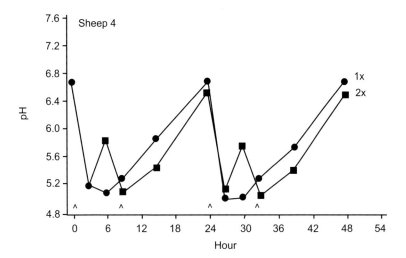

Figure 2.3. Diurnal changes in rumen pH for two sheep fed once a day (1x) at 0 and 24 h or twice a day (2x) at 0, 8, 24 and 32 h (Dehority, unpublished).

for 70% of the day and 5.4 or less for 30% of the day. This latter value is near the minimum pH for a number of rumen bacteria, particularly the cellulolytics. Russell and Dombrowski (1980) have studied the effect of pH on a number of rumen bacteria in continuous culture, and except for the acid-tolerant species *Selenomonas ruminantium* and *Streptococcus bovis*, cell growth is markedly reduced at pH values below 5.5. Growth of the three predominant cellulolytics begins to decrease at about pH 6.5, with washout occurring at pH 5.9, 6.0 and 6.15. It should be noted that the dilution rate for these continuous culture studies was equal to a liquid turnover rate of 4 times per day

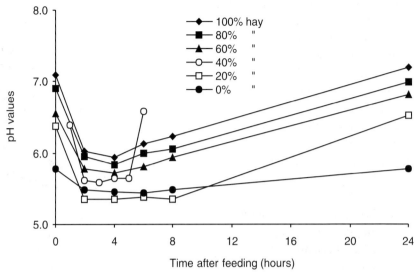

Figure 2.4. Mean rumen pH values for four sheep, each fed diets ranging from 100% corn to 100% orchardgrass hay (Dehority, unpublished).

which is about twice that normally observed *in vivo*. Minimum pH for growth of these three cellulolytics is 5.4, 5.5 and 5.6. Thus, one might expect washout to occur between these two pH values if turnover rate was adjusted to two volume turnovers per day. Hiltner and Dehority (1983) observed that the rate of cellulose digestion for these three species began to decrease markedly at pH values below 6.3-6.4.

BUFFERING CAPACITY

The buffering capacity of rumen contents is quite high, thereby helping to maintain the pH in a range compatible with microbial growth (Hungate, 1966; Church, 1969, 1976, 1988). Those factors affecting the buffering system in the rumen are the amount and composition of parotid saliva secreted and concentration of acid end-products, chiefly VFA and CO_2. Ruminant saliva contains large amounts of bicarbonate and phosphate, and has a pH of 8 or above. These compounds neutralize the VFA produced by the microflora. Salivary production is greater when animals are eating, compared to not eating. Also, the physical nature and moisture content of the feed influence saliva production. With animals fed hay or other dried feeds, it has been estimated that total salivary flow per day will equal the rumen volume. Ruminal infusion of VFA, HCl or H_2O have been reported to have very little effect on salivary flow.

Emmanuel *et al.* (1969) studied the rumen buffering system of sheep fed pelleted roughage-concentrate rations. They found that the buffering capacity of partially neutralized VFA was very high in the pH range of 4-6, exceeding the contribution of bicarbonate and phosphate buffers. Their data also suggested that H_2CO_3 and VFA were both important buffers between pH 5-7. The quantity of phosphate buffers in rumen fluid were inadequate to regulate pH in the 6-8 range.

Rumen buffer systems in dairy cattle under widely different feeding conditions were studied by Counotte et al. (1979). They found bicarbonate and VFA to be the main components in the buffering system, with phosphate having little value as a buffering agent. However, phosphate does neutralize the fermentation acids produced in the rumen.

In the previously mentioned study by Kovacik et al. (1986), three levels of $NaHCO_3$, 1.5, 3.0 and 4.5% were also fed with the 50% hay-50% concentrate diet. The percentage of time per day at pH 5.8 or below decreased from 70% without $NaHCO_3$ to 62, 45 and 15%, respectively, with the three $NaHCO_3$ levels. It is of interest that there were no significant differences in dry matter or organic matter digestibility with addition of $NaHCO_3$. It might be postulated that any difference in rumen digestibility as a result of low pH could have been masked by subsequent fermentation in the hindgut. In a separate study, addition of 4% $NaHCO_3$ significantly increased DM and OM digestibility of an 85% concentrate diet but not with a 70% concentrate diet (Hadjipanayiotou, 1981). Rumen pH, measured 3 h after the morning feeding on the last day of the digestion trial, was not changed by the addition of 4% $NaHCO_3$.

OSMOTIC PRESSURE

Warner and Stacy (1965) have investigated the osmotic pressure of rumen contents and found that prior to feeding, rumen fluid is hypotonic with respect to plasma. Although a good deal of animal variation was observed, rumen fluid osmolality was in the range of 250 mOsm/kg while plasma was around 300 mOsm/kg. Immediately after feeding rumen fluid osmolality rose sharply to values of about 400 mOsm/kg and then gradually decreased to a hypotonic level with respect to plasma in 8-10 hours. Their work indicated that concentration of the potassium ion was primarily responsible for the marked increase in osmolality after feeding. None of their experiments suggested that drinking was regulated to keep the osmotic pressure of either rumen fluid or plasma within specific limits.

Bergen (1972) has studied the possible role of osmotic pressure in altering voluntary feed intake. When rumen osmolality was artificially elevated to above 400 mOsm/kg with NaCl or NaAc, feed intake decreased markedly in sheep. Simultaneous introduction of a local anesthetic with the osmotic load reversed the inhibition of voluntary feed intake. He also found that osmotic pressures greater than 400 mOsm/kg in the medium inhibited *in vitro* cellulose digestion. On the basis of his studies he concluded that although rumen osmotic pressure may affect voluntary feed intake in an experimental model where an osmotic load is introduced, the short duration of elevated osmotic pressure when feeding practical roughage type rations suggests that it is not an important factor in controlling feed intake.

Dehority and Males (1974) studied the effects of osmotic pressure on numbers of holotrich protozoa in sheep, and found a similar rise in osmotic pressure after feeding. Values ranged from about 270 mOsm/kg to a maximum near 400 mOsm/kg about 1 ½ h after feeding. This was followed by a gradual decline back to near normal levels in 5 to 6 h. The increase in osmolality after feeding was reduced during feed restriction. In contrast, marked and prolonged increases in osmolality were observed after feeding when water was restricted. However, after six weeks on water restriction, little, if any, change in osmolality was noted over the five hour postfeeding period. Observation of these animals in the barn revealed that instead of eating their ration within ½ h after feeding as they normally did, they were now spacing their consumption over 12-16 h.

Beauchemin and Buchanan-Smith (1990) measured osmolality of rumen fluid in dairy cows after eating. They observed a rise in osmotic pressure immediately after eating, reaching a peak at about 2 h post feeding and then gradually decreasing. A similar pattern was observed for three methods of feeding, i.e., concentrate (C) followed by silage (S), long hay (H) followed by C and then S, C followed by S and H. In all cases, higher osmotic pressures were recorded when concentrate was fed first. In general, this pattern is quite similar to the previous data reported by Dehority and Males (1974).

DRY MATTER CONTENT

Although one might expect this criteria to be extremely variable, depending on the nature of the feed, when it is measured, drinking behavior, etc., most values reported fall into the range of 10-13%. However, values can range from less than 7% to over 16% (Church, 1969, 1976; Dehority and Purser, 1970; Owens and Goetsch, 1988). In sheep fed at hourly intervals, rumen dry matter was higher, 17.7% ($P < 0.02$), as compared to when they were fed the same amount of feed once daily, 13.2%, or six times daily, 14.6% (Dehority and Tirabasso, 2001).

Thornton and Yates (1968) in studies on water restriction in cattle, found significant differences in dry matter % between water-restricted and unrestricted cattle; however, the magnitude of the difference was quite small and indicated that the dry matter percentage of the rumen was being held quite constant despite large differences in the ratio of total water intake to dry matter intake. In studies by Dehority and Purser (1970) where the ratio of ml water per g of feed varied from approximately 1.7 on unlimited H_2O intake to 1.1 on limited water intake, the dry matter of rumen contents was unchanged.

Studies with tritium-labeled water have shown that there is a rapid exchange of water between rumen contents and blood (Willes et al., 1970). Mean water absorption from the rumen ranged from 37.1 to 70.8 ml/min, insorption into the rumen ranged from 30.5 to 65.0 ml/min, and net water absorption varied from 5.1 to 13.4 ml/min. These values were determined at several postfeeding times. Water exchange from the rumen increased 2-3 h postfeeding and declined after 17 h. Lowering pH of the rumen contents increased the rate of water exchange. In these studies rumen fluid was consistently hypotonic to the blood, thus providing an osmotic gradient for net absorption of water from the rumen. Similar experiments in which rumen fluid was hypertonic to the blood would be of extreme interest.

SURFACE TENSION

Reported values for surface tension of rumen fluid vary from 45-59 dynes per centimeter (Hungate, 1966; Church, 1969, 1976). Surface tension can have a marked affect upon microbial physiology, both beneficial and inhibitory. Low concentrations of surface-active agents are sometimes used in media to enhance bacterial growth; however, several species of rumen bacteria are inhibited by low concentrations of Tween 80 (Minato and Suto, 1978). On the other hand, Dehority and Grubb (1980) found that adding 0.1% of the surfactant Tween 80 to the anaerobic dilution solution increased ($P < 0.05$) the total count of bacteria in rumen contents. Surfactants have also been used in the treatment of bloat; however, some of these agents are anti-protozoal (Church, 1976).

COMPOSITION OF RUMEN GAS

The principal gases in the rumen are CO_2 (65%) and CH_4 (27%), both of which are major end-products of the microbial fermentation in the rumen (Hungate, 1966; Clarke, 1977). Carbon dioxide is also produced from salivary bicarbonate, amino acids and other organic acids. The other gaseous end-product of fermentation is H_2; however, it only occurs at about 0.2% since it is used by the methanogenic bacteria to reduce CO_2 to CH_4. Nitrogen comprises about 7% of the gas mixture with traces of H_2S and CO and low transient quantities of O_2

OXIDATION-REDUCTION POTENTIAL

The oxidation-reduction potential or Eh has the dimension of volts, and a negative Eh is thus an estimate of the reducing intensity or ability to accept hydrogen and electrons. Although the fact that most rumen microorganisms are obligate anaerobes, very little work has been done on the redox potential in rumen contents. Most of the values reported range from about -150 to -350 mv (Clarke, 1977). In a study by Baldwin and Emery (1960), they found that the majority of the reducing substances in rumen contents are associated with feed particles and collodial material, not the bacterial cells. Also, concentration of reducing substances is higher several hours after feeding than at any other time. The addition of limited amounts of oxygen to rumen contents either *in vivo* or *in vitro* does not cause much change in the redox potential or end-products (Church, 1976). Apparently the facultative anaerobes in the rumen, chemical reduction, or both, effectively remove these limited quantities of oxygen. Hungate (1966) suggests that forages, etc., contribute natural reducing substances to the rumen environment, which would agree with the higher concentration of reducing power several hours after feeding. Studies by Males (Ph.D. Thesis, Ohio State University, 1973) would support this conclusion, since the Eh of rumen contents from sheep fed forage was much lower than values observed in animals fed a concentrate type ration.

Aerobic or respiratory microorganisms couple the oxidation of organic substances with the reduction of an inorganic oxidizing agent (electron acceptor) usually oxygen. In anaerobic or fermentative organisms, the energy yielding metabolism of organic substances is accomplished by transfer of hydrogen and electrons to other substrates. The energy obtained from a specific quantity of nutrients is thus much less in anaerobes because oxidation of the substrate is less complete and there is an accumulation of partially oxidized end-products. This concept clearly fits with the normal end-products of rumen fermentation which are chiefly acetate, propionate, butyrate, CO_2 and methane. Most evidence to date suggests that rumen bacteria are able to ferment carbohydrates through the Embden-Myerhoff pathway to pyruvic acid; however, rather than proceeding on through the Krebs tricarboxylic acid cycle which uses molecular oxygen as an electron acceptor, other pathways are employed. For example, two main pathways have been demonstrated in rumen bacteria for the production of acetate from pyruvate. In the first, the clostridial phosphoroclastic type, pyruvate in the presence of coenzyme A and several co-factors is converted to acetyl-phosphate, CO_2 and H_2. Products of the other pathway, the formate phosphoroclastic type, are acetyl-phosphate and formate. Acetyl-phosphate plus ADP yields acetate plus ATP, while formate is converted to CO_2, H_2 and CH_4 (Baldwin, 1965).

Although the toxicity of oxygen to obligate anaerobic bacteria and protozoa is well documented, its mode of toxic action to the cell is unclear. The presence of oxygen in culture media generally causes an increase in redox potential (Morris, 1976); however, Marounek and Wallace (1984) found that oxygen itself and not Eh is the toxic factor in "oxidized" anaerobic growth medium. In pH-controlled anaerobic batch cultures, three species of rumen obligate anaerobic bacteria were able to grow over a wide of Eh values: *Fibrobacter* (*Bacteroides*) *succinogenes*, -290 to +175 mV; *Ruminobacter* (*Bacteroides*) *amylophilus*, -320 to +250 mV and *Selenomonas ruminantium*, -360 to +360 mV. The facultative anaerobe, *Streptococcus bovis* grew over a much wider range, -340 to +414 mV. The authors do point out that their results do not preclude the possibility that the toxic factor could be a product produced in the medium by reaction with oxygen.

Morris (1976) has reviewed the subject of oxygen and the obligate anaerobe in considerable detail. He defines an obligate anaerobe as an organism which is capable of generating energy and synthesizing its substance without recourse to molecular oxygen, and demonstrates a singular degree of adverse sensitivity to oxygen which renders it unable to grow in air at 1 atmosphere. One additional point of interest to this definition is that there is considerable difference between organisms in their sensitivity to oxygen poisoning. Loesche (1969) investigated the growth of a group of anaerobes, including several rumen species, on spread agar plates incubated in artificial atmospheres containing different concentrations of oxygen. His results suggested the occurrence of three subgroups: (a) strict anaerobes which would grow only when the atmosphere contained less than 0.5% O_2; (b) moderate anaerobes which were capable of growth in the presence of oxygen levels as high as 2 to 8%; and (c) microaerophiles which actually require a low concentration of O_2 for growth but cannot grow in air. Classification of anaerobes into one of these groups can be confounded because of different nutrient requirements and resulting differences in media used for oxygen sensitivity tests.

Two main hypotheses have been proposed to explain the toxicity of oxygen to obligate anaerobes (Morris, 1976). The first is that oxygen is toxic because of its excellence as an oxidant. This could inhibit growth as follows: (a) oxygen in the medium interferes with the attainments and maintenance of the proper Eh value required for growth; (b) preferential reduction of exogenous oxygen depletes the organism of reducing power required for biosynthesis; and (c) essential compounds within the cell are subject to "autoxidation". These would include SH compounds, iron sulfur proteins, flavoproteins, etc. Since several moderate anaerobes can withstand exposure to air for considerable periods and then recover completely when anaerobic conditions are restored, oxygenation for short terms appears to be bacteriostatic rather than bactericidal. The second hypothesis contends that oxygen itself is not toxic, but its toxicity results from products of the interaction of oxygen with the organisms and/or components of the culture media. It would follow that aerobes are capable of detoxifying these substances, whereas anaerobes cannot. Toxic products could accumulate in nutrient media exposed to oxygen, i.e., organic peroxides, aldehydes, free radicals, etc. Interaction of oxygen with reduced cell constituents (flavoproteins and iron sulfur proteins) along with the action of certain oxidases produces hydrogen peroxide, superoxide anion, hydroxyl radical and singlet oxygen, all of which are extremely toxic.

Hydrogen peroxide, or the organic peroxides formed in culture media, probably exert their toxic effect through oxidation of free sulfhydral groups of some of the respiratory enzymes to render them inactive. Strong support for this theory would be the observation that strict anaerobes are either lacking or deficient in the enzymes catalase and/or peroxidase, which can decompose hydrogen peroxides and organic peroxides, respectively.

The superoxide anion, a highly reactive free radical produced by the univalent reduction of the oxygen molecule, is produced through interaction of molecular oxygen with reduced flavins, flavoproteins, etc., as well as by the action of enzymes. Several metalloprotein enzymes have been discovered, whose function is to catalyze the "safe" dismutation of the superoxide anion to yield hydrogen peroxide and oxygen. These enzymes, called superoxide dismutases, served as the basis for the superoxide dismutase (SOD) theory of obligate anaerobiosis, which states that the total lack of this enzyme is the prime cause of the aero-intolerance in obligate anaerobes. In general, the aerobic organisms contain SOD and catalase, whereas the strict anaerobes are devoid of these enzymes.

However, low levels of SOD have been found in strict anaerobes along with low levels of catalase activity (Gregory *et al.*, 1978; Rolfe *et al.*, 1978). Superoxide dismutase has also been shown to be inducible, in that the amount of activity increases with higher partial pressures of O_2 (Privalle and Gregory, 1979). This would suggest that the line between aero-tolerant and aero-intolerant organisms cannot be clearly defined on this basis. In a recent study, Jenney *et al.* (1999) measured very high SOD activity in cell-free extracts of an obligate anaerobe, using the standard SOD assay; however, further purification revealed that it's activity was different than SOD. The enzyme, named superoxide reductase (SOR), reduces the superoxide anion to hydrogen peroxide, which is then reduced to water by peroxidases. This contrasts to SOD which generates hydrogen peroxide and oxygen, thus propagating the problem of oxygen toxicity.

The rumen bacterium *Selenomonas ruminantium* possesses an oxygen-inducible NADH oxidase which can be coupled to glucose catabolism to scavenge oxygen from the environment (Wimpeny and Samah, 1978). However, if this system is overloaded, an accumulation of the toxic superoxide anion will result.

Morris (1976) concluded that "no unitary hypothesis predicated on the total absence from the organism of any single protective agent can wholly explain the toxic effects of oxygen on all obligate anaerobes in all media". Even with the information obtained in more recent studies, this would still appear to be a valid conclusion.

Summary

Based on the previous information, we can summarize the physical environment which exists within the rumen as follows:

1. Temperature - 39°C
2. pH - In the general range of 6.4 to 6.6, and fairly well buffered between 5.5 and 7.0.
3. Osmotic pressure - Hypotonic to blood plasma except shortly after feeding. Normally around 250 mOsm/kg, increasing to a peak of 400 mOsm/kg after ingestion of feed.
4. Dry matter content - relatively constant under most feeding conditions, generally in the range of 10-13%.
5. Redox potential - anaerobic, ranging between -150 to -350 mv.

Within the limits of this environment, a diverse population of bacteria, protozoa and fungi live under symbiotic conditions with the host. Although the microorganisms are rather specific for this ecological location, some species of bacteria and protozoa have been found in other sites and will be discussed later.

References

Abe, M., T. Iriki, K. Kondoh and H. Shibui. (1979) Effects of nipple or bucket feeding of milk-substitute on rumen by-pass and on rate of passage in calves. *British Journal of Nutrition,* **41,** 175-181.

Balch, C. C. and R. C. Campling. (1962) Regulations of voluntary food intake in ruminants. *Nutrition Abstracts and Reviews,* **32,** 669-686.

Baldwin, R. L. (1965) Pathways of carbohydrate metabolism in the rumen. In: *Physiology of Digestion in the Ruminant.* Edited by R. W. Dougherty. Butterworth, Inc., Washington, DC. USA. pp. 379-389.

Baldwin, R. L. and R. S. Emery. (1960) The oxidation-reduction potential of rumen contents. *Journal of Dairy Science,* **43,** 506-511.

Beauchemin, K. A. and J. G. Buchanan-Smith. (1990) Effects of fiber source and method of feeding on chewing activities, digestive function, and productivity of cows. *Journal of Dairy Science,* **73,** 749-762.

Bergen, W. G. (1972) Rumen osmolality as a factor in feed intake control of sheep. *Journal of Animal Science,* **34,** 1054-1060.

Church, D. C. (1969) *Digestive Physiology and Nutrition of Ruminants.* Vol. 1. O.S.U. Book Stores Inc., Corvallis, OR. USA.

Church, D. C. (1976) *Digestive Physiology and Nutrition of Ruminants.* Vol. 1. Second Edition. O.S.U. Book Stores, Inc., Corvallis, OR. USA.

Church, D. C. (1988) Salivary function and production. In: *The Ruminant Animal, Digestive Physiology and Nutrition.* Edited by D. C. Church. Prentice Hall, Englewood Cliffs, NJ. USA. pp. 117-124.

Clarke, R. T. J. (1977) The gut and its micro-organisms. In: *Microbial Ecology of the Gut.* Edited by R. T. J. Clarke and T. Bauchop. Academic Press, New York, NY. USA. pp. 36-71.

Counotte, G. H. M., A. Thy. van't Klooster, J. van der Kuilen and R. A. Prins. (1979) An analysis of the buffer system in the rumen of dairy cattle. *Journal of Animal Science,* **49,** 1536-1544.

Dehority, B. A. (1997) Foregut fermentation. In: *Gastrointestinal Microbiology, Vol 1.* Edited by R. I. Mackie and B. A. White. Chapman and Hall, New York, NY. USA. pp. 39-83.

Dehority, B. A. and J. A. Grubb. (1980) Effect of short-term chilling of rumen contents on viable bacterial numbers. *Applied and Environmental Microbiology,* **39,** 376-381.

Dehority, B. A. and J. R. Males. (1974) Rumen fluid osmolality: evaluation of its influence upon the occurrence and numbers of holotrich protozoa in sheep. *Journal of Animal Science,* **38,** 865-870.

Dehority, B. A. and D. B. Purser. (1970) Factors affecting the establishment and numbers of Holotrich protozoa in the ovine rumen. *Journal of Animal Science,* **30,** 445-449.

Dehority, B. A. and P. A. Tirabasso. (2001) Effect of feeding frequency on bacterial and fungal concentrations, pH, and other parmeters in the rumen. *Journal of Animal Science*, **79,** 2908-2912.

Ehle, F. R. and M. D. Stern. (1986) Influence of particle size and density on particulate passage through alimentary tract of Holstein heifers. *Journal of Dairy Science*, **69,** 564-568.

Ehle, F. R., M. R. Murphy and J. H. Clark. (1982) *In situ* particle size reduction and the effect of particle size on degradation of crude protein and dry matter in the rumen of dairy steers. *Journal of Dairy Science*, **65,** 963-971.

Emmanuel, B., M. J. Lawlor and D. M. McAleese. (1969) The rumen buffering system of sheep fed pelleted roughage-concentrate rations. *British Journal of Nutrition*, **23,** 805-811.

Gerson, T., A. S. D. King, K. E. Kelly and W. J. Kelly. (1988) Influence of particle size and surface area on *in vitro* rates of gas production, lipolysis of triacylglycerol and hydrogenation of linoleic acid by sheep rumen digesta or *Ruminococcus flavefaciens*. *Journal of Agricultural Science*, **110,** 31-37.

Gordon, J. G. (1968) Rumination and its significance. *World Review of Nutrition and Dietetics*, **9,** 251-273.

Gregory, E. M., W. E. C. Moore and L. V. Holdeman. (1978) Superoxide dismutase in anaerobes: survey. *Applied and Environmental Microbiology*, **35,** 988-991.

Grubb, Jean A. and B. A. Dehority. (1975) Effects of an abrupt change in ration from all roughage to high concentrate upon rumen microbial numbers in the ovine. *Applied Environmental Microbiology*, **30,** 404-412.

Haaland, G. L. and H. F. Tyrrell. (1982) Effects of limestone and sodium bicarbonate buffers on rumen measurements and rate of passage in cattle. *Journal of Animal Science*, **55,** 935-942.

Hadjipanayiotou, M. (1981) Effect of sodium bicarbonate and of roughages on milk yield and milk composition of goats and on rumen fermentation of sheep. *Journal of Dairy Science*, **65,** 59-64.

Hiltner, P. and B. A. Dehority. (1983) Effect of soluble carbohydrates on digestion of cellulose by pure cultures of rumen bacteria. *Applied and Environmental Microbiology*, **46,** 642-648.

Hofmann, R. R. (1988) Anatomy of the gastrointestinal tract. In: *The Ruminant Animal, Digestive Physiology and Nutrition*. Edited by D. C. Church. Prentice Hall, Englewood Cliffs, NJ. USA. pp. 14-43.

Hooper, A. P. and J. G. Welch. (1985a) Effects of particle size and forage composition on functional specific gravity. *Journal of Dairy Science*, **68,** 1181-1188.

Hooper, A. P. and J. G. Welch. (1985b) Change of functional specific gravity of forages in various solutions. *Journal of Dairy Science*, **68,** 1652-1658.

Hungate, R. E. (1966) *The Rumen and Its Microbes*. Academic Press, New York, NY. USA.

Jenney, F. E., Jr., M. F. J. M. Verhagen, X. Cui and M. W. W. Adams. (1999) Anaerobic microbes: oxygen detoxification without superoxide dismutase. *Science*, **286**, 306-309.

Johnson, R. R. (1966) Techniques and procedures for *in vitro* and *in vivo* rumen studies. *Journal of Animal Science*, **25**, 855-875.

Kovacik, A. M., S. C. Loerch and B. A. Dehority. (1986) Effect of supplemental sodium bicarbonate on nutrient digestibilities and ruminal pH measured continuously. *Journal of Animal Science*, **62**, 226-234.

Loesche, W. J. (1969) Oxygen sensitivity of various anaerobic bacteria. *Applied and Environmental Microbiology*, **18**, 723-727.

McLeod, M. N. and D. J. Minson. (1988) Large particle breakdown by cattle eating ryegrass and alfalfa. *Journal of Animal Science*, **66**, 992-999.

Marounek,M. And R. J. Wallace. (1984) Influence of culture Eh on the growth and metabolism of the rumen bacteria *Selenomonas ruminantium, Bacteroides amylophilus, Bacteroides succinogenes* and *Streptococcus bovis* in batch culture. *Journal of General Microbiology*, **130**, 223-229.

Minato, H. and T. Suto. (1978) Techniques for fractionation of bacteria in rumen microbial ecosystem. II. Attachment of bacteria isolated from bovine rumen to cellulose powder *in vitro* and elution of bacteria attached therefrom. *Journal of General Microbiology*, **24**, 1-16.

Morris, J. G. (1976) Oxygen and the obligate anaerobe. *Journal of Applied Bacteriology*, **40**, 229-244.

Ørskov, E. R. and D. Benzie. (1969) Studies on the oesophogeal groove reflex in sheep and on the potential use of the groove to prevent the fermentation of food in the rumen. *British Journal of Nutrition*, **23**, 415-420.

Ørskov, E. R., D. Benzie and R. N. B. Kay. (1970) The effects of feeding procedure on closure of the oesophageal groove in young sheep. *British Journal of Nutrition*, **24**, 785-795.

Owens, F. N. and A. L. Goetsch. (1988) Ruminal fermentation. In: *The Ruminant Animal, Digestive Physiology and Nutrition*. Edited by D. C. Church. Prentice Hall, Englewood Cliffs, NJ. USA. pp. 145-171.

Potter, E. L., D. B. Purser and W. G. Bergen. (1972) A plasma reference index for predicting limiting amino acids of sheep and rats. *Journal of Animal Science*, **34**, 660-670.

Prigge, E. C., B. A. Stuthers and N. A. Jacquemet. (1990) Influence of forage diets on ruminal particle size, passage of digesta, feed intake and digestibility by steers. *Journal of Animal Science*, **68**, 4352-4360.

Privalle, C. T. and E. M. Gregory. (1979) Superoxide dismutose and O_2 lethality in *Bacteroides fragilis*. *Journal of Bacteriology*, **138**, 139-145.

Rolfe, R. D., D. J. Hentges, B. J. Campbell and J. T. Barrett. (1978) Factors related to the oxygen tolerance of anaerobic bacteria. *Applied and Environmental Microbiology*, **36**, 306-313.

Ruckebusch, Y. (1988) Motility of the gastrointestinal tract. In: *The Ruminant Animal,*

Digestive Physiology and Nutrition. Edited by D. C. Church. Prentice Hall, Englewood Cliffs, NJ. USA. pp. 64-107.

Russell, J. B. and D. B. Dombrowski. (1980) Effect of pH on the efficiency of growth by pure cultures of rumen bacteria in continuous culture. *Applied and Environmental Microbiology*, **39,** 604-610.

Shaver, R. D., A. J. Nytes, L. D. Satter and N. A. Jorgensen. (1988) Influence of feed intake, forage physical form, and forage fiber content on particle size of masticated forage, ruminal digesta and feces of dairy cows. *Journal of Dairy Science,* **71,** 1566-1572.

Siciliano-Jones, J. and M. R. Murphy. (1991) Specific gravity of various feedstuffs as affected by particle size and *in vitro* fermentation. *Journal of Dairy Science,* **74,** 896-901.

Smith, L. W., B. T. Weinland, D. R. Waldo and E. C. Leffel. (1983) Rate of plant cell wall particle size reduction in the rumen. *Journal of Dairy Science,* **66,** 2124-2136.

Thornton, R. F. and N. G. Yates. (1968) Some effects of water restriction on apparent digestibility and water excretion of cattle. *Australian Journal of Agricultural Research,* **19,** 665-672.

Ulyatt, M. J., D. W. Dellow, A. John, C. S. W. Reid and G. C. Waghorn. (1986) Contribution of chewing during eating and rumination to the clearance of digesta from the ruminoreticulum. In: *Control of Digestion and Metabolism in Ruminants.* Edited by L. P. Milligan, W. L. Grovum and A. Dobson. Prentice-Hall, Englewood Cliffs, NJ. USA. pp. 498-515.

Varga, G. A. and E. C. Prigge. (1982) Influence of forage species and level of intake on ruminal turnover rates. *Journal of Animal Science,* **55,** 1498-1504.

Warner, A. C. I. and B. D. Stacy. (1965) Solutes in the rumen of the sheep. *Quarterly Journal of Experimental Physiology,* **50,** 169-184.

Wattiaux, M. A., D. R. Mertens and L. D. Satter. (1991) Effect of source and amount of fiber on kinetics of digestion and specific gravity of forage particles in the rumen. *Journal of Dairy Science,* **74,** 3872-3883.

Wattiaux, M. A., L. D. Satter and D. R. Mertens. (1992) Effect of microbial fermentation on functional specific gravity of small forage particles. *Journal of Animal Science*, **70,** 1262-1270.

Welch, J. G. (1986) Physical parameters of fiber affecting passage from the rumen. *Journal of Dairy Science,* **69,** 2750-2754.

Welch, J. G. and A. M. Smith. (1968) Influence of fasting on rumination activity in sheep. *Journal of Animal Science*, **27,** 1734-1737.

Welch, J. G. and A. M. Smith. (1969a) Influence of forage quality on rumination time in sheep. *Journal of Animal Science,* **28,** 813-818.

Welch, J. G. and A. M. Smith. (1969b) Effect of varying amounts of forage intake on rumination. *Journal of Animal Science,* **28,** 827-830.

Welch, J. G. and A. M. Smith. (1970) Forage quality and rumination time in cattle. *Journal of Dairy Science,* **53,** 797-800.

Welch, J. G., A. M. Smith and K. S. Gibson. (1970) Rumination time in four breeds of dairy cattle. *Journal of Dairy Science,* **53,** 89-91.

Willes, R. F., V. E. Mendel and A. R. Robblee. (1970) Water transfer from the reticulo-rumen in sheep. *Journal of Animal Science,* **31,** 85-91.

Wimpenny, J. W. T. and O. A. Samah. (1978) Some effects of oxygen on the growth and physiology of *Selenomonas ruminantium. Journal of General Microbiology,* **108,** 329-332.

CHAPTER 3

CLASSIFICATION AND MORPHOLOGY OF RUMEN PROTOZOA

The rumen protozoa were first observed by Gruby and Delafond in 1843, and have subsequently intrigued biologists with regard to both their specificity for this habitat and functional role in the rumen fermentation. Identification of the rumen protozoa is based primarily on cell morphology, since the organisms are large enough to distinguish many cellular features microscopically at low magnifications. The majority of protozoa in the rumen are ciliate species, although flagellate species do occur. In general, the flagellate protozoa have been observed to occur in relatively low numbers in adult ruminants and are quite small in size as compared to the ciliates (Eadie, 1962; Hungate, 1966; Warner, 1966; Clarke, 1977). Occasionally the number of flagellates will increase markedly in animals without ciliates (Eadie, 1962; Hungate, 1966, 1978). Reliability of these early observations on the concentration of flagellate protozoa has been seriously questioned since Orpin (1977) found that many of the "flagellates" were in reality fungal zoospores. Obviously additional studies are needed which differentiate between the true flagellates and zoospores.

The rumen ciliates have evolved into a highly specialized group fitted to survive only in the rumen or a closely related habitat. They are anaerobic, can ferment plant materials for energy, and can grow at rumen temperatures in the presence of billions of accompanying bacteria (Hungate, 1966). The rumen protozoa vary considerably in size, ranging from approximately 15 to 250 μm in length and 10 to 200 μm in width for the different species. The protozoa can be considered as the simplest form of animal life and thus have many of the features common to all animals. The organism is bounded by a skin (cuticle or pellicle), has a mouth, a digestive tract (reduced to one cavity), a rectum and an anus. Between the digestive tract and the cuticle are located the controlling "organs" and the body fluid. Also present are a macronucleus, micronucleus and one or more contractile vacuoles, presumably which function in the excretion of gasses as well as liquid and soluble waste products (Hungate, 1978; Kofoid and MacLennan, 1930, 1932, 1933). The organisms propagate by binary fission; however, conjugation occasionally has been observed, particularly in the genus *Dasytricha* (Warner, 1966).

Classification

The ciliate protozoa which occur in the rumen are all classified in the phylum Ciliophora; however, detailed ultrastructural studies, molecular techniques such as ribosomal RNA sequencing and the use of sophisticated cladistic analyses have resulted in numerous changes in the system of classification below the phylum level (Corliss, 1994). As new information becomes available, additional changes will undoubtedly be made. Based on the most recent revisions, the classification of rumen protozoa to the genus level is shown in Table 3.1. This classification is according to the 1985 revision published by the Society of Protozoologists (Lee *et al.*, 1985). Subfamilies under Ophryoscolecidae follow the scheme proposed by Lubinsky (1957c) and genera under Diplodiniinae follow the proposal of Latteur (1966). For purposes of uniformity, the classification scheme shown in Table 3.1 will be used throughout this text.

Table 3.2 presents the classification scheme proposed in 1980 by Levine *et al.* and subsequently used by Ogimoto and Imai (1981) and Dehority (1993). In 1966, Latteur proposed dividing the family Ophryoscolcidae into six subfamilies. Essentially he kept two of Lubinsky's subfamilies and divided the subfamily Ophryoscolecinae into four new subfamilies. Grain (1994) modified Latteur's classification of the family Ophryoscolecidae by elevating the subfamily Entodiniinae to family status, which he named Entodiniidae (Table 3.3). Table 3.4 presents an even earlier system by Honigberg *et al.*, (1964). These tables of the various classification schemes are helpful when looking up descriptions in the literature. Other references useful for classification of gastrointestinal tract ciliates are Hsiung (1930a) and Hungate (1978).

Essentially classification down to the species level under the families Isotrichidae, Paraisotrichidae, Blepharocorythidae and Buetschliidae is agreed upon by most workers, probably because the morphological criteria used for classification are quite distinctive and stable. These four families were originally classified in the subclass Holotricha (Table 3.4) and are commonly referred to in the literature as "holotrichs". Williams and Coleman (1992) use this term in their book *The Rumen Protozoa*. The remaining ciliate protozoa, which are in the majority as far as numbers in the rumen are concerned, are in the order Entodiniomorphida, family Ophryoscolecidae (Table 3.1). Based on previous classifications, they have been called "oligotrichs," which referred to their having tufts of cilia on one end as opposed to the holotrichs which are mostly covered with cilia (Kudo, 1947), "spirotrichs" (Table 3.4) and more recently "entodiniomorphs". However, to follow the most recently accepted classification they would be called "ophryoscolecids". Awareness of these different names can be helpful in reading some of the older literature.

The subfamily Entodiniinae contains only one genus, *Entodinium*, and classification is quite straight forward, being based on the feature that they have only a single ciliary zone located at the anterior end of the cell. However, over the years some confusion has arisen over classification of ophryoscolecid protozoa in the subfamily Diplodiniinae. Dogiel (1927) established the genus *Diplodinium*, which he distinguished from *Entodinium* by the presence of a second ciliary zone, located at the anterior end of the cell in the same transverse plane as the oral ciliary zone. In the higher genera, i.e., *Epidinium*, *Epiplastron*, *Opisthotrichum*, *Ophryoscolex* and *Caloscolex*, the dorsal or left ciliary zone is no longer at the anterior end of the cell and lies in a different transverse plane

Table 3.1 CLASSIFICATION OF RUMEN CILIATE PROTOZOA BASED ON LEE *et al.* (1985)

Kingdom PROTOZOA Goldfuss, 1818
  Phylum Ciliophora Doflein, 1901
    Subphylum Rhabdophora Small, 1976
      Class Litostomatea Small and Lynn, 1981
        Subclass Trichostomatia Bütschli, 1889
          Order Vestibuliferida de Puytorac *et al.*, 1974
            Family Isotrichidae Bütschli, 1889
              Genus *Isotricha* Stein, 1859
              Genus *Dasytricha* Schuberg, 1888
              Genus *Oligoisotricha* Imai, 1981
            Family Paraisotrichidae da Cunha, 1917
              Genus *Paraisotricha* Fiorentini, 1890
          Order Entodiniomorphida Reichenow, in Doflein and Reichenow, 1929
            Suborder Blepharocorythina Wolska, 1971
              Family Blepharocorythidae Hsiung, 1929
                Genus: *Charonina* Strand, 1928
            Suborder Archistomatina de Puytorac *et al.*, 1974
              Family Buetschliidae Poche, 1913
                Genus *Buetschlia* Schuberg, 1888
                Genus *Blepharoprosthium* Bundle, 1895
                Genus *Blepharoconus* Gassovsky, 1919
                Genus *Polymorphella* Dogiel, 1929
                Genus *Parabundleia* Imai and Ogimoto, 1983
            Suborder Entodiniomorphina Reichenow in Doflein and Reichenow, 1929
              Family Ophryoscolecidae Stein, 1858
                Subfamily Entodiniinae Lubinsky, 1957
                  Genus: *Entodinium* Stein, 1858
                Subfamily Diplodiniinae Lubinsky, 1957
                  Genus: *Diplodinium* Schuberg, 1888
                  Genus: *Eudiplodinium* Dogiel, 1927
                  Genus: *Ostracodinium* Dogiel, 1927
                  Genus: *Metadinium* Awerinzew and Mutafowa, 1914
                  Genus: *Enoploplastron* Kofoid and MacLennan, 1932
                  Genus: *Elytroplastron* Kofoid and MacLennan, 1932
                  Genus: *Polyplastron* Dogiel, 1927
                Subfamily Ophryoscolecinae Lubinsky, 1957
                  Genus: *Epidinium* Crawley, 1923
                  Genus: *Epiplastron* Kofoid and MacLennan, 1933
                  Genus: *Opisthotrichum* Buisson, 1923
                  Genus: *Ophryoscolex* Stein, 1858
                  Genus: *Caloscolex* Dogiel, 1926
              Family Cycloposthiidae Poche, 1913
                Genus: *Parentodinium* Thurston and Noirot-Timothée, 1973

Table 3.2 CLASSIFICATION OF RUMEN CILIATE PROTOZOA BASED ON LEVINE et al. (1980)

Subkingdom PROTOZOA
  Phylum CILIOPHORA Doflein, 1901
    Class 1. KINETOFRAGMINOPHOREA de Puytorac et al., 1974
      Subclass 1. GYMNOSTOMATIA Bütschli, 1889
        Order 1. PROSTOMATIDA Schewiakoff, 1896
          Suborder 1. ARCHISTOMATINA de Puytorac et al., 1974
            Family BUETSCHLIIDAE Poche, 1913
      Subclass 2. VESTIBULIFERIA de Puytorac et al., 1974
        Order 1. TRICHOSTOMATIDA Bütschli, 1889
          Suborder 1. TRICHOSTOMATINA Bütschli, 1889
            Family ISOTRICHIDAE Bütschli, 1889
            Family PARAISOTRICHIDAE da Cunha, 1916
          Suborder 2. BLEPHAROCORYTHINA Wolska, 1971
            Family BLEPHAROCORYTHIDAE Hsiung, 1929
        Order 2. ENTODINIOMORPHIDA Reichenow, in Doflein and Reichenow, 1929
          Family OPHRYOSCOLECIDAE Stein, 1858
            Subfamily ENTODINIINAE Lubinsky, 1957
            Subfamily DIPLODINIINAE Lubinsky, 1957
            Subfamily OPHRYOSCOLECINAE Lubinsky, 1957
          Family CYCLOPOSTHIIDAE Poche, 1913

Table 3.3 CLASSIFICATION OF RUMEN CILIATE PROTOZOA IN THE FAMILY OPHRYOSCOLECIDAE AS PROPOSED BY LATTEUR (1966) AND MODIFIED BY GRAIN (1994)

Order Entodiniomorphida Reichenow, in Dofelin and Reichenow, 1929
  Family Entodiniidae Grain, 1994
    Genus: *Entodinium* Stein, 1858
    Genus: *Parentodinium* Thurston and Noirot-Timothée, 1973
  Family Ophryoscolecidae Stein, 1858
    Subfamily Diplodiniinae Lubinsky, 1957
      Genus: *Diplodinium* Schuberg, 1888
      Genus: *Eudiplodinium* Dogiel, 1927
      Genus: *Ostracodinium* Dogiel, 1927
      Genus: *Metadinium* Awerinzew and Mutafowa, 1914
      Genus: *Enoploplastron* Kofoid and MacLennan, 1932
      Genus: *Elytroplastron* Kofoid and MacLennan, 1932
      Genus: *Polyplastron* Dogiel 1927
    Subfamily Epidiniinae Latteur, 1966
      Genus: *Epidinium* Crawley, 1923
      Genus: *Epiplastron* Kofoid and MacLennan, 1933
    Subfamily Opisthotrichinae Latteur, 1966
      Genus: *Opisthotrichum* Buisson, 1923
    Subfamily Ophryoscolecinae Latteur, 1966
      Genus: *Ophryoscolex* Stein, 1858
    Subfamily Caloscolecinae Latteur, 1966
      Genus: *Caloscolex* Dogiel, 1926

Table 3.4 CLASSIFICATION OF RUMEN CILIATE PROTOZOA BASED ON HONIGBERG et al. (1964)

Phylum PROTOZOA Goldfuss, 1845
  Subphylum Ciliophora Doflein, 1901
    Class Ciliatea Perty, 1852
      Subclass Holotricha Stein, 1859
        Order Trichostomatida Bütschli, 1889
          Family Isotrichidae Bütschli, 1887
          Family Blepharocorythidae Hsiung, 1930
        Order Gymnostomatida Bütschli, 1889
          Family Buetschliidae Poche, 1913
      Subclass Spirotricha
        Order Entodiniomorphida Reichenow, in Doflein and Reichenow, 1929
          Family Ophryoscolecidae Stein, 1859
          Family Cycloposthidae Poche, 1913

---

than the oral ciliary zone. Under the genus *Diplodinium*, Dogiel then established four subgenera. These subgenera, *Anoplodinium*, *Eudiplodinium*, *Ostracodinium* and *Polyplastron*, were distinctly different with respect to nuclear structure and skeletal plates. In 1932, Kofoid and MacLennan revised the classification of *Diplodinium* by raising the four subgenera of Dogiel to the generic level and used such morphological features as body size, complexity of caudal projections and the size and number of skeletal plates to erect six new genera for a total of 10 genera, all of which have two ciliary zones on the anterior end of the cell. These 10 genera are: *Eodinium, Diplodinium, Eremoplastron, Eudiplodinium, Ostracodinium, Diploplastron, Metadinium, Enoploplastron, Elytroplastron* and *Polyplastron*. However, most investigators concluded that the revision of *Diplodinium* by Kofoid and MacLennan (1932) was not practical and in reality was "splitting hairs". Since considerable variation has been observed in caudal projections with clonal cultures (Hungate, 1966) and cell size differed between individual hosts of the same and different ruminant species, these characteristics did not appear to be suitable criteria for taxonomic purposes. Noirot-Timothée (1960) recommended subdivision of the genus *Diplodinium* into six subgenera with a system based primarily on skeletal plates. This provided distinct separation and reduced splitting. However, the use of subgeneric names can be somewhat confusing in that three names are required for accurate identification, i.e., genera (subgenera) species, with the generic name always the same.

    Lubinsky (1957c) proposed establishment of three subfamilies of Ophryoscolecidae, based on number and location of ciliary zones as follows: Entodiniinae - one zone at the anterior end of cell; Diplodiniinae - two ciliary zones (oral and left or dorsal) situated in one transverse plane at the anterior end of the cell; Ophryoscolecinae - two ciliary zones situated in different transverse planes, the oral zone is always located at the anterior end of the cell. However, Lubinsky retained all ten of the *Diplodinium* genera proposed by Kofoid and MacLennan (1932). Latteur (1966) suggested that the six subgenera of the genus *Diplodinium*, as established by Noirot-Timothée (1960), be raised to the generic level under the subfamily Diplodiniinae and that one of the genera of Kofoid and MacLennan also be included. Division into these seven genera is then based solely upon the number of skeletal plates. This classification scheme, as shown in Table 3.1, is quite logical, easy to understand and will be described in detail later in the chapter.

Latteur (1966) also proposed that the subfamily Ophryoscolecinae be replaced by four subfamilies (Table 3.3) However, in the author's opinion, since only one of these four subfamilies contains more than one genus, the establishment of additional subfamilies seems redundant.

Rument ciliates in the families Isotrichidae, Blepharocorythidae and Buetschliidae

Except for several species in the families Buetschliidae and Blepharocorythidae, protozoa in these three families have cilia over most of their body surface. Each of the cilia is inserted singly and they are not fused except in the region of the mouth (Hungate, 1966). Definitions of the three families and the genera which commonly occur in the rumen are as follows:

> Isotrichidae Bütschli, 1889 - Body ellipsoidal; cilia cover the entire body surface except in one genus (*Oligoisotricha*) which lacks cilia on posterior one-sixth of body surface (genera: *Isotricha, Dasytricha, Oligoisotricha*).
>
> Buetschliidae Poche, 1913 - Body rounded; cilia cover the entire body surface or are on the anterior end with tufts on both lateral and posterior surfaces; concretion vacuoles present (genera: *Buetschlia, Blepharoconus, Blepharoprosthium, Polymorphella* and *Parabundleia*).
>
> Blepharocorythidae Hsiung, 1929 - Body elongated; ciliary zones present only on anterior end and in one or two tufts on posterior end (genus: *Charonina*).

Diagrammatic sketches illustrating their morphological features are shown in Figure 3.1. The common species occurring in the rumen are in the genera *Isotricha* and *Dasytricha*, of the family Isotrichidae. For descriptive purposes, the term isotrichid has been suggested to refer to protozoa in the family Isotrichidae (Dehority and Tirabasso, 1989).

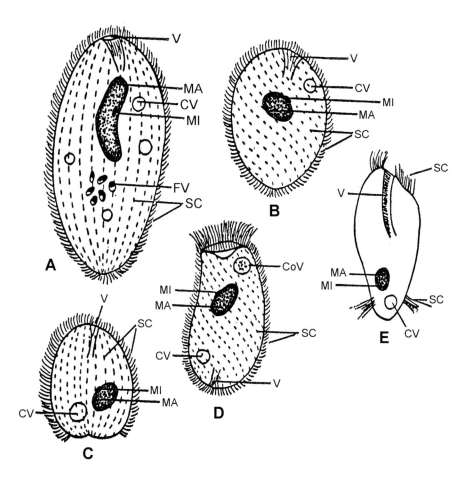

Figure 3.1. Diagrammatic sketches of rumen ciliates in the families Isotrichidae, Buetschliidae and Blepharocorythidae. (a) *Isotricha prostoma*; (b) *Dasytricha ruminantium*; (c) *Oligoisotricha bubali*; (d) *Buetschlia parva*; (e) *Charonina ventriculi*. Key: (CV) contractile vacuole; (CoV) concretion vacuole; (FV) food vacuole; (Ma) macronucleus; (Mi) micronucleus; (SC) somatic cilia; (V) vestibulum (from Dehority, 1993).

ISOTRICHIDAE

Isotricha. One of the distinguishing characteristics of the genus *Isotricha*, which contains two species commonly found in the rumen, *I. intestinalis* and *I. prostoma*, is that the cilia covering the body surface run in longitudinal rows, i.e., rows parallel to the long body axis (Ogimoto and Imai, 1981). This can be seen in the line drawing, Figure 3.1a and photomicrograph, Figure 3.2.

50 Rumen microbiology

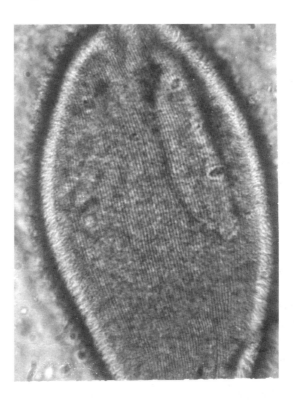

Figure 3.2 Photomicrograph of *Isotricha prostoma* showing longitudinal lines of cilia.

The mean body size for *I. intestinalis* is 60 x 110 µm as compared to 70 x 135 µm for *I. prostoma* (Dehority, 1993). Although the two species differ slightly in size and overall body shape, the distinguishing characteristic between them is the location of the so-called "mouth" or vestibulum. In *I. prostoma* the "mouth" is located at the posterior end of the cell, or that end which is towards the rear when the protozoon is in motion (Figure 3.1a). In *I. intestinalis* the "mouth" is located on the side of the cell (Hungate, 1966), approximately half-way between the middle and end which is to the rear in locomotion. In both species of *Isotricha*, the macronucleus and micronucleus are enclosed within a membrane which is supported by a fibrillar nucleo-suspensory apparatus (Williams and Coleman, 1988). Plant particles are not observed in the endoplasm.

Imai *et al*. (1995) have reported on the occurrence of an new species of *Isotricha, I jalaludinii,* which they found in the rumen of the lesser mouse deer in Malaysia. *I jalaludinii* resembles *I. Intestinalis,* but is considerably shorter in length. The location of the vestibular opening is much nearer to the posterior end of the body and also the vestibulum differs in relative size and direction. To date, this species has not been observed in any other host or location.

Dasytricha. For many years, the only species described in this genus was *D. ruminantium*. However, in 1954, Hukui and Nisada described *D. hukuokaensis*, which is similar to *Isotricha intestinalis* in size and location of the mouth, but lacks a nucleo-suspensory apparatus. Distribution of this latter species is extremely limited. A line drawing of *D. ruminantium* is shown in Figure 3.1b. The overall size of *D. ruminantium* is considerably smaller than that of *Isotricha*; the mean length is 58 µm with a range of 46-100 µm (Dehority, 1993). The so-called mouth is located at the posterior end. In some cases extremely large cells of *Dasytricha* have been encountered, in which case differentiation between *Dasytricha* and *Isotricha* can be difficult. However, the rows of cilia in *Dasytricha* spiral around the long body axis (Ogimoto and Imai, 1981) and are clearly distinguishable from the longitudinal rows in *Isotricha*.

A new species of *Dasytricha*, *D. kabanii*, has now been described from forestomach contents of the dromedary camel (Selim *et al.*, 1996). It differs from *D. ruminantium* in that it lacks somatic cilia on the posterior one-fifth of the body. It is also slightly larger in body size. More recently, Kubesy and Dehority (2002) observed *D. kabanii* in forestomach contents of camels living in a different region of Egypt.

Microscopically, the endoplasm in both the isotrichs and dasytrichs appears quite granular and the macronucleus is generally seen without much difficulty. With animals fed once daily, the isotrichids will be almost transparent just prior to feeding; however, within an hour after feeding they become somewhat enlarged and quite opaque as a result of carbohydrate storage within the cell. In fresh mounts of rumen fluid the isotrichids are readily noticed because of the speed with which they move across the field and their relatively large size (Hungate, 1966).

Oligoisotricha. In 1928, Dogiel described a new species of *Isotricha*, *Isotricha bubali*, which he observed in rumen contents of two water buffalo from Russia. No additional observations of this species were made until 1981, when Imai detected its presence in water buffalo from Taiwan. Imai noted several morphological differences between this species and the genus *Isotricha*, i.e., lack of somatic cilia on the posterior one-sixth of the body surface and the absence of a nucleo-suspensory apparatus. On this basis he proposed a new genus for this species, *Oligoisotricha* (Figure 3.1c).

This organism was subsequently found to occur in relatively high concentrations in the rumen of domestic cattle from two different areas in Tennessee (Dehority *et al.*, 1983). It is difficult to explain the very limited and sporadic observation of this species; however, the organism is quite small (about 14 x 20 µm) and could have easily been overlooked in some studies.

BUETSCHLIIDAE

Buetschlia. With a few minor exceptions, only one rumen species has been described in the family Buetschliiidae, *Buetschlia parva*, which occurs sporadically and generally in very low numbers (Figure 3.1d). *B. parva* was first described by Schuberg in 1888. In 1914, Sharp observed *B. parva* in the rumen of both cattle and sheep along the Pacific Coast of the U.S. Subsequently it was observed in Indian cattle by Kofoid and MacLennan (1933); more recently, Clarke (1964) observed this species in New Zealand cattle and Dehority has reported its occurrence in sheep (1970), musk-ox (1974), reindeer (1975), water buffalo (1979) and Brazilian cattle (1986). *B. parva* ranges in length from 30-67 µm, has a convex anterior end where the vestibulum is located and the rows of cilia wind around the long body axis, similar to *Dasytricha* (Dehority, 1993).

Several other species of Buetschliidae have been reported in rumen contents of cattle from China and Thailand. In 1932, Hsiung described the species *Pingius minutus*, *Buetschlia triciliata* and *Blepharoprosthium parvum* from Chinese cattle. Imai and Ogimoto (1983) described a new genus and species, *Parabundleia ruminantium*, from rumen contents of zebu cattle in Thailand. Other than the original description of this species, no further observations have been reported. In 1984, Imai reported the presence of another new genus and species, *Polymorphella bovis*, from the same Thailand cattle. This species has since been observed in cattle from Kenya (Imai, 1988) as well as from camels in Egypt and Inner-Mongolia (Imai and Gui Rung, 1988; Selim *et al.*,1996; Kubesy and Dehority, 2002).

Blepharoconus krugerensis was identified in rumen contents from a zebu cow in Brazil (Dehority, 1986). This species had previously been observed only in the cecum of the elephant (Eloff and van Hoven, 1980).

BLEPHAROCORYTHIDAE

Charonina. *Charonina ventriculi*, was first observed and described from the rumen of cattle and sheep by Jameson in 1925. *Charonina* differs from the other rumen species in the families Isotrichidae and Buetschliidae, in that most of the body surface is not covered with cilia. A schematic drawing is shown in Figure 3.1e. *C. ventriculi* is also a relatively small ciliate, with a range of 24-41 µm in length (Dehority, 1993). Two other species of *Charonina* have been described, *C. nuda* from Chinese cattle (Hsiung, 1932) and *C. equi* in cattle from New Zealand (Clarke, 1964). *C. equi* was originally described from the colon of the horse (Hsuing, 1930b). To this time, neither of these latter two species have been observed again in ruminants.

PARAISOTRICHIDAE

Paraisotricha - An unknown species of *Paraisotricha* was observed in rumen contents from a single cow in Brazil (Dehority, 1986). Previously, Kleynhans and van Hoven (1976) described an unknown ciliate in the rumen of the giraffe which resembled *Paraisotricha minuta*. It would appear that the occurrence of this family in the rumen is extremely rare.

OPHRYOSCOLECIDAE

Lubinsky (1958) proposed a new system of orientation of ophryoscolecid cells for descriptive purposes (Figure 3.3).

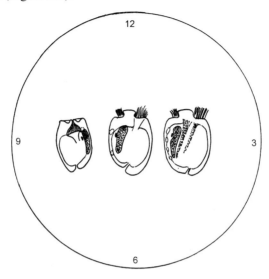

Figure 3.3. Orientation of rumen protozoa for description of morphological features. Assuming the circle is a clock face, when the oral or anterior end is directed towards 12:00 o'clock and the micronucleus is to the left of the macronucleus, the surface closest to the observer is the upper side and the opposite surface is the lower side. The posterior end is directed towards 6:00 o'clock; the right side towards 3:00 o'clock; and the left side towards 9:00 o'clock (from Dehority, 1993).

Although several investigators are now using this system, it differs from the terminology used by older workers and can thus cause some confusion in identification studies. A comparison of this system with the terminology used by previous investigators is shown in Table 3.5

Table 3.5 RELATIONSHIP BETWEEN THE TERMINOLOGY USED BY LUBINSKY, DOGIEL AND KOFOID AND MACLENNAN

Nomenclature of Lubinsky[a]	Nomenclature of Dogiel[b] and Kofoid & MacLennan[c]	
	For Entodinium	For higher genera
Upper side	Left side	Right side
Lower side	Right side	Left side
Right side	Dorsal side	Ventral side
Left side	Ventral side	Dorsal side

[a] Lubinsky (1958)
[b] Dogiel (1927)
[c] Kofoid and MacLennan (1930)

54 Rumen microbiology

Division of the Ophryoscolecidae into three subfamilies, Table 3.1, is based on the occurrence and location of ciliary zones (Figure 3.4).

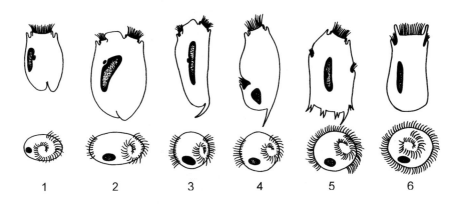

Figure 3.4 Ciliary zones in the family Ophryoscolecidae. Top row — side view; Bottom row — top view. (1) Subfamily Entodiniinae; (2) Subfamily Diplodiniinae; (3—6) Subfamily Ophryoscolecinae: 3, genus *Epidinium*; 4, genus *Opisthotrichum;* 5, genus *Ophryoscolex;* 6, genus *Caloscolex* (from Dehority, 1993).

These three subfamilies are described as follows:

> Subfamily Entodiniinae Lubinsky, 1957 — One ciliary zone; one contractile vacuole; in side view, the macronucleus lies between the micronucleus and nearest body side (Figure 3.4-1).

> Subfamily Diplodiniinae Lubinsky, 1957 — Two ciliary zones located in one transverse plane at anterior end of cell; two or more contractile vacuoles; in side view, micronucleus lies between macronucleus and nearest body side; skeletal plates absent or present; body more or less flattened (Figure 3.4-2).

> Subfamily Ophryoscolecinae Lubinsky, 1957 — Two ciliary zones, located in different transverse planes; two or more contractile vacuoles; in side view the micronucleus situated between the macronucleus and nearest body side; skeletal plates present; body more or less cylindrical (Figures 3.4-3,-4,-5,-6).

SUBFAMILY ENTODINIINAE

Entodinium is the only genus classified in the subfamily Entodiniinae. Figure 3.5 shows the general morphology of a typical *Entodinium* cell.

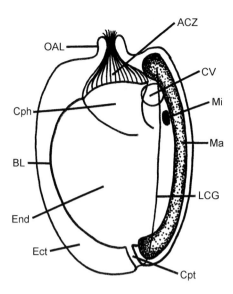

Figure 3.5. Schematic drawing of *Entodinium longinucleatum.* Key: (ACZ) adoral ciliary zone; (BL) boundary layer; (Cph) cytopharynx or esophagus; (Cpt) cytoproct or rectum; (CV) contractile vacuole; (Ect) ectoplasm; (End) endoplasm; (LCG) longitudinal cuticular groove; (Ma) macronucleus; (Mi) micronucleus; (OAL) outer adoral lip.

Early studies showed that caudal spines are environmentally plastic in the family Ophryoscolecidae, particularly in the genus *Entodinium*, and thus not a good criteria for taxonomic purposes. A single cell of *E. caudatum* forma *caudatum* can give rise to a culture which contains *E. caudatum* cells of all three forms shown in Figure 3.6 (Hungate, 1966; Lubinsky, 1957a).

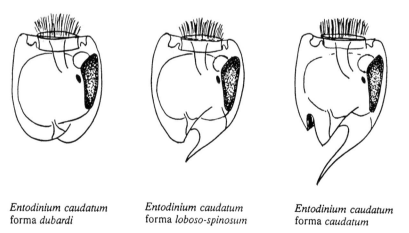

Figure 3.6. Variation in caudal spinution within a single species of *Entodinium* (from Dehority, 1993).

The genus *Entodinium* is primarily characterized by having a single ciliary band which encircles the mouth. In living cells the individual cilia appear to be joined together in membranelles or small tufts called syncilia; however, after the cells are fixed they are visible as individual cilia. The oral ciliary band is generally referred to as the adoral ciliary zone. The ciliary zone is thought to have a function in both locomotion and food ingestion. All *Entodinium* species known to date contain one macronucleus, one micronucleus and one contractile vacuole. In 1992, Williams and Coleman listed 100 different species of *Entodinium*, and numerous new species have been described since then (a few representative references are: Dehority, 1995; Göçmen *et al.*, 2001; Guirong *et al.*, 2000).

The type species for the genus *Entodinium* is *Entodinium bursa*, described by Stein in 1858. He described it as the largest entodinial species and none have been subsequently found any larger. The oral cilia are slightly displaced to one side. The off-center adoral cilia, position of the contractile vacuole on the left side, size and overall shape resembles a *Diplodinium* species more than the other species of *Entodinium*. Few reports have appeared on the occurrence of *E. bursa* as originally described by Stein and pictured by Schuberg in 1888. Dogiel has suggested that the species *E. bursa* Stein is not a single species and that it probably contains the species *E. simplex, E. ovinium, E. dubardi dubardi, E. parvum* and *E. vorax*. His evidence for this is the considerable variation in size (55-114 x 37-78 µm) of individuals of the supposed species, whereas he considers a true species of *Entodinium* to vary little in size. Kofoid and MacLennan (1930) considered *E. vorax vorax* Dogiel as a synonym for the type species *E. bursa* Stein.

The contracted form of *E. longinucleatum* is shown in Figure 3.5, while Figure 3.6 illustrates the appearance of an *Entodinium* cell when the adoral ciliary zone is open or expanded. This retraction or enclosure of the adoral ciliary zone by the adoral lips is believed to be the organisms response to adverse conditions (Hungate, 1978). If one observes a single *Entodinium* cell in a live preparation, the ciliary zone may open and close several times while under observation. In retracted living cells the oral cilia may show considerable movement inside the cell.

SUBFAMILY DIPLODINIINAE

Protozoa in the subfamily Diplodiniinae possess a left or dorsal zone of cilia in addition to the oral ciliary zone. The left zone is located at the anterior end of the cell and is in the same transverse plane as the adoral ciliary zone (Figure 3.4-2). The principal feature used to distinguish the various genera are the size, number and position of skeletal plates (Figure 3.7).

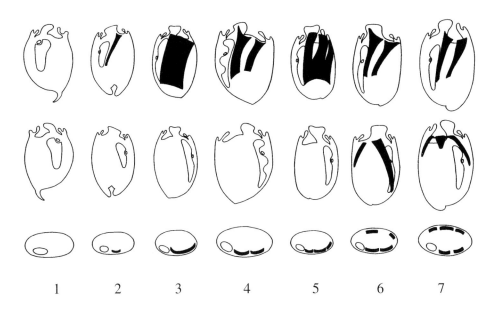

Figure 3.7 Location and shape of the skeletal plates which are the basis for generic classification of rumen protozoa in the subfamily Diplodiniinae. Top, middle and bottom rows are upper, lower and cross-sectional views, respectively. (1) *Diplodinium*; (2) *Eudiplodinium*; (3) *Ostracodinium*; (4) *Metadinium*; (5) *Enoploplastron*; (6) *Elytroplastron*; (7) *Polyplastron* (from Dehority, 1993).

Other characteristics used for species identification include body size, shape of the cell, position and shape of the macro- and micronucleus, number and location of contractile vacuoles, and spination. However, Hungate (1966) observed the offspring from an individual cell of *D. dentatum* having six spines and found daughter cells having none, one, or two spines but none like the original type. Thus, it appears that spination in Diplodiniinae, as in the genus *Entodinium*, is not a stable characteristic. General morphology of the Diplodiniinae cell is shown in Figure 3.8. The left ciliary zone does not have an opening into the interior of the cell and is generally regarded as an organ of locomotion.

The seven genera in the subfamily Diplodiniinae are described below. Estimates of the number of species in each genus are from Williams and Coleman (1992); however, a considerable number of additional species have subsequently been described.

> ***Diplodinium.*** The main characteristic of this genus is the lack of any skeletal plates (Figure 3.7-1). Species in this genus have a large range in size, i.e. from *D. polygonale* with a mean length of 35 μm up to *Diplodinium Africanum*, which ranges from 150 to 250 μm in length(40 plus species have been identified).

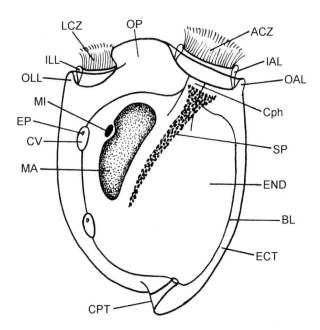

Figure 3.8. Schematic drawing of Diplodiniinae species. Key: (ACZ) adoral ciliary zone; (BL) boundary layer; (Cph) cytopharynx or esophagus; (Cpt) cytoproct or rectum; (CV) contractile vacuole; (Ect) ectoplasm; (End) endoplasm; (EP) excretory pore; (IAL) inner adoral lip; (ILL) inner left lip; (LCZ) left ciliary zone; (Ma) macronucleus; (Mi) micronucleus; (OAL) outer adoral lip; (OLL) outer left lip; (OP) operculum; (SP) skeletal plate (from Dehority, 1993).

Eudiplodinium. The genus is identified by having one narrow skeletal plate on the upper side (Figure 3.7-2) which angles from a point near the mouth caudally and to the left, along the right side of the macronucleus and usually diminishes in width (30 plus species have been reported).

Ostracodinium. The distinctive characteristic of the genus *Ostracodinium* is a single large skeletal plate which covers about half the upper side of the cell, Figure 3.7-3 (at least 30 species described).

Metadinium. Species with two skeletal plates on the upper side are classified in the genus *Metadinium* (Figure 3.7-4). In some species, the skeletal plates may be fused in the posterior region (about 12 species).

Enoploplastron. Protozoa classified in the genus *Enoploplastron* have three skeletal plates on the upper side which can either be separate or partially fused, Figure 3.7-5 (only four species described).

Elytroplastron. The genus *Elytroplastron* is represented by a single species, *Elytroplastron bubali*. This species is quite similar in size and morphology to *Polyplastron*. Two distinct skeletal plates are located on the upper side, the same as in *Polyplastron*; however, it has one well developed skeletal plate and one small plate on the lower side, in contrast to the three small plates on the lower side of *Polyplastron multivesiculatum* (Figure 3.7-6). Occurrence of this species is quite rare in the U.S., but it occurs commonly in humped cattle (*Bos indicus*) and water buffalo.

Polyplastron. The last genus in the subfamily Diplodiniinae is *Polyplastron* with five skeletal plates (Figure 3.7-7). Two large plates are on the upper side and three small plates are on the lower side. Only one species, *Polyplastron multivesiculatum* occurs in domestic ruminants. However, three additional species of *Polyplastron* have been described from wild ruminants: *P. alaskum* Dehority, 1974, from Dall sheep; *P. arcticum* Lubinsky, 1958, from reindeer; and *P. californiense* Bush and Kofoid, 1948, from Sierra Nevada bighorn sheep.

SUBFAMILY OPHRYOSCOLECINAE.

The subfamily Ophryoscolecinae contains a total of five genera, *Epidinium, Epiplastron, Opisthotrichum, Ophryoscolex* and *Caloscolex*. The left ciliary zone is more posterior and lies in a different transverse plane than the oral zone. Location of the left ciliary zone, Figures 3.4-3,-4,-5,-6 and location and shape of skeletal plates (Figure 3.9) are the principal criteria used for classification of genera in this subfamily. General morphology of cells in this subfamily is illustrated in Figure 3.10

Epidinium. In addition to the slightly posterior location of the left ciliary zone (Figure 3.4-3), this genus is characterized by three slightly curved skeletal plates on the upper side (Figures 3.9-1 and 3.10). The primary species of *Epidinium* which occur in domestic ruminants are *E. ecaudatum*, which has no caudal spines and *E. caudatum*, having one spine. Other species, which generally occur in low numbers are *E. bicaudatum* (two spines); *E. tricaudatum* (three spines); *E. quadricaudatum* (four spines); *E. parvicaudatum* (five spines) and *E. cattanei* (five large spines of the same size). Five or six additional species of *Epidinium* have been described; however, their occurrence appears to be quite limited or restricted to a specific animal host (Williams and Coleman, 1992).

Epiplastron. Only two species of *Epiplastron* have been described, *E. africanum* and *E. spinosum*, both occurring only in African antelope (Kofoid and MacLennan, 1933). This genus resembles *Epidinium*, except it has five skeletal plates, Figure 3.9-2.

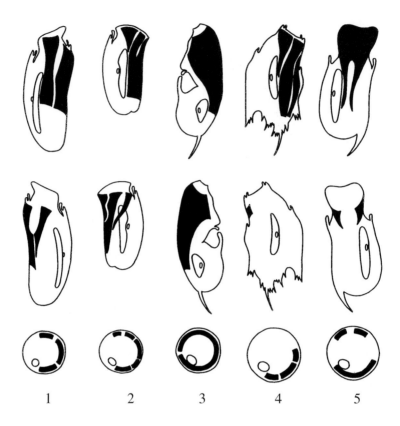

Figure 3.9. Location and shape of skeletal plates for protozoa classified in the subfamily Ophryoscolecinae. Top, middle and bottom rows are upper side, lower side and cross-sectional views, respectively. (1) *Epidinium*; (2) *Epiplastron*; (3) *Opisthotricum*; (4) *Ophryoscolex*; (5) *Caloscolex* (from Dehority, 1993).

Opisthotrichum. This genus is represented by a single species, *Opisthotrichum janus*, which has been observed in several species of African antelope (reedbuck, impala, blesbok, steinbok, etc.). The left ciliary zone is located near the middle of the cell on the left side, Figures. 3.4-4 and 3.9-3(Buisson, 1924; Dogiel, 1927). Figure 3-11 is a photomicrograph of this relatively rare protozoa.

Ophryoscolex. The genus *Ophryoscolex* is described as the most complex of the genera in domestic ruminants. In this genus the left ciliary zone is displaced about one-third the length of the body towards the posterior end. Also, the left ciliary zone is increased in length so that it forms a band which encircles about three-fourths of the body (Figures. 3.4-5; 3.9-4 and 3.10). Although protozoa in the genus *Ophryoscolex* are generally quite easy to recognize, identification to the species level can be difficult (Kofoid and MacLennan, 1993). Eight species have been described.

Classification and morphology of rumen protozoa 61

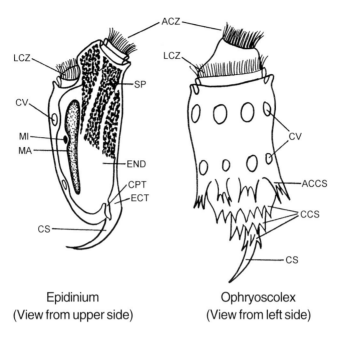

Figure 3.10. Diagrammatic sketches of two genera in the subfamily Ophryoscolecinae. Key: (ACCS) anterior circlet of secondary caudal spines; (ACZ) adoral ciliary zone; (CCS) additional circlets of secondary caudal spines; (CPT) cytoproct or rectum; (CS) caudal spine; (CV) contractile vacuole; (Ect) ectoplasm; (End) endoplasm; (LCZ) left ciliary zone; (Ma) macronucleus; (Mi) micronucleus; (SP) skeletal plate (from Dehority, 1993).

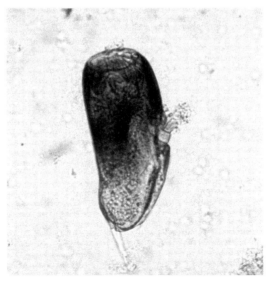

Figure 3.11. Photomicrograph of *Opisthotrichum janus* found in rumen contents taken from a hartebeest in Africa.

62 Rumen microbiology

Caloscolex. In *Caloscolex*, the left ciliary zone is actually a girdle which lies just below the anterior end of the cell and completely encircles the body. There are three skeletal plates, one large plate on the upper side and two small anterior plates, one on the right and one on the left side. To date, this genus has only been observed in the camel. Caudal spination in *Caloscolex* is similar to that observed in the genus *Epidinium* in that the number of spines can range from zero to five. Whether these morphologically different cells should be classified as species or forms is still uncertain. Schematic drawings of *Caloscolex camelinus* forma *laevis* and forma *cuspidatus* are shown in Figures 3.4-6 and 3.9-5, respectively (Dogiel, 1926).

CYCLOPOSTHIIDAE

Until just recently, protozoa in this family had not been observed to occur in the rumen. Primarily they were found in the cecum and colon of hindgut fermenting herbivores; however, two new genera (three species total) were described by Thurston and Noirot-Timothée (1973) from stomach contents of the hippopottamus. One of these species *Parentodinium africanum*, was subsequentially observed to occur in the rumen contents of four Brazilian cattle (Dehority, 1986). This was the first observation of Cycloposthiidae in the rumen habitat. More recently, *P. africanum* was found in rumen contents of domestic cattle (*Bos taurus*) in Montana, with concentrations ranging from 4.6 to 80.3% (Dehority *et al.*, 1999). *Parentodinium* is the simplest genus in the family Cycloposthiidae, possessing no caudalia or skeletal plates (Figure 3.12). Its adoral zone of cilia is borne on an anterior retractile cone, which when protruded extends beyond the anterior body limit. However, when the cone is retracted it lies deep inside the body. Thurston and Noirot-Timothée (1973) considered it to be the ancestral form of the family, similar to *Entodinium* in the family Ophryoscolecidae. However, its limited occurrence compared to *Entodinium* is difficult to explain.

Ultrastructure of rumen protozoa

The availability of the electron microscope (EM) has prompted numerous investigations on ultrastructure of the rumen protozoa (Stern *et al.*, 1977a; Stern *et al.*, 1977b; Ogimoto and Imai, 1981; Imai *et al.*, 1983; Furness and Butler, 1985a,b). One particularly interesting report was that of Imai *et al.* (1983), who studied the adoral ciliary zone of *Entodinium* by scanning electron microscopy. They found that it is divided into at least two zones, an outer zone with long cilia and an inner zone with short cilia. The outer ciliary zone has membranelle-like structures each of which contains two rows of about eight cilia each. The inner zone has ciliary aggregates arranged irregularly. The cilia are in the same horizontal plane, not arranged spirally and start on the left side of the vestibulum, go around the lower side and enter the vestibulum opening on the right side proceeding

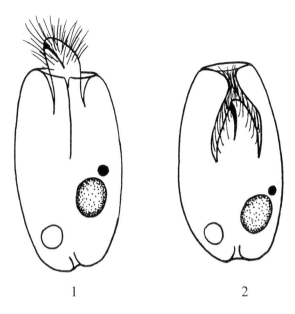

Figure 3.12 Schematic drawings of *Parentodinium africanum*. (1) Anterior cone extended; (2) Anterior cone retracted (from Dehority, 1993).

downward a short distance into the vestibulum. The left side of the vestibulum is without cilia. An open or non-ciliated area occurs on the upper side of the cell so that the cilia do not form a complete circle around the vestibulum. The authors suggest that the outer ciliary zone is primarily concerned with locomotion while the inner ciliary zone is responsible for ingestion of food.

Phylogeny of rumen ophryoscolecid protozoa

Both Dogiel (1947) and Lubinsky (1957b,c) have proposed an evolutionary lineage for the rumen ciliates, progressing from the simplest genus, *Entodinium* to the most complex, *Ophryoscolex* and *Caloscolex*. Figure 3.13 illustrates the evolutionary relationship suggested by Lubinsky (1957c).

The criteria used were: number of skeletal plates; number of contractile vacuoles; the number and size of ciliary zones; and overall body size. All of these increased in the direction of advancement. Lubinsky (1957b,c) further suggested that changes in location of the nuclear apparatus, left (upper) lateral groove and the contractile vacuole were the result of torsional displacement from the right to the left side. He postulated that torsional displacement resulted from selective pressure of locomotion, i.e., a persistent rotational swimming movement.

Imai (1998) has suggested several modifications to the phylogenetic tree proposed by Lubinsky (1957c). His scheme differs as follows:

1. Ophryoscolecinae species branch off immediately after *Diplodinium*, before the species of Diplodiniinae with skeletal plates.
2. *Enoploplastron* branches off with *Ostracodinium* rather than in the Ophryoscolecinae line.
3. *Elytroplastron* and *Polyplastron* branch off with *Metadinium* rather than directly from the Diplodiniinae line.

The main difference in these two proposals would appear to be in the origin of the more complex species of Diplodiniinae. Göçmen *et al.* (2001) just reported a new species of *Eudiplodinium*, *E. dehorityi*, which shows definite similarities or evolutionary trends toward the genera *Elytroplastron* and *Polyplastron*. This new species generally has a single narrow skeletal plate, but occasionally two plates are observed. They may be separate or fused. The number of contractile vacuoles varies between 7-8 with 2-3 occurring to the right of the macronucleus. This might suggest that the genera *Elytroplastron* and *Polyplastron* are on a continuous line from *Eudiplodinium*.

Furness and Butler (1988) studied three genera of protozoa, *Entodinium*, *Eudiplodinium* and *Epidinium*, which are progressively more complex. They found that the infraciliature, nuclei, contractile vacuoles, cortex and cytoplasm are very similar between the three genera and in many instances indistinguishable. However, the cytoalimentary system (cytopharynx, esophagus and cytoproct) shows considerable variation, which appears to have allowed some forms to use food sources not available to other forms and resulted in the emergence of the more complex genera. The most simple genus, *Entodinium*, readily ingests small particles such as bacteria, chlorplasts and starch grains. *Eudiplodinium* can ingest larger particles, which includes whole cells, whereas *Epidinium* attaches itself onto large food particles via the oral aperture and actually appears to physically remove portions by force. The esophagus is rudimentary in *Entodinium*, sac-like in *Eudiplodinium* and tube-like in *Epidinium* with a structure suggesting an expansion-contraction capability. This increasingly complex cytoalimentary system, which shows a progressive ability to ingest food sources, parallels the evolutionary lineage originally proposed on the basis of morphological studies with light microscopy (Dogiel, 1947; Lubinsky, 1957b,c). Additional observations by Furness and Butler (1988) suggested that the cytoalimentary systems of *Diplodinium* and *Polyplastron* are similar to that of *Eudiplodinium*, while *Ophryoscolex* resembles *Epidinium*. This relationship is clearly consistent with their relative positions in the proposed evolutionary lineage.

Our knowledge about the phylogeny of rumen ciliates has been dramatically increased in recent years, based on results obtained with molecular techniques. Using small subunit ribosomal RNA sequences (SsrRNA), the ophryoscolecid protozoa fall into three distinct groupings which correspond to the three subfamilies proposed by Lubinsky (1957c) on the basis of morphological characteristics (Wright and Lynn, 1997a). Analyses of both

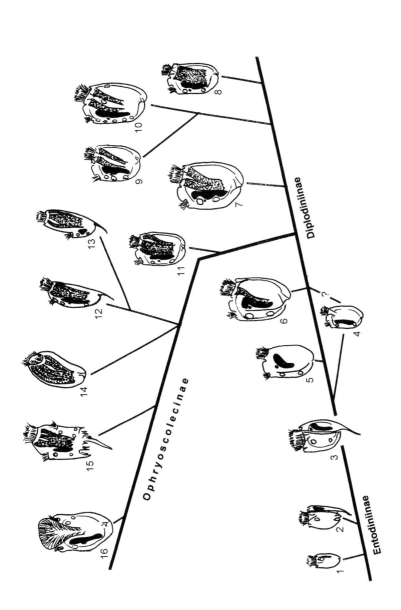

Figure 3.13 Adaptation of the dendrogram of the family Ophryoscolecidae proposed by Lubinsky (1957c). No. 1. *Entodinium nanellum* (Dogiel, 1923). No. 2. *Entodinium simulans* (Lubinsky, 1957). No. 3. Hypothetical transition form between *Entodinium* and the higher Ophryoscolecidae. No. 4. *Diplodinium lobatum* (Kofoid and MacLennan, 1932). No.5. *Diplodinium minor* (Dogiel, 1925). No.6. *Eudiplodinium maggii* (Fiorentini, 1889). No. 7 *Metadinium tauricum* (Dogiel and Fedorowa, 1925). No. 8 *Ostracodinium gracile* (Dogiel, 1925). No. 9. *Elytroplastron bubali* (Dogiel, 1928). No. 10. *Polyplastron multivesiculatum* (Dogiel and Fedorowa, 1925). No. 11. *Enoploplastron triloricatum* (Dogiel, 1925). No. 12. *Epidinium caudatum* (Fiorentini, 1889). No. 13. *Opisthotrichum janus* (Dogiel, 1923). No. 14. *Epiplastron africanum* (Dogiel, 1925). No. 15. *Ophryoscolex caudatus* (Eberlein, 1895). No. 16. *Caloscolex camelinus* (Dogiel, 1926).

parsimony and distance matrix trees strongly support the ophryoscolecid ciliates as a monophyletic group and a sister group to the vestibulifered ciliates *Isotricha* and *Dasytricha* (Wright and Lynn, 1997a,b; Wright *et al.*, 1997). *Entodinium* is the earliest branching ciliate, basal to a clade consisting of the other ophryoscolecids. Within this latter clade, the more complex Ophryoscolecinae (*Epidinium* and *Ophryoscolex*) group together while the intermediary Diplodiniinae (*Diplodinium, Eudiplodinium, Polyplastron* and presumably the other four genera in this subfamily which were not analyzed) form a monophyletic sister-group to the Ophryoscolecinae. The data obtained by Wright and Lynn in their 1997a study suggested that *Eudiplodinium* branched first in Diplodiniinae. However, this positioning was not strongly supported by all three phylogenetic methods employed. The authors did suggest that if this were the case, *Diplodinium* would have subsequently lost its skeletal plate(s). This was a possibility which Lubinsky suggested earlier (Fig. 3.13). Analysis of the new species of *Eudiplodinium* described by Göçmen *et al.* (2001) would determine whether there is a direct line from *Eudiplodinium* to *Elytroplastron* and *Polyplastron*. The location of exactly where *Ostracodinium, Metadinium* and *Enoploplastron* branch awaits analysis of the SsrRNA sequences for these genera.

Rumen flagellate protozoa

Prior to the study by Orpin (1977), reports on flagellate protozoa in the rumen were confounded by the presence of fungal zoospores. Most values reported for the concentration of flagellates in the rumen were taken in the 1960's and studies need to be repeated to differentiate between the protozoa and zoospores. Seven species of flagellate protozoa in five different genera, have been described in the rumen. They are *Monocercomonas ruminantium, Monocercomonoides caprae, Monocercomoides bovis, Chilomastix caprae, Tetratrichomonas buttreyi, Pentatrichomonas hominis* and *Trichomonas ruminantium*, all in the class Zoomastigophorea, subphylum Mastigophora, phylum Sarcomastigophora (Ogimoto and Imai, 1981). A key for the identification of the rumen flagellate protozoa is shown in Figure 3.14.

Essentially the characteristics used for classification are shape and the presence or absence of an undulating membrane, axostyle and cytostomal groove. The rumen flagellates are rather small, ranging from 4-15 µm in length. Body shape is elliptical to piriform with 3-5 anterior flagella and a nucleus located at the anterior end of the body. A posterior flagellum is present in one species, *Pentatrichomonas hominis*. Since the flagellates appear to occur in relatively low numbers and utilize only soluble substrates, their contribution to the overall rumen fermentaiion is probably minimal (Clarke, 1977).

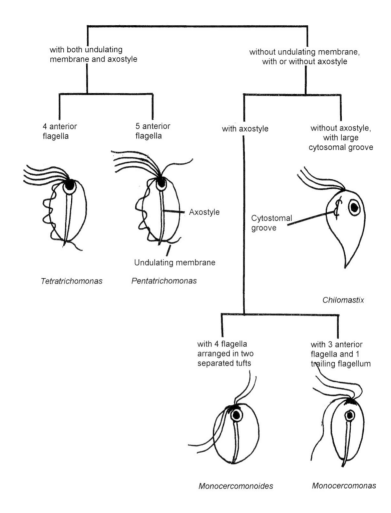

Figure 3.14. Key to the identification of rumen flagellate protozoa to the generic level (redrawn from Ogimoto and Imai, 1981).

References

Bush, M. and C. A. Kofoid. (1948). Ciliates from the Sierra Nevada bighorn *Ovis canadensis sierrae* Grinnel. *University of California Publications in Zoology*, **53**, 237-262.

Buisson, J. (1924). Quelques infusoires parasites d'antilopes africaines. *Annales de Parasitologie Humaine ey Comparee*, **2**, 155-160.

Clarke, R.T.J. (1964). Ciliates of the rumen of domestic cattle. (*Bos taurus* L.). *New Zealand Journal of Agricultural Research*, **7**, 248-257.

Clarke, R.T.J. (1977). Protozoa in the rumen ecosystem. In: *Microbial Ecology of the Gut.* Edited by R.T.J. Clarke and T. Bauchop. Academic Press, New York, NY. USA. pp. 251-276.
Corliss, J. O. (1994). An interim utilitarian ("user-friendly") hierarchical classification and characterization of the protists. *Acta Protozoologica* **33**, 1-51.
Dehority, B. A. (1970). Occurrence of the ciliate protozoa *Buetschlia parva* Schuberg in the rumen of the ovine. *Applied Microbiology*, **19**, 179-181.
Dehority, B. A. (1974). Rumen ciliate fauna of Alaskan moose (*Alces americana*), musk-ox (*Ovibos moschatus*) and Dall mountain sheep (*Ovis dalli*). *Journal of Protozoology*, **21**, 26-32.
Dehority, B. A. (1975). Rumen ciliate protozoa of Alaskan reindeer and caribou (*Rangifer tarandus* L.). In: *Proceedings of the 1st International Reindeer and Caribou Symposium*, Special Report No. 1, Biological Papers of the University of Alaska, Fairbanks, Alaska. pp. 241-250.
Dehority, B. A. (1979). Ciliate protozoa in the rumen of Brazilian water buffalo, *Bubalus bubalis* Linnaeus. *Journal of Protozoology*, **26**, 536-544.
Dehority, B. A. (1986). Rumen ciliate fauna of some Brazilian cattle: occurrence of several ciliates new to the rumen including the Cycloposthid *Parentodinium africanum. Journal of Protozoology*, **33**, 416-421.
Dehority, B. A. (1993). *Laboratory Manual for Classification and Morphology of Rumen Ciliate Protozoa.* CRC Press, Inc. Boca Raton, FL. USA.
Dehority, B. A. (1995). Rumen ciliates of the pronghorn antelope (*Antilocapra americana*), mule deer (*Odocoileus hemionus*), white-tailed deer (*Odocoileus virginianus*) and elk (*Cervus canadensis*) in the northwestern United States. *Archiv für Protistenkunde*, **146**, 29-36.
Dehority, B. A. and P. A. Tirabasso. (1989). Factors affecting the migration and sequestration of rumen protozoa in the family Isotrichidae. *Journal of General Microbiology*, **135**, 539-548.
Dehority, B. A., W. S. Damron and J. B. McLaren. (1983). Occurrence of the rumen ciliate *Oligoisotricha bubali* in domestic cattle (*Bos taurus*). *Applied and Environmental Microbiology*, **45**, 1394-1397.
Dehority, B. A., E. E. Grings and R. E. Short. (1999). Effects of cross-inoculation from elk and feeding pine needles on the protozoan fauna of pregnant cows: occurrence of *Parentodinium africanum* in domestic U. S. cattle (*Bos taurus*). *Journal of Eukaryotic Microbiology*, **46**, 632-636.
Dogiel, V. (1926). Sur quelques infusoires nouveaux habitant l'estomac du dromadaire (*Camelus dromedarius*). *Annales de Parasitologie*, **4**, 241-271.
Dogiel, V. (1927). Monographie der Familie Ophryoscolecidae. *Archiv für Protistenkunde*, **59**, 1-288.
Dogiel, V. A. (1928). La faune d'infusoires habitant l'estomac du buffle et du dromadaire. *Annales de Parasitologie*, **6**, 328-338.
Dogiel, V. (1947). The phylogeny of the stomach-infusoriens of ruminants in the light of

palaeontological and parasitological data. *Quarterly Journal of Microscopical Science*, **88**, 337-343.

Eadie, J. M. (1962). The development of rumen microbial populations in lambs and calves under various conditions of management. *Journal of General Microbiology*, **29**, 563-578.

Eloff, A. K. and W. van Hoven. (1980). Intestinal protozoa of the African elephant *Loxodonta africana* (Blumenbach). *South African Journal of Zoology*, **15**, 83-90.

Furness, D. N. and R. D. Butler. (1985a). The cytology of sheep rumen ciliates. II. Ultrastructure of *Eudiplodinium maggii*. *Journal of Protozoology*, **32**, 205-214.

Furness, D. N. and R. D. Butler. (1985b). The cytology of sheep rumen ciliates. III. Ultrastructure of the genus *Entodinium* (Stein). *Journal of Protozoology*, **32**, 699-707.

Furness, D. N. and R. D. Butler. (1988). The functional and evolutionary significance of the ultrastructure of the Ophryoscolecidae (Order Entodiniomorphida). *Journal of Protozoology*, **35**, 34-38.

Göçmen, B., M. Tosunoğlu and B. Falakali. (2001). New rumen ciliates from Turkish domestic cattle (*(Bos taurus* L.): 3. *Entodinium oektemae* n. sp. and *Entodinium imaii* n. sp. (Entodiniinae, Entodiniomorphida). *Turkish Journal of Zoology*, **25**, 269-274.

Göçmen, B., B. Falakali Mutaf and M. Tosunoğlu. (2001). New rumen ciliates from Turkish domestic cattle (*Bos taurus* L.): IV. *Eudiplodinium dehorityi* n. sp. *Acta Parasitologica Turcica,* **25**, 305-307.

Grain, J. (1994). Infusoires ciliés (Ordre des Entodiniomorphida). In: *Traite de Zoologie* 2. Edited by P. Grassé. Masson, Paris. pp. 327-364.

Gruby, D. and O. Delafond. (1843). Recherches sur des animalcules se développant dans L'estomac et dans les intestins pendant la digestion des animaux herbivores et carnivores. *Comptes Rendus Hebdomadaire des Seances de l'Academie des Sciences,* **17**, 1304-1308.

Guirong, N., Z. Hua, S. Zhu and S. Imai. (2000). Rumen ciliated protozoan fauna of the yak (*Bos grunniens*) in China with the description of *Entodinium monuo* n. sp. *Journal of Eukaryotic Microbiology,* **47**, 178-182.

Honigberg, B. M., W. Balamuth, E. C. Bovee, J. O. Corliss, M. Gojdics, R. P. Hall, R. R. Kudo, N. D. Levine, A. R. Loeblich, Jr., J. Weiser and D. H. Wenrich. (1964). A revised classification of the phylum protozoa. *Journal of Protozoology,* 11, 7-20.

Hsiung, T. S. (1930a). A monograph on the protozoa of the large intestine of the horse. *Iowa State College Journal of Science,* **4**, 359-423.

Hsiung, T. S. (1930b). Some new ciliates from the large intestine of the horse. *Transactions of The American Microscopical Society*, **49**, 34-41.

Hsiung, T. S. (1932). A general survey of the protozoan fauna of the rumen of the

Chinese cattle. *Bulletin of the Fan Memorial Institute of Biology*, **3**, 87-107.

Hukui, T. and K. Nisada. (1954). On *Dasytricha hukuokaensis* sp.n. *Zoological Magazine (Tokyo)*, **63**, 367-369.

Hungate, R. E. (1966). *The Rumen and its Microbes*. Academic Press, New York, NY. USA.

Hungate, R. E. (1978). The rumen protozoa. In: *Parasitic Protozoa*, Vol. II. Edited by J. P. Kreier. Academic Press, Inc., New York, NY. pp. 655-695.

Imai, S. (1981). Four new rumen ciliates, *Entodinium ogimotoi* sp.n., *E. bubalum* sp.n., *E. fujitai* sp.n. and *E. tsunodai* sp.n. and *Oligoisotricha bubali* (Dogiel, 1928) n. comb. *Japanese Journal of Veterinary Science*, **43**, 201-209.

Imai, S. (1984). New rumen ciliates, *Polymorphella bovis* sp.n. and *Entodinium longinucleatum* forma *spinolobum* f.n., from the zebu cattle in Thailand. *Japanese Journal of Veterinary Science*, **46**, 391-395.

Imai, S. (1988). Ciliate protozoa in the rumen of Kenyan zebu cattle, *Bos taurus indicus*, with the description of four new species. *Journal of Protozoology*, **35**, 130-136.

Imai, S. (1998). Phylogenetic taxonomy of rumen ciliate protozoa based on their morphology and distribution. *Journal of Applied Animal Research*, **13**, 17-36.

Imai. S. and Gui Rung. (1990). Ciliate protozoa in the forestomach of the bactrian camel in Inner-Mongolia, China. *Japanese Journal of Veterinary Science*, **52**, 1069-1075.

Imai, S. and K. Ogimoto. (1983). *Parabundleia ruminantium* gen. n., sp.n., *Diplodinium mahidoli* sp.n. with two formae, and *Entodinium parvum* forma *monospinosum* forma n. from the zebu cattle (*Bos indicus* L., 1758) in Thailand. *Japanese Journal of Veterinary Science*, **45**, 585-591.

Imai, S., H. Tashiro and T. Ishii. (1983). Scanning electron microscopy of the adoral ciliary zone of *Entodinium* Stein (Ciliophora, Entodiniomorphida). *Journal of Protozoology*, **30**, 466-472.

Imai, S., H. Kudo, K. Fukuta, N. Abudullah, Y. Ho and R. Onodera. (1995). *Isotricha jalaludinii* n. sp. found from the rumen of lesser mouse deer, *Tragulus javanicus*, in Malaysia. *Journal of Eukaryotic Microbiology*, **42**, 75-77.

Jameson, A. P. (1925). A new ciliate, *Charon ventriculi* n.g., n.sp., from the stomach of ruminants. *Parasitology*, **17**, 403-405.

Kleynhans, C. J. and W. van Hoven. (1976). Rumen protozoa of the giraffe with a description of two new species. *East African Wildlife Journal*, **14**, 203-214.

Kofoid, C. A. and R. F. MacLennan. (1930). Ciliates from *Bos indicus* Linn. I. The genus *Entodinium* Stein. *University of California Publications in Zoology*, **33**, 471-544.

Kofoid, C. A. and R. F. MacLennan. (1932). Ciliates from *Bos indicus* Linn. II. A revision of *Diplodinium* Schuberg. *University of California Publications in Zoology*, **37**, 53-152.

Kofoid, C. A. and R. F. MacLennan. (1933). Ciliates from *Bos indicus* Linn. III.

Epidinium Crawley, *Epiplastron* gen. nov., and *Ophryoscolex* Stein. *University of California Publications in Zoology*, **39**,1-34.

Kubesy, A. and B. A. Dehority. (2002). Forestomach ciliate protozoa in Egyptian dromedary camels (*Camels dromedarius*). *Zootaxa*, **51**:1-12.

Kudo, R. R. (1947). *Protozoology*. Charles C. Thomas. Springfield, IL. USA.

Latteur, Bernard. (1966). Contributions a la systematique de la Famille du Ophryoscolecidae Stein. *Annales de la Societe Royal Zoologique de Belgique*, **96,** 117-144.

Lee, J. J., S. H. Hutner and E. C. Bovee (Eds). (1985). *An Illustrated Guide to the Protozoa*. Society of Protozoologists, Lawrence, Kansas. USA.

Levine, N. D., J. O. Corliss, F. E. G. Cox, G.. Deroux, J. Grain, B. M. Honigberg, G. F. Leedale, A. R. Loeblich, III, J. Lom, D. Lynn, E. G. Merinfeld, F. C. Page, G. Poljansky, V. Sprague, J. Vavra, and F. G. Wallace, (1980). A newly revised classification of the protozoa. *Journal of Protozoology*, **27**, 37-58.

Lubinsky, G. (1957a). Studies on the evolution of the Ophryoscolecidae (Ciliata:Oligotricha). I. A new species of *Entodinium* with "caudatum", "lobosospinosum", and "dubardi" forms, and some evolutionary trends in the genus *Entodinium*. *Canadian Journal of Zoology*, **35**, 111-133.

Lubinsky, G. (1957b). Studies on the evolution of the Ophryoscolecidae (Ciliata:Oligotricha). II. On the origin of the higher Ophryoscolecidae. *Canadian Journal of Zoology*, **35**, 135-140.

Lubinsky, G. (1957c). Studies on the evolution of the Ophryoscolecidae (Ciliata:Oligotricha). III. Phylogeny of the Ophryoscolecidae based on their comparative morphology. *Canadian Journal of Zoology*, **35**, 141-159.

Lubinsky, G. (1958). Ophryoscolecidae (Ciliata:Entodiniomorphida) of reindeer (*Rangifer tarandus* L.) from the Canadian arctic. I. Entodiniinae. *Canadian Journal of Zoology*, **36**, 819-835.

Noirot-Timothée, C. (1960). Etude d'une famille de cilies:Les Ophryoscolecidae. Structures et ultrastructures. *Annales des Sciences Naturelles Zoologie et Biologie Animale*, **2**, 527-718.

Ogimoto, K. and S. Imai. (1981). *Atlas of Rumen Microbiology*. Japan Scientific Societies Press, Tokyo, Japan.

Orpin, C. G. (1977). The occurrence of chitin in the cell walls of the rumen organisms *Neocallimastix frontalis, Piromonas communis* and *Sphaeromonas communis*. *Journal of General Microbiology*, **99**, 215-218.

Schuberg, A. (1888). Die Protozoen des Wiederkauermagens. 1. *Buetschlia, Isotricha, Dasytricha, Entodinium*. *Zoologische Jahrbücher Abteilung für Systematik Oekologie und Geographie der Tiere*, **3**, 365-418.

Selim, H. M., S. Imai, O. Yamato, E. Miyagawa and Y. Maede. (1996). Ciliate protozoa in the forestomach of the dromedary camel (*Camelus dromedarius*) in Egypt, with description of a new species. *Journal of Veterinary Medical Science*, **58,** 833-837.

Sharp, R. G. (1914). *Diplodinium ecaudatum* with an account of its neuromotor apparatus. *University of California Publications in Zoology*, **13**, 43-122.

Stein, F. (1858). Über mehrere neve in Pansen der wiederkauer lebende Infusionsthiere. *Abhandlungen der k, Bohmischen Gesellschaft des Wissenschaften*, **10**, 69-70.

Stern, M. D., W. H. Hoover and J. B. Leonard. (1977a). Ultrastructure of rumen holotrichs by electron microscopy. *Journal of Dairy Science*, **60**, 911-918.

Stern, M. D., W. H. Hoover, R. G. Summers, Jr. and J. H. Rittenburg. (1977b). Ultrastructure of rumen entodiniomorphs by electron microscopy. *Journal of Dairy Science*, **60**, 902-910.

Thurston, J. P. and C. Noirot-Timothée. (1973). Entodiniomorph ciliates from the stomach of *Hippopotamus amphibius* with descriptions of two new genera and three new species. *Journal of Protozoology*, **20**, 562-565.

Warner, A.C.I. (1966). Diurnal changes in the concentrations of microorganisms in the rumens of sheep fed limited diets once daily. *Journal of General Microbiology*, **45**, 213-235.

Williams, A. G. and G. S. Coleman. (1988). The rumen protozoa. In: *The Rumen Microbial Ecosystem*. Edited by P. N. Hobson. Elsevier Applied Science, London. pp. 77-128.

Williams, A. G. and G. S. Coleman. (1992). *The Rumen Protozoa*. Springer-Verlag New York, Inc. New York, NY. USA

Wright, A.-D. G. and D. H. Lynn. (1997a). Phylogenetic analysis of the rumen ciliate family Ophryoscolecidae based on 18S ribosomal RNA sequences from *Diplodinium, Eudiplodinium* and *Ophryoscolex*. *Canadian Journal of Zoology*, **75**, 963-970.

Wright, A.-D. G. and D. H. Lynn. (1997b). Monophyly of the trichostome ciliates (phylum Ciliophora: class Litostomatea) tested using new 18S rRna sequences from the vestibuliferids, *Isotricha intestinalis* and *Dasytricha ruminantium*, and the haptorian, *Didinium nasutum*. *European Journal of Protistology*, **33**, 305-315.

Wright, A.-D. G., B. A. Dehority and D. H. Lynn. (1997). Phylogony of the rumen ciliates *Entodinium, Epidinium* and *Polyplastron* (Litostomatea: Entodiniomorphida) inferred from small subunit ribosomal RNA sequences. *Journal of Eukaryotic Microbiology*, **44**, 61-67.

CHAPTER 4

ESTABLISHMENT, NUMBERS AND DIURNAL CHANGES IN THE CONCENTRATION OF RUMEN PROTOZOA

Faunation

Before considering numbers and diurnal changes in concentration of rumen protozoa, it would seem desirable to briefly discuss the establishment of a ciliate protozoal population in the rumen. Two factors appear to be of prime importance in the development of a rumen fauna; first, that the animal is exposed to an adult or faunated animal, and second, that the environmental conditions within the rumen are satisfactory for survival of the protozoa (Hungate, 1966; Dehority, 1986; Dehority and Orpin, 1988). All studies conducted to date have indicated that a young animal can become faunated only by inoculation from another ruminant. This can be accomplished by several means, some more subtle than others. Primarily, if the mother grooms a young animal the protozoa present in her mouth from rumination are passed on via her saliva. Salivation on the feed or even on pasture plants by a faunated animal, followed by ingestion of the contaminated material by a young animal also leads to faunation. Observations by Eadie (1962a) even suggested that some of the smaller ciliate protozoa might be transmitted short distances between animals in airborne droplets from the mouth or nose. In general, the exposure of a young animal to older faunated animals is of no problem; however, under experimental conditions or possibly adverse normal conditions, inoculation of a young animal with rumen contents from an older animal can be used to establish a fauna.

Bryant and co-workers (1958, 1960) and Eadie (1962b) have demonstrated experimentally that calves isolated from other ruminants at birth do not become faunated. In one study by Bryant and Small (1960), the calves were raised to 24 weeks of age without any ciliate protozoa appearing in the rumen. In studies conducted by Dehority (1978), sheep obtained by hysterectomy and reared in isolation remained ciliate protozoa-free for nearly a year, at which time they were inoculated with rumen contents from another animal. Under the isolation conditions employed, it seems probable they could have remained free of protozoa indefinitely.

Eadie (1962a), concluded that flagellated protozoa just seem to appear in isolated animals, as originally observed by Becker and Everett (1930). Presumably the flagellated species are more resistant and can survive long enough to be transmitted by means other than direct contact. However, further studies are needed to determine whether these organisms are truly flagellate protozoa or zoospores of anaerobic rumen fungi (Dehority and Orpin, 1988). In general, anaerobic fungi have been found to only survive for short periods of time in moist feces and saliva stored in air (Milne *et al.*, 1989). However, some storage conditions such as allowing feces to dry at 20°C or 39°C in air apparently induces the formation of resistant structures such as cysts or spores, since viable fungi could be isolated from fecal pellets after periods as long as 128 days.

Following inoculation, establishment of the protozoa then becomes dependent on conditions within the rumen itself. Both Bryant and Small (1960) and Eadie (1962a) have shown that the pH in the rumen is quite acid in young animals, presumably due to the fermentation of soluble sugars in their diet of milk or starter ration. The pH rises as forage and less fermentable feeds are consumed and alkaline salivary production is increased. Using inoculation methods these workers concluded that the *Entodinium* become established at about pH 6, while the holotrichs and remaining entodiniomorphs did not establish until the rumen pH reached the vicinity of 6.5.

Rumen ciliate protozoa free calves were inoculated with different types and numbers of protozoa by Williams and Dinusson (1972). Using a micromanipulator, an inoculum of 2 to 50 cells of either entodiniomorphs or holotrichs resulted in establishment of ciliate densities by 5 to 7 weeks equal to densities obtained in 1-2 weeks by inoculating with 10,000 to 94,000 cells. About 16 weeks were required to establish similar protozoal densities when protozoa-free calves were allowed to run with mature ruminants. These authors were able to establish holotrichs in calves free of entodiniomorphs and suggested that the sequence of establishment noted earlier may be a result of the numbers of the particular genera normally occurring in rumen contents, i.e., *Entodinium* occurring in the highest density. Although this conclusion may be quite valid, the authors seem to have overlooked the possibility that pH may also be involved as suggested by the previously cited studies. Unfortunately they either did not measure or did not report pH of the rumen in their animals.

In the study conducted by Dehority (1978), six sheep, free of ciliate protozoa from birth, were each inoculated with 300 ml of rumen contents containing 16.7×10^4 protozoa per ml. In five of the six sheep, protozoan concentrations increased rapidly and leveled off after 7 days. The protozoan concentration continued to increase between 7 and 14 days in the other animal, leveling off after 14 days. Adjusting for differences in rumen volumes, total protozoan numbers in the rumen increased from 9.5 to 121 fold the 7 days following inoculation.

Concentrations

Table 4.1 is a compilation of rumen ciliate protozoa concentrations in domestic ruminants. These values are in a range similar to earlier data summarized by Hungate (1966). As an overall estimate, a protozoan concentration of about 1×10^6 per ml of rumen contents appears to be "normal" across most rations for both cattle and sheep.

Most of the information on protozoan numbers reported in the literature is based on the concentration of protozoa per ml of rumen contents; however, in some cases these values may be misleading (Dehority, 1978). Table 4.2 shows that the concentration of protozoa per ml was statistically different between two group of sheep which were fed alfalfa and concentrate, respectively. Rumen volumes were determined on these animals and when the total number of protozoa in the rumen was calculated, there was no difference between the groups. Obviously this factor should be kept in mind when studying protozoan data reported on a concentration basis.

Another factor which should be considered is the rate at which the protozoa pass out of the rumen. We can determine both fluid and dry matter turnover times in the rumen, but as yet we have been unable to accurately determine the relationship between these values and protozoan turnover rate.

Table 4.1 CONCENTRATIONS OF PROTOZOA IN RUMEN CONTENTS

Animal	Diet	Protozoa per ml ($\times 10^4$)	Reference
Sheep	1500 g orchardgrass hay	12.4 - 19.5	Nakamura and Kanegasaki
	1500 g orchardgrass hay plus 600 g concentrate	73.7 - 102.4	(1969)
Cattle	50% alfalfa hay, 42% barley plus supplement	48.4	Ibrahim et al. (1970)
Sheep	90 g alfalfa pellets every 2 hr	49.8	Hungate et al. (1971)
	540 g alfalfa pellets twice a day	23.7	
Sheep	Bromegrass hay	20.4 - 41.8	Dehority (1975)
Goat	Bromegrass hay	53.7	Dehority (1975)
Cattle	Equal parts rice straw and alfalfa meal pellets plus 0.5 parts conc.	25.3 - 44.8	Abe et al. (1973)
Sheep	45% corn cobs, 35% alfalfa meal, 12.6% oats plus supp. (650 g/day)	74	Potter and Dehority (1973)
Sheep	40% alfalfa, 28% corn, 25% corn cobs plus supplement	85.7	Dearth et al. (1974)
Sheep	Orchardgrass hay (800 g/day)	40 - 53	Grubb and Dehority (1975)
	60% corn plus 40% orchardgrass hay (800 g/day)	101 - 163	
Cattle	Varied	63.5	Towne and Nagaraja (1990)
Sheep	Varied	180.9	Towne and Nagaraja (1990)
Bison	Varied	174.8	Towne and Nagaraja (1990)

Diet effects

Studies by Nakamura and Kanegasaki (1969) and Grubb and Dehority (1975), both with sheep, demonstrate the influence of the type of diet on protozoan

76 Rumen microbiology

Table 4.2 EFFECT OF RUMEN VOLUME ON TOTAL PROTOZOA NUMBERS[a]

Sheep	Ration	Rumen volume (ml)	Protozoa per ml ($\times 10^4$)	Total protozoa ($\times 10^9$)
2	Alfalfa	8960	36.6	3.28
5	"	5360	27.9	1.50
6	"	4790	52.2	2.50
Mean ± SE			38.9 ± 7.1[b]	2.43 ± 0.52[b]
3	Concentrate	2090	139.6	2.92
4	"	2710	132.8	3.60
8	"	2950	82.8	2.44
Mean ± SE			118.4 ± 17.9[c]	2.98 ± 0.34[b]

[a] Data from Dehority (1978)
[b,c] Means within a column followed by different superscripts are significantly different at $P < 0.025$

concentrations under well controlled experimental conditions. Nakamura and Kanegasaki (1969) fed two sheep, A and B, a diet of 1500 g orchardgrass hay plus 600 g concentrate per day for three months (Period 1); 1500 g straight hay for four weeks (Period 2); then in Period 3, animal A continued on the hay while animal B was again given the hay plus concentrate diet. The diets were fed in equal portions twice a day. A dramatic decrease in protozoan concentrations occurred in Period 2 when the hay diet was fed. In Period 3, concentrations remained about the same in Animal A who remained on the hay diet, while concentrations increased back to those observed in Period 1 for Animal B, who was again fed the hay-concentrate diet. Total protozoan concentrations ranged between 7-12 x 10^5/ml on the hay-concentrate diet and between 2-4 x 10^5 on hay alone. These changes were broken down to the species level and in general, the major effect observed was a sharp drop in *Entodinium* numbers when concentrate was removed from the diet.

The graph shown in Figure 4.1 summarizes the data obtained by Grubb and Dehority (1975) on protozoan numbers when an animal is abruptly changed from an all roughage diet to a 60% corn-40% roughage diet. Concentrations ranged between 4-6 x 10^5 protozoa per ml on 100% orchardgrass hay, rose markedly during the five days following the ration change and then stabilized between 10-18 x 10^5 protozoa per ml. The sheep were fed once daily 800 g of both diets. No obvious relationship between the two rations and generic distribution was observed. Although there are some differences in the experimental design of the two experiments just cited, basically they both used similar type diets and when the amount of available energy in the diet increased, the concentration of protozoa increased. Similar results were obtained in studies with cattle (Abe *et al.*, 1973; Puch, 1977, M.S. Thesis, Ohio State University; Dehority and Mattos, 1978), and water buffalo (Michalowski, 1975) when concentrates were added to the diet.

Dennis *et al.* (1983) studied the effects of energy level (30%, 50% and 70% concentrate) in protein-free semipurified diets on the number and types of rumen protozoa. Nitrogen sources were urea or soybean meal (SBM). Protozoan concentrations increased as the percentage concentrate in the diet increased, i.e., 1.5, 2.5 and 4.1 x 10^5/ml for the 30, 50 and 70% concentrate diets, respectively. Concentrations of all genera except *Dasytricha* increased with increased concentrate feeding. These data clearly support previous studies. Urea supported higher concentrations of ciliates than did SBM; however, *Isotricha* and *Dasytricha* concentrations were higher with SBM. The authors concluded that diets free of natural protein can support a large and complex protozoan fauna, which presumably uses bacteria as its nitrogen source.

Nour *et al.* (1979) studied the effect of substituting urea for 0, 36, 55 or 100% of cottonseed cake protein on protozoan concentrations and generic compositions in sheep, goats, cattle and buffalo. Concentrations were highest on the 0 and 100% urea-N diets and sheep and goats had higher protozoan concentrations than buffalo and cattle. When total protozoa in the rumen were calculated, using rumen volume measurements, sheep had higher numbers than goats and buffalo were higher than cattle. Generic composition was similar across all animal species, and percent *Entodinium* increased from 91.4 to 99.7 on the 0 and 100% urea-N diets, respectively.

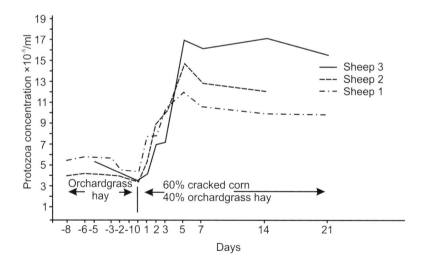

Figure 4.1. Concentrations of protozoa in rumen contents of three sheep abruptly changed from an all hay to a hay-concentrate diet (from Grubb and Dehority, 1975).

pH

Purser and Moir (1959) investigated the possible effects of pH on numbers and growth of rumen protozoa. It is worth noting that the protozoa in their animals were principally *Entodinium* species, with other genera never exceeding 13% of the total. By introducing varying concentrations of glucose through the fistula they established lower ruminal pH values. A distinct diurnal cycle was evident, concentrations falling off markedly in the first hour after feeding and continuing downward for an additional 6 to 8 hours. After this time concentrations began to increase gradually to the prefeeding level. A correlation of the minimum daily pH with mean daily concentration of protozoa was highly significant. Counts were also made of dividing protozoa at each sampling time and a marked inhibition in division was observed at the period of lowest pH in the rumen. Thus, both sampling time and pH would certainly influence the numbers of protozoa.

Based on the observations of Bryant and Small (1960) and Eadie (1962a), pH appears to be important in the establishment and maintenance of rumen protozoa. Feeding of high concentrate diets with a corresponding marked decrease in rumen pH is commonly thought to essentially eliminate the protozoa. Latham *et al.* (1971) changed cows from all hay to 80% grain - 20% hay, and noted considerable reduction in protozoan numbers. When corn was the grain, holotrichs were eliminated within 3-6 weeks; however, the holotrichs remained with barley as the grain. For the same three cows, rumen pH values after 6 weeks on ration were 6.67, 5.95 and 6.00 with corn and 6.30, 5.75 and 6.10 with barley. Abe *et al.* (1973) observed a marked decrease in protozoan concentrations within 7 days when cows were fed 12 kg conc. plus 1 kg alfalfa pellets. The pH of the rumen contents fell to 5.5. Ciliate protozoan concentrations were observed to increase as the percentage concentrate in the diet of sheep increased from 10 to 60%, but decreased when the level of concentrate increased to 71% (Mackie *et al.*, 1978). The hours per day that pH of the rumen contents was below 6.0 increased markedly with length of time on the diet (Mackie and Gilchrist, 1979). Towne *et al.* (1988) measured protozoan concentrations in 81 bison. They were divided into three groups on the basis of diet, i.e., those fed forage, forage plus concentrate and a feedlot-concentrate diet. Protozoan concentrations were 27, 210 and 169 x 10^4/g, respectively. These data would substantiate the above observations of Mackie *et al.* (1978).

Not all studies would completely agree with the above listed conclusions. Slyter *et al.* (1970) fed steers all concentrate diets ad libitum, containing either 90% corn or 90% wheat. Average protozoan concentrations between 6 and 12 weeks were 6.5 and 8.0 x 10^3 per g of rumen contents for corn and wheat, respectively. Only entodiniomorph protozoa were observed and especially important, pH values were as low as 5.0 - 5.2. In a 4 x 4 Latin square experiment with steers, all concentrate rations containing 90% corn, wheat, barley or milo were fed at a restricted level of 1.5% body weight (Slyter *et al.*, 1970). Protozoal numbers/g of rumen contents were 30.8, 9.8, 36.2 and 26.7 x 10^3, while pH values were 6.0, 5.2, 5.8 and 6.1 for corn, wheat, barley and milo, respectively.

Fifteen of the 16 steers contained only entodiniomorphs; however, one steer fed wheat with the correspondingly lower pH contained holotrichs. Vance et al. (1972) fed all concentrate rations to steers using whole shelled corn or crimped corn. Protozoa disappeared within 14 days but reappeared after about 112 days on feed, concentrations rising to 5.5 x 10^3 in the crimped corn fed animals by 140 days. Rumen pH values were 5.5 on crimped corn and 5.6 on whole corn. Primarily *Entodinium* species were present.

Franzolin and Dehority (1996) studied the effect of prolonged high-concentrate feeding on the concentration of rumen protozoa. In general, feeding high-concentrate diets results in a lowering of rumen pH below 6.0 with a marked decrease in protozoal concentrations. However, as mentioned previously, some discrepancies have been observed and might suggest that factors in addition to low pH may be involved in lowering protozoal concentration. When they sequentially fed steers an all forage, 50% concentrate and 75% concentrate diet, protozoal numbers increased from 3.61 to 6.42 and 8.03 x 10^5 per ml, respectively. The all forage and 75% concentrate values were different ($P <$ 0.05). The overall average rumen pH decreased from 6.33 to 5.89 and 5.67, respectively. Figure 4.2 shows the average rumen pH for each steer individually, on all three diets. Steers 3 and 5 had a lower average ruminal pH ($P <0.05$) when fed the all forage and 50% concentrate diets.

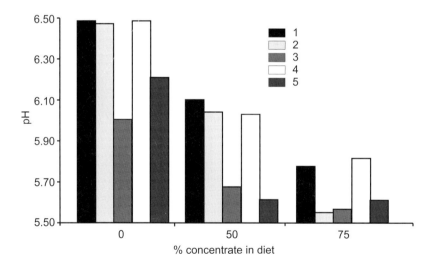

Figure 4.2. Average ruminal pH for five steers when fed diets containing 0, 50, or 75% concentrate. The pH value for each steer was the average of measurements taken at 0, 3, 6, 9, 12, 15, and 24 h after feeding. (from Franzolin and Dehority, 1996).

The steers were then divided into two groups: steers 1, 2, and 4, which had the highest average rumen pH values in the initial study, were fed an all-concentrate diet for 17 weeks followed by feeding a 90% concentrate-10% forage diet for 11 weeks; the other two steers were fed the same diets in the reverse order. In general, based on protozoal concentrations, steers 1, 2 and 4 had relatively high concentrations of ruminal protozoa on both diets while steers 3 and 5 were defaunated most of the time. Across both diets, rumen protozoal concentrations were lower in steers 3 and 5 ($P<0.05$). Two diurnal pH curves were measured for each steer on each of the two diets, and the average curves are shown in Figure 4.3. For all sampling times, mean pH values were 5.75, 5.71, 5.56, 5.88, and 5.34 in steers 1-5, respectively. The mean ruminal pH in steer 3 was lower ($P < 0.05$) than in steer 4 and mean ruminal pH in steer 5 was lower ($P < 0.05$) than in steers I, 2, and 4. The authors concluded that in addition to the lowering of rumen pH in all animals as a result of feeding high concentrate diets, other factors are involved. These could include rate of feed consumption, rate of passage, salivary production and ruminating activity. These so-called "other factors" seem to vary between individual animals and may contribute to lower ruminal pH values.

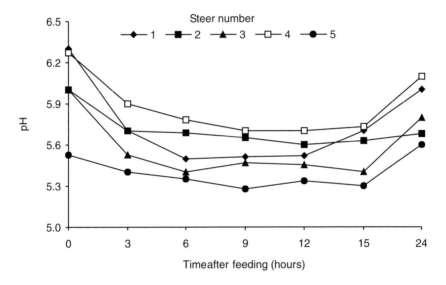

Figure 4. 3. Average diurnal pH curves for all steers during the final 22 weeks on high-concentrate diets. Four curves for each animal, two on all-concentrate and two on 10% forage diets. (from Franzolin and Dehority, 1996).

It would appear that rations containing between 40-60% concentrate will support maximal protozoan numbers with a diverse fauna containing species in most of the genera. When high- or all-concentrate rations are fed and ruminal pH decreases to below 6.0, numbers are decreased and primarily *Entodinium* species are present. However, the discrepancies between the different studies suggest that additional factors not measured may also be involved.

Frequency of feeding

The data of Moir and Somers (1956), presented in Table 4.3, clearly shows the effects of frequency of feeding on protozoan concentrations. The experiment was conducted as a 5 x 5 Latin square and samples for protozoa counts were taken on the final day of a 4-week period immediately before the 9:00 a.m. feeding. Feeding the same quantity of feed four times daily versus once a day resulted in a doubling of protozoan concentrations. Protozoan concentrations on the four times daily feeding schedule were significantly higher ($P< 0.05$) than all other treatments, while the three, twice daily, feeding treatments were significantly higher ($P< 0.01$) than the single feeding. Their protozoal population was primarily small entodiniomorphs. Rumen pH was measured over a 24 h period for all treatments and only in those animals fed once daily did the pH fall below 6.0.

Table 4.3. EFFECT OF FEEDING FREQUENCY ON PROTOZOAN CONCENTRATIONS IN SHEEP[a]

Ration	Feeding time	% of total ration at each feeding	Protozoa (10^6/ml)
Roughage and sheep cubes	0900	100%	1.15[b]
Roughage and sheep cubes	0900, 1100, 1300 & 1500	25%	3.14[c]
Roughage and sheep cubes	0900 & 1700	50%	2.26
Roughage	0900		
Sheep cubes	1700		2.34
Sheep cubes	0900		
Roughage	1700		2.26

[a] Data from Moir and Somers (1956)
[b] Significantly lower than all other concentrations ($P<0.01$)
[c] Significantly higher than all other concentrations ($P<0.05$)

Similar results on the effect of feeding frequency on protozoan concentrations were obtained in a study by Froetschel et al. (1990). Mean protozoan concentrations increased from 2.18×10^6/ml in steers fed once a day to 3.51×10^6/ml in steers fed 12 times daily (every 2 h over a 24 h period). One of the factors previously believed to be responsible for the increased concentration of protozoa was a higher rumen pH with less fluctuation. However, in this study, the mean pH in steers fed 12 times daily was .24 units lower than the mean pH in those animals fed only once (6.69 and 6.45; SE = .03).

Clarke et al. (1982) have studied the variation in protozoan concentrations of sheep fed two different levels of chopped alfalfa hay (1000 or 700 g/day) at two feeding frequencies (hourly or once a day). The authors also calculated volume and assuming a specific gravity of 1.1 and 10% DM, calculated total mass of ciliates in the rumen. Level of feed, frequency of feeding and sampling time markedly affected protozoan concentrations, weight of rumen contents and mass of ciliates. In addition, differences between sheep on the same regime and feeding frequency were very large. The authors concluded that animals must be considered individually in studies on the contribution of protozoa to the overall rumen fermentation, i.e., ciliate concentrations, generic distribution and size of the individual cells must all be taken into account.

Feed level

The effect of feed level on protozoan concentrations was first investigated by Christiansen *et al.* (1964). A pelleted diet containing 32% alfalfa hay, 48.5% corn, 7% cobs, 7% molasses and supplements was fed to lambs in a switch-back design to compare the effects of a full feed versus a 1/3 restriction. Protozoan concentrations rapidly decreased in the full-fed lambs and in most animals the protozoa disappeared completely within 2-3 weeks. The effect of physical form of the diet on protozoan concentrations was also studied and the protozoa decreased in number or disappeared when finely ground or pelleted diets were fed. Very little decrease was noted the first week, followed by a rapid decline and complete disappearance in 2-3 weeks. The authors concluded that the decrease in protozoan concentrations was probably the result of increased rate of passage of digesta from the rumen.

In a study by Dearth *et al.* (1974) protozoan concentrations were determined to the generic level for sheep receiving diets at the maintenance and 1.8 x maintenance energy level. The 1.8 x maintenance level of intake was very near maximum voluntary intake for the animals. The experimental design was a 4 x 4 Latin square with an extra period. The pelleted diet, fed once daily, contained 40% dehydrated alfalfa meal, 28% shelled corn, 26% ground corn cobs, 5% soybean meal plus minerals and vitamins, which was a higher roughage diet than that fed by Christiansen *et al.* (1964). The concentration of total protozoa, *Dasytricha, and Ophryoscolex* all decreased ($P < 0.01$) when the sheep were fed at 1.8 x maintenance. *Entodinium* concentrations also decreased ($P < 0.05$). These data would in general agree with the observations of Christiansen *et al.* (1964); however, the magnitude of the decrease in protozoan concentrations was far less. This may have been the result of using a higher roughage diet.

Warner (1962) has reported some very interesting data on the variability of protozoan concentrations with season, between animals on the same diet, effects of level of feed intake, and effects of changing the diet. He also concluded that the quantity of a given ration fed above a certain minimum level (50% of normal intake) has little effect on numbers. However, his data were obtained from just two animals and in view of the results cited previously from the study by Dearth *et al.* (1974), his conclusion that all of the fluctuation is of the same kind noted in his seasonal experiments may not be warranted.

Warner (1962) also investigated the time required for the reappearance of protozoa following a 4-day period of starvation. The entodinia appear to be quite hardy, disappearing in only one instance and reappearing within one day. In contrast, the holotrichs were markedly affected by starvation, requiring 2 to 3 weeks to reappear in minimal concentrations. In a study by Dehority (unpublished), five sheep in isolation were starved for 10 days and numbers decreased drastically, ranging from .24 x 10^4 to 2 x 10^4 per ml. Almost all the protozoa were two species of *Entodinium*, but an occasional cell of *Metadinium affine* or *Polyplastron* was seen. Concentrations had increased considerably after three days back on feed and by 7 to 14 days were very high. Both *M. affine* and *Polyplastron* were also present. In a separate experiment a lamb was fed I.V. for 51 days, at which time there were still 13.6 x 10^3 protozoa per ml rumen contents. About 99.9% were four species of *Entodinium* but several cells of *M. affine* were also present.

Potter and Dehority (1973) studied the effects of starvation upon concentrations of rumen protozoa in sheep. Figure 4.4 shows diurnal cycles of mean protozoan concentrations in four sheep either fed 650 g once daily or not fed. By witholding feed for 24 h, protozoan concentrations were reduced 80%.

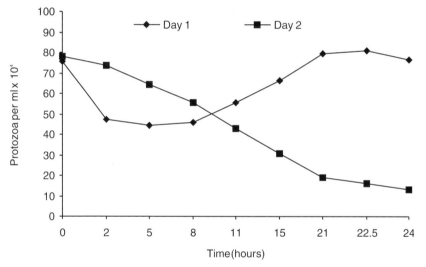

Figure 4.4. Mean protozoan concentrations determined in four lambs (from Potter and Dehority, 1973). On day 1 the animals received 650 g and on day 2 feed was withheld. Samples were taken at 0, 2, 5, 8, 11, 15, 21 and 24 h after the normal feeding time.

Diurnal variation

In their studies on pH effects, Purser and Moir (1959) noted a distinct diurnal cycle for *Entodinium*. Concentrations decreased for 6 to 8 h after feeding and then gradually rose to prefeeding levels by 20 to 24 h. Subsequent work by Purser (1961) established that a diurnal cycle also existed for the holotrichs; however, it differed from the cycle for the entodiniomorphs. He observed a peak concentration at feeding time (animals fed once daily), gradually diminishing until 20 h after feeding and then a rapid increase up to feeding.

84 Rumen microbiology

Warner (1966a,b,c) conducted a series of studies in sheep in which the diurnal changes in protozoal concentrations were followed for three different feeding practices. These were feeding a limited diet once daily, feeding to appetite in pens or pasture, and feeding a limited ration every three hours. For sheep fed a limited diet once daily (Warner, 1966a), the diurnal curves obtained for *Entodinium, Polyplastron, Epidinium, Diplodinium* and the holotrichs were very similar to the curves reported previously by Purser and Moir (1959) and Purser (1961). After suitable measurements of dilution, etc., Warner (1966a) concluded that the diurnal fluctuation in entodiniomorph concentrations was the end result of changes in the dilution rate due to eating and growth rate in response to incoming nutrients. The only discrepancy would appear to be in the curve he obtained for *Diplodinium*, in which there was no decrease in concentration due to the dilution effects of feeding. Studies by Dehority and Potter (1974) on *D. flabellum* concentrations in sheep gave very similar results in several animals. Dehority and Mattos (1978) subsequently noted this same pattern for *Diplodinium* concentrations in cattle. On this basis it might be concluded that division or growth of *Diplodinium* is extremely rapid immediately after feeding. In contrast to the entodiniomorphs, the diurnal cycle for holotrichs consisted of a gradual decrease in concentration for 18-20 h after feeding, with a gradual to marked increase just prior to or at the next feeding (Warner, 1966a). The diurnal cycles shown in Figure 4.5 were drawn from the data reported by Michalowski (1975) and represent the typical shape found for these two groups of ciliates when concentration is plotted against time after feeding.

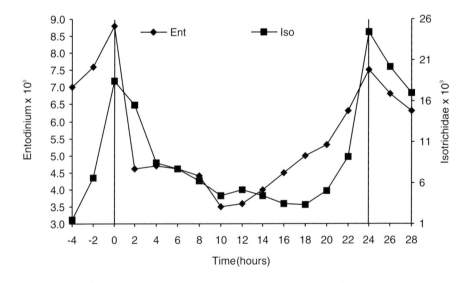

Figure 4.5. Diurnal variation of protozoan concentrations in the genus *Entodinium* (Ent) and family Isotrichidae (Iso) in water buffalo fed once daily (drawn from data of Michalowski, 1975).

In general, Warner (1966c) obtained similar results in his animals fed to appetite, probably because the eating behavior of his animals was such that almost all of the ration was consumed during one major period. His studies on limited feeding every three hours (Warner, 1966b) indicated a slight 3-hour rhythm cycle for most of the protozoa; however, superimposed on this was a gradual decline in numbers presumably due to the repeated sampling. Of the three studies, the latter is much less conclusive.

Clarke (1965) studied the diurnal cycle of rumen protozoa in cattle and his results are shown in Figures 4.6 and 4.7. His procedure differed from other workers in that at each sampling time the entire contents of the reticulo-rumen were removed, weighed, mixed and sampled, and the remainder returned to the animal. Although it seems that such a rigorous treatment might upset or alter normal rumen function, he did not see any indication to support this contention. In Figure 4.6, total protozoa in the rumen are compared to

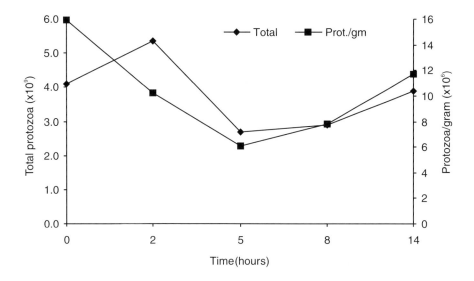

Figure 4.6. Comparison of diurnal changes in total numbers and concentration (number/gram) of rumen protozoa in a cow fed fresh red clover (drawn from data of Clark, 1965).

protozoan concentrations. The protozoan concentration curve is similar to that observed by both Warner (1966a) and Michalowski (1975). However, it differs markedly from the curve for total protozoa in the five hour period immediately after feeding. Figure 4.7 presents the curves for total protozoa, entodiniomorphs and isotrichids. These values are for the total numbers occurring in the rumen, and the initial rise can thus be ascribed solely to the holotrichs. A differential count of the isotrichids revealed that the dasytrichs were responsible for the marked increase after feeding. Based on the data in Figure 4.6, Clarke (1965) concluded that the differences between his curves in Figure 4.7 and the previous results of Purser and Moir (1959), Purser (1961) and Warner (1966a,b,c) are based on the fact that he determined total numbers in the rumen, thereby eliminating the dilution effect of feeding. He suggested that if their data were corrected for the dilution effect, it would lie on a similar curve to those which he reports. Feeding fresh clover once or twice daily gave very similar shaped diurnal cycles.

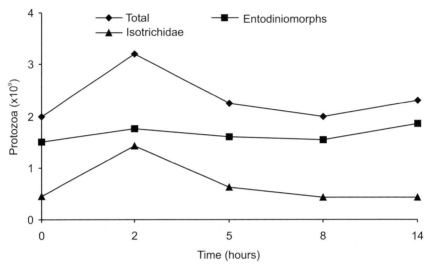

Figure 4.7. Diurnal variation in the numbers of total protozoa, entodiniomorphs and Isotrichidae in cattle fed red clover hay once a day (drawn from data of Clarke, 1965).

The growth cycle of holotrich protozoa in sheep has been studied by the author (unpublished), and even though only concentration was measured, results were slightly different than those of Clarke (1965). On a ration of 45% ground corn cobs, 35% dehydrated alfalfa leaf meal, 12.5% rolled oats, 5% molasses and 0.4% urea, a sharp increase in holotrich numbers was observed in the first half hour after feeding, followed by a sharp decline to prefeeding levels in about two hours. For example, in one experiment the holotrich numbers (x 10^3 per ml) increased from 2.8 at 1½ h before feeding to 17 at feeding, to 26.4 at ½ h after feeding and then dropped to 16 and 8 at 1 and 2 h after feeding. The same cycle was noted for both *Dasytricha* and *Isotricha*. The animals consumed their ration in less than ½ h, thus the sharp increase in numbers at the ½ h sampling time is undoubtedly even larger than estimated. Since dilution would not be involved between the ½, 1 and 2 h samples, one must conclude that some other factor, possibly sequestration or increased rate of passage in response to feeding must be involved. Very similar data were obtained by Dehority and Mattos (1978) in Brazilian cattle fed grass hay (Table 4.5). By not sampling between 0 and 2 h Clarke (1965) may have missed some important changes.

Clarke (1965) suggested that the decrease in holotrichs was the result of overfeeding and subsequent bursting of the cells. The author investigated this possibility by taking samples of rumen contents from sheep immediately after the entire ration had been consumed (about ½ h) and incubating them *in vitro* (unpublished). Numbers decreased

Table 4.5. CHANGES IN *ENTODINIUM, ISOTRICHA* AND *DASYTRICHA* CONCENTRATIONS ASSOCIATED WITH FEEDING[a]

Day	Time after feeding (h)	% of concentration at feeding		
		Entodinium	Isotricha	Dasytricha
1	0.5	148	600	740
	1.5	141	475	828
	3	102	125	352
2	0.5	124	462	458
	1.5	119	300	528
	3	76	312	228

[a]Data from Dehority and Mattos (1978)

as usual *in vivo* but were maintained *in vitro*, indicating that some other mechanism must be involved. Whether the holotrichs actually undergo a rapid stage of growth and multiplication when energy becomes available is not known for certain, since no one has observed high nos. of dividing cells. When feeding is delayed for several hours, or only a small portion, 1/5 of the daily ration is fed, the holotrichs increase in concentration slightly or maintain their numbers and then respond to feeding the remaining 4/5 of the diet with a sharp increase in numbers (Dehority, 1970). This increase in numbers after feeding could be chemotactic, assuming the cells detach and migrate to a soluble energy source. The rapid decrease in number after feeding cannot readily be explained, but it would appear that sequestration must be involved.

Several reports have now been published on sequestration of holotrich protozoa in the rumen. Abe *et al.* (1981) observed an approximate four-fold increase in the concentration of holotrichs within one hour after the commencement of feeding. Their data suggested that the fluctuation in holotrich numbers was related to the type or composition of the feed, as well as the quantity or volume of feed and possibly the physical act of ingestion. A differential response of the holotrichs and entodiniomorphs to feeding was observed, the entodiniomorphs decreasing in concentration as expected, while the holotrich concentrations increased markedly. Holotrich numbers increased in response to either feeding or direct additions of feed into the rumen. Reduced, but definite, fluctuations were noted in holotrich concentrations when the daily ration was fed in 8 equal portions at 3 h intervals. In general, those data supported the previous findings of Warner (1966a), Dehority (1970) and Dehority and Mattos (1978).

When these authors physically observed the walls of the rumen and reticulum, they noted that in a number of animals a thick protozoal mass could be seen on the walls of the reticulum. This mass consisted of 75% holotrichs and 25% small entodiniomorphs. They concluded that the holotrichs sequester on the wall of the reticulum, migrating into the rumen contents at feeding in a chemotactic response to incoming soluble nutrients (Orpin and Letcher, 1978) or possibly being dislodged as a result of strong reticular contractions associated with feeding. The factors or stimulus for the rather rapid return of the holotrichs to the reticulum wall is unclear. The authors also point out that the reduction in holotrich concentrations with frequent feeding might suggest that the more frequently migration occurs, the more holotrichs are washed out of the rumen.

In a subsequent study by Murphy, Drone and Woodford (1985), similar responses of holotrich concentrations to nutrients were observed. When glucose was infused directly into the reticulum at the normal feeding time, a marked increase in holotrich numbers occurred. However, infusion of water, saliva, NaCl or starch had no effect on holotrich concentrations. These authors suggested that rapid utilization of the soluble carbohydrate available immediately after feeding would lower the concentration below the chemotactic threshold and the holotrichs would return to the reticulum wall. However, it would seem that some other factors must be involved. For example, as the holotrichs feed they store intercellular polysaccharide, thus because of an increase in specific gravity they may simply settle into the reticulum area.

In the studies on diurnal changes in the concentration of isotrichids by Abe *et al.* (1981) and Murphy *et al.* (1985), it was concluded that *Isotricha* and *Dasytricha* sequester on the wall of the reticulum and migrate back into the rumen contents when the animal is fed. The stimulus for this migration was thought to be a chemotactic response to soluble sugars in the incoming feed. However, this explanation would not be satisfactory for those instances where isotrichid numbers begin to increase prior to actual feeding. This increase in concentrations before feeding was investigated by Dehority and Tirabasso (1989). Their approach was to establish a standardized routine for handling and feeding the animals, i.e. enter the barn and take a sham sample from all sheep at 0800 h; return to barn at 0850 h, empty feed bunks and weigh-out feed; feed sheep at 0900 h. Marked variation occurred in isotrichid concentrations among the four sheep studied, with two animals exhibiting increases prior to feeding (Figure 4.8). When feeding was delayed for 4.5 h, all animals showed some increase in concentration before they were fed (Figure 4.9).

Additional experiments were conducted, which were designed to determine possible effects of other stimuli on isotrichid concentrations. Sampling the animal 1, 2 or 3 times (1, 2 or 3 h before feeding) did not appear to be responsible for an increase in concentration; however, a chemotaxis to incoming feed was observed by feeding 3 h before the normal feeding time. Additional experiments with feeding at 0700 or 0900 h and sampling at these two times, substantiated that concentrations increased prior to feeding and increased without any prior handling or stimulation of the animals.

The extent to which concentrations decreased after feeding was related to feed level, i.e., the higher the feed level the greater the decrease. Chemotaxis to incoming feed was of a greater magnitude for those animals fed at reduced levels. Most of these points are illustrated in the data shown in Figure 4.10. Animals were fed at levels varying from 25% to 125% at 0900 h, then 50% of daily ration 4 and 8 h later and 25% after 24 h. A chemotactic response in protozoan concentrations was noted at 4 h with the two sheep initially fed at 25 and 50%, with essentially no response for any sheep at

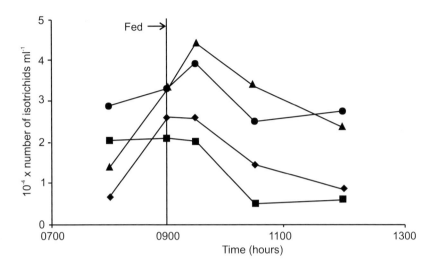

Figure 4.8. Effect of feeding upon the concentration of isotrichids in rumen contents (four separate sheep) (data from Dehority and Tirabasso, 1989).

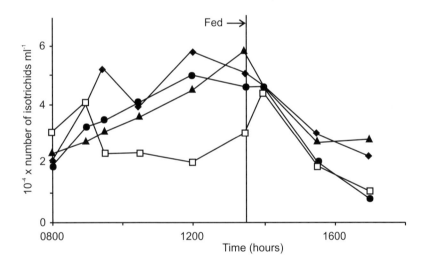

Figure 4.9. Effect of delayed feeding upon the concentration of isotrichids in rumen contents (four sheep). Normal feeding time was at 0900 h (data from Dehority and Tirabasso, 1989).

8 h. By 24 h, the sheep initially fed 25% increased prior to feeding and both it and the sheep initially fed 50% showed a chemotaxis to 25% of the ration. The sheep initially fed 100% and 125% showed only a slight chemotactic response at 24 h. In similar experiments, feeding the same levels as above at 0900 h (25%, 50%, 100% and 125%) and then 50% of the diet after 12 h resulted in an increase in concentration inversely proportional to the original diet level, i.e., highest response for the sheep fed 25% of diet,

90   Rumen microbiology

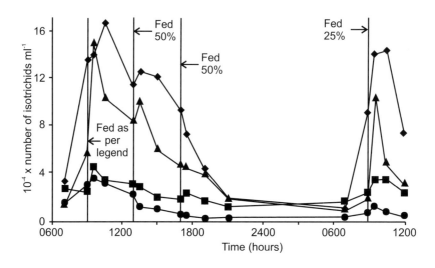

Figure 4.10. Effect of initial feed level on changes in the concentration of isotrichids where 50% of daily ration is fed 4 and 8 h after the normal feeding time and 25% after 24 h (four separate sheep). Initial feed levels at 0900 h were: ♦, 25% of daily ration, ▲ 50%; ■ 100%; ● 125% (data from Dehority and Tirabasso, 1989).

etc. When the normal ration was fed in two equal quantities at 0800 and 1800 h, two peaks in protozoan concentration were observed. In general, the largest increase was noted after the 0800 h feeding. In a separate experiment, 35% of the daily ration was fed at 0800 h, and 800 ml of rumen contents were removed and replaced with anaerobic buffer and 35% of the daily diet about 30 min after feeding. There was an immediate to sharp decrease in protozoan concentrations and essentially no increase when the animal was fed at 1700 h. The concentrations remained low even when the animal was fed normally the next morning and sampled between 0700 and 1400 h.

This experiment was repeated in two other sheep with similar results. The total number of isotrichids removed from the three sheep at 0830 h was 9.1, 14.5 and 12.6 x 10^7. In contrast, when 1900 ml of rumen contents were removed and replaced with anaerobic buffer 6 h after the morning feeding, no change in the normal diurnal pattern or decrease in concentrations was observed. It was of interest that in this experiment, the first 1800 ml of contents removed contained 2 x 10^4 isotrichs/ml, while the last 100 ml removed contained 13.7 x 10^4 isotrichids/ml. In this experiment, when the contents were removed 6 h after feeding, a total of only 5.0 x 10^7 isotrichids were removed, half or less the number previously removed from the three sheep at 0830 h. This would clearly suggest some sequestration of the isotrichids in the ventral part of the rumen.

It was also concluded from these studies that the isotrichids which sequester after feeding at 0800 h are the same ones which respond to incoming nutrients and migrate back into the rumen at 1800 h.

These results suggest that feeding level probably controls the level of storage polysaccharide in the isotrichid cell, which in turn may be the controlling factor in sequestration and migration. After the isotrichids have sequestered they apparently begin to utilize the stored polysaccharide. When this is depleted to a given level about 10-12 h later, depending on the previous feed intake, the cells will exhibit chemotaxis to incoming soluble sugars. If the animal is not fed, utilization continues and eventually the stored polysaccharide is depleted to the extent that migration into the rumen contents occurs without feeding. These two types of migration might be termed as a chemotactic response and a depletion response.

Additional studies on sequestration and migration of protozoa were subsequently carried out in this same laboratory (Ankrah et al., 1990). Rumen contents were placed into a container which allowed passage of bacteria and soluble substrate, but not protozoa, and the container was incubated for different time periods in the rumen. Rumen contents were placed into the container 40 min after feeding, and at 4 h after feeding isotrichid numbers had decreased only slightly in the container compared to the drastic decrease observed in the rumen (Table 4.6). The concentration of isotrichids decreased 88% in the rumen but only 32% inside the container. In contrast, the concentration of ophryoscolecids was essentially unchanged both in the rumen and container. Presumably, lysis and multiplication of the isotrichids would be similar inside and outside the container. The decrease in isotrichid concentration in the rumen itself could then be explained either by dilution from water intake or sequestration. Since the ophryoscolecid concentration remained the same, sequestration appears to be the probable cause for the decrease in isotrichid concentration.

Table 4.6 OBSERVATIONS ON THE DECREASE IN RUMEN PROTOZOAN CONCENTRATIONS BETWEEN 40 MINUTES AND 4 HOURS AFTER FEEDING (FROM ANKRAH et al., 1990)

			Protozoa/ml x 10^4		
Site	Time after feeding	pH	Total	Ophryoscolecidae	Isotrichidae
Rumen	0 h	6.90^a	11.96^a	11.08	0.88^a
Rumen when container was filled	40 min	6.49^{ab}	18.52^b	10.92	7.62^b
Rumen	4 h	6.51^{ab}	11.32^a	10.40	0.92^a
Container	4 h	6.01^b	15.38^c	10.18	5.20^c
SE		0.12	0.66	0.55	0.29

[abc]Means in the same column with different superscripts differ at $P < 0.05$.

In the reverse of this experiment, rumen contents were added to the container 6 h after feeding and isotrichid concentrations were determined at 24 h in the rumen and at 24 h and 40 min in both the rumen and container (Table 4.7). Isotrichid concentrations in the rumen increased significantly between 24 h and 24 h and 40 min, whereas no increase occurred inside the container. The increase of isotrichids in the rumen was thus attributed to migration of sequestered Isotrichidae. On the other hand, a similar increase in Ophryoscolecidae concentrations occurred both in the rumen and container. These data clearly support the previous study of Dehority and Tirabasso (1989).

Table 4.7 INCREASE IN RUMEN PROTOZOAN CONCENTRATIONS IMMEDIATELY AFTER FEEDING (FROM ANKARAH et al., 1990)

Site	Time after feeding	pH	Protozoa/ml x 10^4		
			Total	Ophryoscolecidae	Isotrichidae
Rumen when container was filled	6 h	6.32^a	9.36^a	8.60	0.76^{ac}
Rumen	24 h	7.08^b	14.48^b	13.16	1.32^c
Rumen	24 h 40 min	6.35^a	20.68^c	13.32	7.36^b
Container	24 h 40 min	6.02^c	13.12^b	12.56	0.56^a
SE		0.03	0.79	0.98	0.44

[abc]Means in the same column with different superscripts differ at $P<0.05$.

Diurnal variation has also been studied in the concentration of several less numerous holotrich species, *Buetschlia parva* (Dehority, 1970) and *Charonina ventriculi* (Dehority and Mattos, 1978). In general, the diurnal cycle for *B. parva* was very similar to that for *Isotricha* and *Dasytricha*, while concentration changes after feeding for *C. ventriculi* appeared to be more closely related to the entodiniomorphs.

Orpin and Mathiesen (1986) reported the occurrence of a small species of isotrichid in rumen contents of Norwegian Red cattle. Although quite similar in size to *Oligoisotricha bubali*, they concluded it was a new species and suggested it be named *Microcetus lappus*. However, their description was somewhat incomplete. This species was subsequently reported to occur in American bison (Towne et al., 1988) and cattle (Towne and Nagaraja, 1989). Diurnal changes in the concentration of this organism were similar to those normally observed for entodiniomorphs, rather than the holotrichs.

Evidence for sequestration of protozoa within the particulate matter was also obtained by Nakamura and Kurihara (1978). Using an agitated continuous *in vitro* fermentation system, with the substrate added in nylon bags, protozoa (primarily *Entodinium*) rapidly migrated from the old bag to the new bag. Similar concentrations were reached in both bags within 2 h, while less than 10% of the number in the bags occurred in the free fluid. Bauchop (1979a) has been able to show a definite chemotactic response of the entodiniomorph *Epidinium ecaudatum* toward physically damaged areas of alfalfa and grass stems; however, no such chemotaxis has been noted for *Entodinium*.

Establisment of *Isotricha* and *Dasytricha*

In the study reported by Dehority and Purser (1970) on the establishment and maintenance of *Isotricha* and *Dasytricha in vivo*, it did not seem logical that in two sheep penned next to each other and fed the same diet at the same level, that one should have large numbers of isotrichids and the second be isotrichid-free or have only very low numbers. Since earlier workers had noted some association between protozoal numbers and water intake or level of feed intake, these two variables plus inoculation were chosen as factors to be studied. When water intake was restricted, an initial small increase in holotrich concentrations was noted in some animals; however, a gradual decrease occurred over time. Feed restriction increased isotrichid concentrations when starting populations were quite low. Under normal conditions, inoculations were unsuccessful, but establishment by inoculation was very successful in conjunction with restricted water or feed intake.

Warner and Stacy (1965) observed that two out of 18 sheep had fasting rumen fluid osmotic pressures above 280 mOsmoles/kg, and these two animals were the only ones without holotrich protozoa. Fasting, as defined in their work, was without food or water 18-24 h before sampling. The studies discussed above on establishment and numbers of isotrichids (Dehority and Purser, 1970) were continued with emphasis on the effects of osmotic pressure (Dehority and Males, 1974). Feed and water restriction were again included as variables. In general, results of these studies indicated that within both the normal ranges of osmotic pressure and extremes caused by manipulation of feed and water intake, osmolality was not associated with the occurrence or numbers of isotrichid protozoa. It was of interest that in this study the results of inoculation in conjunction with feed or water restriction were the same as observed previously, i.e., isotrichids became established and were able to persist when feed and water intake were returned to normal levels.

Results of these two studies (Dehority and Purser, 1970, Dehority and Males, 1974) suggest that some change or alteration must be made in the overall rumen environment before the isotrichids and possibly other genera can become established in a previously existing fauna. After establishment, they apparently contribute to and thus change the environment so they can be maintained.

Antagonism

One last area to be covered with regard to numbers and growth of rumen protozoa is concerned with the antagonistic relationships which apparently exist between certain rumen ciliate species. Eadie (1962b) observed that two general types of rumen ciliate populations seemed to occur. Type A contained entodinia and isotrichid species plus *Polyplastron multivesiculatum* as the predominant large entodiniomorph. Type B contained entodinia and isotrichid species together with a large entodiniomorph, *Eudiplodinium* and/or *Epidinium*, together or separately. She found that both type A or B could be present in sheep; however, type A was most prevalent. Inoculation of an animal with a type B fauna with type A rumen fluid almost always resulted in an irreversible change to the type A population. In contrast, type B populations appeared to be the most frequent type in cattle. Changes from B to A were also observed with calves when inoculated with type A rumen contents. It was of interest, that on only one occasion in which *Polyplastron* was observed in either a calf or lamb, did it not become predominant. Her results indicated that food competition or gross bacterial change did not appear to be responsible; and that the *Entodinium* and holotrich species did not appear to be involved.

In a later, more detailed study Eadie (1967) investigated establishment of species in young animals plus additional experiments on antagonism. She broke her populations down into Type A organisms - *Polyplastron multivesiculatum, Metadinium affine* and *Ophryoscolex tricoronatus;* Type B organisms - *Eudiplodinium maggi* and other *Eudiplodinium* spp., *Epidinium* spp., and *Ostracodinium* spp.; and those species common to both type populations: *Entodinium* spp., *Isotricha* spp., and *Dasytricha ruminantium*. In a series of inoculation experiments, animal species differences were noted. With cattle, inoculation of a B type animal with type A organisms resulted in a mixed population of A plus giant sized *Eudiplodinium* for a period of about 2 months and then A type was dominant. In goats the change required only about 10 days, but again the large *Eudiplodinium* were observed. A mixed population could not be obtained in sheep and a type A population readily and irreversibly removed type B organisms from a sheep rumen fauna. She then investigated this phenomena of antagonism using a container in vivo which was permeable to fluids and bacteria but not protozoa. On the basis of her results, she concluded that: (1) Antagonism between type A and B populations was not caused by a diffusible toxic substance. Type B population of ciliates within the container were unaffected when placed in the rumen of sheep with either A or B type faunas; (2) competition for food did not appear to be the primary cause of the disappearance of type B organisms. Type B organisms survived in the container while they were eliminated from the fauna outside; and (3) predation of type B organisms by *Polyplastron* appeared to be the major means by which this organism predominates. Ingested type B organisms were observed inside *Polyplastron*, and then the *Polyplastron* became very dense. The very dense appearance of *Polyplastron* was similar to their appearance *in vivo* under conditions of mixed types A and B. The smaller type B organisms were removed first, and *Epidinium* before *Eudiplodinium*, which was always the last to be removed. This predation could even be observed in the container. It was interesting to note that starvation of the *Polyplastron* appeared to prevent predation rather than stimulate it. Moderately full, apparently healthy Polyplastron were necessary. Cannibalism was also observed in *Polyplastron* cultures inside the container when they were moderately starved; however, it was shown to be less effective nutritionally than predation. *Polyplastron* will eliminate *Epidinium, Eudiplodinium maggi* plus many other *Eudiplodinium* spp. and *Ostracodinium* spp. from a protozoal population. This predation by *Polyplastron* differs from "accidental" predation in that it leads to the complete removal from the population of those species which form the prey.

Ophryoscolex proved to be rather difficult to establish in young ciliate-free sheep and goats, requiring as many as 5 or 6 inoculations (Eadie, 1967). However, *Ophryoscolex* was successfully established in animals with only one other large Ophryoscolecid, either *Polyplastron* (type A) or *Eudiplodinium* (type B). It was not possible to establish *Ophryoscolex* plus *Epidinium* in the same animal. *Epidinium* consistently appeared to develop in preference to *Ophryoscolex*.

Imai *et al.*(1978, 1979), described two additional fauna types which occur with some regularity. Type O, which contains only *Entodinium* and holotrichs, and type K (cattle only) which is characterized by the presence of *Elytroplastron bubali*. A general summary of the different fauna types is given in Table 4.8

Table 4.8. DIFFERENT POPULATION TYPES WHICH OCCUR IN RUMINANTS

Type A	*Type B*	*Type O*	*Type K*
Entodinium	*Entodinium*	*Entodinium*	*Entodinium*
Isotrichids[a]	Isotrichids	Isotrichids	Isotrichids
Polyplastron multivesiculatum	*Eudiplodinium maggii*		*Elytroplastron bubali*
Metadinium affine	*Epidinium* spp.		
Ophryoscolex	*Ostracodinium* spp.		
Diplodiniinae	Diplodiniinae		Diplodiniinae

[a]Includes *Isotricha* and *Dasytricha*.

References

Abe, M., T. Iriki, N. Tobe and H. Shibui. (1981). Sequestration of holotrich protozoa in the reticulo-rumen of cattle. *Applied and Environmental Microbiology*, **41**, 758-765.

Abe, M., H. Shibui, T. Iriki and F. Kumeno. (1973). Relation between diet and protozoal population in the rumen. *British Journal of Nutrition*, **29**, 197-202.

Ankrah, P., S. C. Loerch and B. A. Dehority. (1990). Sequestration, migration and lysis of protozoa in the rumen. *Journal of General Microbiology*, **136**, 1869-1875.

Bauchop, T. (1979). The rumen ciliate *Epidinium* in primary degradation of plant tissues. *Applied and Environmental Microbiology*, **37**, 1217-1223.

Becker, E. R. and R. C. Everett. (1930). Comparative growth of normal infusoria-free lambs. *American Journal of Hygiene*, **11**, 362-370.

Bryant, M. P. and N. Small. (1960). Observations on the ruminal microorganisms of isolated and inoculated calves. *Journal of Dairy Science*, **43**, 654-667.

Bryant, M. P., N. Small, C. Bouma and I. Robinson. (1958). Studies on the composition of the ruminal flora and fauna of young calves. *Journal of Dairy Science*, **41**, 1747-1767.

Christiansen, W.C., W. Woods and W. Burroughs. (1964). Ration characteristics influencing rumen protozoal populations. *Journal of Animal Science*, **23**, 984-988.

Clarke, R.T.J. (1965). Diurnal variation in the numbers of rumen ciliate protozoa in cattle. *New Zealand Journal of Agricultural Research*, **8**, 1-9.

Clarke, R.T.J., M. J. Ulyatt and A. John. (1982). Variation in numbers and mass of ciliate protozoa in the rumens of sheep fed chaffed alfalfa (*Medicago sativia*). *Applied and Environmental Microbiology*, **43**, 1201-1204.

Dearth, R.N., B.A. Dehority and E.L. Potter. (1974). Rumen microbial numbers in lambs as affected by level of feed intake and dietary diethylstilbestrol. *Journal of Animal Science*, **38**, 991-996.

Dehority, B. A. (1970). Occurrence of the ciliate protozoa *Bütschlia parva* Schuberg in the rumen of the ovine. *Applied Microbiology*, **19**, 179-181.

Dehority, B. A. (1975). Rumen ciliate protozoa of Alaskan reindeer and caribou (*Rangifer tarandus* L.) In: *Proceedings of the 1st International Reindeer and Caribou Symposium.* Edited by J.R. Luick, P.C. Lent, D.R. Klein and R.G. White. Biological papers of the University of Alaska, Special Report No. 1, pp 241-250.

Dehority, B.A. (1978). Specificity of rumen ciliate protozoa in cattle and sheep. *Journal of Protozoology*, **25**, 509-513.

Dehority, B.A. (1986). Protozoa of the digestive tract of herbivorous mammals. *Insect Science and its Application*, **7**, 279-296.

Dehority, B.A. and J.R. Males. (1974). Rumen fluid osmolality: Evaluation of its influence upon the occurrence and numbers of holotrich protozoa in sheep. *Journal of Animal Science*, **38**, 865-870.

Dehority, B.A. and W.R.S. Mattos. (1978). Diurnal changes and effect of ration on concentrations of the rumen ciliate *Charon ventriculi*. *Applied and Environmental Microbiology*, **36**, 953-958.

Dehority, B.A. and C.G. Orpin. (1988). Development of, and natural fluctuations in, rumen microbial populations. In: *The Rumen Microbial Ecosystem.* Edited by P. N. Hobson. Elsevier Applied Science, London. pp. 151-184.

Dehority, B.A. and E.L. Potter. (1974). *Diplodinium flabellum*: occurrence and numbers in the rumen of sheep with a description of two new subspecies. *Journal of Protozoology*, **21**, 686-693.

Dehority, B. A. and D. B. Purser. (1970). Factors affecting the establishment and numbers of holotrich protozoa in the ovine rumen. *Journal of Animal Science*, **30**, 445-449.

Dehority, B.A. and P.A. Tirabasso. (1989). Factors affecting the migration and sequestration of rumen protozoa in the family Isotrichidae. *Journal of General Microbiology*, **135**, 539-548.

Dennis, S.M., M. J. Arambel, E.E. Bartley and A. D. Dayton. (1983). Effect of energy concentrations and source of nitrogen on numbers and types of rumen protozoa. *Journal of Dairy Science*, **66**, 1248-1254.

Eadie, J.M. (1962a). The development of rumen microbial populations in lambs and calves under various conditions of management. *Journal of General Microbiology*, **29**, 563-578.

Eadie, J.M. (1962b). Interrelationships between certain rumen ciliate protozoa. *Journal of General Microbiology*, **29**, 579-588.

Eadie, J.M. (1967). Studies on the ecology of certain rumen ciliate protozoa. *Journal of General Microbiology*, **49**, 175-194.

Franzolin, R. and B.A. Dehority. (1996). Effect of prolonged high-concentrate feeding on ruminal protozoa concentrations. *Journal of Animal Science*, **74**, 2803-2809.

Froetschel, M.A., A.C. Martin, H.E. Amos and J.J. Evans. (1990). Effects of zinc sulfate concentration and feeding frequency on ruminal protozoal numbers, fermentation patterns and amino acid passage in steers. *Journal of Animal Science*, **68**, 2874-2884.

Grubb, J.A. and B.A. Dehority. (1975). Effects of an abrupt change in ration from all roughage to high concentrate upon rumen microbial numbers in sheep. *Applied Microbiology*, **30**, 404-412.

Hungate, R.E. (1966). *The Rumen and Its Microbes*. Academic Press, Inc. New York, NY. USA.

Hungate, R.E., J. Reichland and R. Prins. (1971). Parameters of rumen fermentation in a continuously fed sheep: Evidence of a microbial rumination pool. *Applied Microbiology*, **22**, 1104-1113.

Ibrahim, E.A., J.R. Ingalls and N.E. Stanger. (1970). Effect of dietary diethylstilbestrol on populations and concentrations of ciliate protozoa in dairy cattle *Canadian Journal of Animal Science*, **50**, 101-106.

Imai, S., M. Katsuno and K. Ogimoto. (1978). Distribution of rumen ciliate protozoa in cattle, sheep and goat and experimental transfaunation of them. *Japanese Journal of Zootechnical Science*, **49**, 494-505.

Imai, S., M. Katsuno and K. Ogimoto. (1979). Type of the pattern of the rumen ciliate composition of the domestic ruminants and the predator-prey interaction of the ciliates. *Japanese Journal of Zootechnical Science*, **50**, 79-87.

Latham, M.J., M. Elizabeth Sharpe and J.D. Sutton. (1971). The microbial flora of the rumen of cows fed hay and high cereal rations and its relationship to the rumen fermentation. *Journal of Applied Bacteriology*, **34**, 425-434.

Mackie, R.I. and F.M.C. Gilchrist. (1979). Changes in lactate-producing and lactate-utilizing bacteria in relation to pH in the rumen of sheep during stepwise adaptation to a high-concentrate diet. *Applied and Environmental Microbiology*, **38**, 422-430.

Mackie, R.I., F.M.C. Gilchrist, A.M. Robberts, P.E. Hannah and H.M. Schwartz. (1978). Microbiological and chemical changes in the rumen during the stepwise adaptation of sheep to high concentrate diets. *Journal of Agricultural Science*, **90**, 241-254.

Michalowski, T. (1975). Effect of different diets on the diurnal concentrations of ciliate protozoa in the rumen of water buffalo. *Journal of Agricultural Science*, **85**, 145-150.

Milne, A., M.K. Theodorou, M.G.C. Jordan, C. King-Spooner and A.P.J. Trinci. (1989). Survival of anaerobic fungi in feces, in saliva, and in pure culture. *Experimental Mycology*, **13**, 27-37.

Moir, R.J. and M. Somers. (1956). A factor influencing the protozoal population in sheep. *Nature*, **178**, 1472.

Murphy, M. R., P. E. Drone, Jr. and S.T. Woodford. (1985). Factors stimulating migration of holotrich protozoa into the rumen. *Applied and Environmental Microbiology*, **49**, 1329-1331.

Nakamura, K. and S. Kanegasaki. (1969). Densities of ruminal protozoa of sheep established under different dietary conditions. *Journal of Dairy Science*, **52**, 250-255.

Nakamura, F. and Y. Kurihara. (1978). Maintenance of a certain rumen protozoal population in a continuous *in vitro* fermentation system. *Applied and Environmental Microbiology*, **35**, 500-506.

Nour, A.M., A.R. Abou Akkada, K. el-Shazly, M.A. Naga, B.E. Borhami and M.A. Abaza. (1979). Effect of increased levels of urea in the diet on ruminal protozoal counts in four ruminant species. *Journal of Animal Science*, **49**, 1300-1305.

Orpin, C.G. and Letcher, A.J. (1978). Some factors controlling the attachment of the rumen holotrich protozoa *Isotricha intestinalis* and *I. prostoma* to plant particles *in vitro*. *Journal of General Microbiology*, **106**, 33-40.

Orpin, C.G. and S.D. Mathiesen. (1986). *Microcetus lappus* gen. nov., sp. nov.: new species of ciliated protozoon from the bovine rumen. *Applied and Environmental Microbiology*, **55**, 527-530.

Potter, E.L. and B.A. Dehority. (1973). Effects of changes in feed level, starvation, and level of feed after starvation upon the concentration of rumen protozoa in the ovine. *Applied Microbiology*, **26**, 692-698.

Purser, D.B. (1961). A diurnal cycle for holotrich protozoa of the rumen. *Nature*, **190**, 831-832.

Purser, D.B. and R.J. Moir. (1959). Ruminal flora studies in the sheep. IX. The effect of pH on the ciliate population of the rumen *in vivo*. *Australian Journal of Agrcultural Research*, **10**, 555-564.

Slyter, L.L., R.R. Oltjen, D.L. Kern and F.C. Blank. (1970). Influence of type and level of grain and diethylstilbestrol on the rumen microbial population of steers fed all-concentrate diets. *Journal of Animal Science*, **31**, 996-1002.

Towne, G. and T.G. Nagaraja. (1989). Occurrence and diurnal population fluctuations of the ruminal protozoan *Microcetus lappus*. *Applied and Environmental Microbiology*, **55**, 91-94.

Towne, G. and T.G. Nagaraja. (1990). Omasal ciliated protozoa in cattle, bison and sheep. *Applied and Environmental Microbiology*, **56**, 409-412.

Towne, G.,T. G. Nagaraja and K.K. Kemp. (1988). Ruminal ciliated protozoa in bison. *Applied and Environmental Microbiology*, **54**, 2733-2736.

Vance, R.D., R.L. Preston, E.W. Klosterman and V.R. Cahill. (1972). Utilization of whole shelled and crimped corn grain with varying proportions of corn silage by growing-finishing steers. *Journal of Animal Science*, **35**, 598-605.

Warner, A.C.I. (1962). Some factors influencing the rumen microbial population. *Journal of General Microbiology*, **28**, 129-146.

Warner, A.C.I. (1966a). Diurnal changes in the concentrations of microorganisms in the rumen of sheep fed limited diets once daily. *Journal of General Microbiology*, **45**, 213-235.

Warner, A.C.I. (1966b). Periodic changes in the concentrations of microorganisms in the rumen of a sheep fed a limited ration every three hours. *Journal of General Microbiology*, **45**, 237-242.

Warner, A.C.I. (1966c). Diurnal changes in the concentrations of microorganisms in the rumens of sheep fed to appetite in pens or pasture. *Journal of General Microbiology*, **45**, 243-251.

Warner, A.C.I. and B.D. Stacy. (1965). Solutes in the rumen of sheep. *Quarterly Journal of Experimental Physiology*, **50**, 169-184.

Williams, P.P. and W.E. Dinusson. (1972). Composition of the ruminal flora and establishment of ruminal ciliated protozoal species in isolated calves. *Journal of Animal Science*, **34**, 469-474.

CHAPTER 5

METABOLISM, NUTRITION AND GROWTH OF RUMEN PROTOZOA

Early studies on the metabolic activities of rumen protozoa were severely hampered by difficulties in culturing these organisms in a purified medium *in vitro*. However, considerable advancement has been made along these lines in recent years. The primary difficulty in studying the utilization of various carbohydrates and end-products produced is the concomitant bacterial fermentation which occurs. Two general approaches have been employed to bypass this difficulty, and a large amount of experimental data has been obtained. Physical washing techniques to remove as many of the bacteria as possible plus adding antibiotics to control subsequent bacterial growth has been a fairly successful method. The protozoa do not appear to be affected by antibiotic concentrations which are inhibitory to the bacteria. However, the possible effects of the antibiotic on the metabolism of the protozoa cannot be fully assessed. The second method involves cell-free enzyme preparations obtained from washed disrupted protozoal cells, which provides information on the metabolic capabilities of the protozoa.

Metabolism of the isotrichids

Early studies by Oxford (1951), Masson and Oxford (1951) Sudgen and Oxford (1952), Heald *et al*. (1952) and Guiterrez (1955) established that *Isotricha* and *Dasytricha* are able to ferment many of the simple sugars (glucose, fructose, sucrose, etc.), with the corresponding deposition of an iodophilic intracellular polysaccharide. This storage polysaccharide has properties similar to amylopectin. Both species of *Isotricha*, *intestinalis* and *prostoma*, but not *Dasytricha*, can ingest small vegetable starch grains, particularly rice starch.

In more recent studies, Prins and Van Hoven (1977), studied the fermentation of a number of soluble carbohydrates by starved, antibiotic treated suspensions of *Isotricha prostoma*. *Isotricha prostoma* fermented fructose, sucrose, glucose, raffinose and pectin most rapidly while galactose and melibiose were used at a slower rate. Little, if any fermentation was observed with xylose, arabinose, maltose, cellobiose, lactose or polymers of galacturonic acid. In general, these results agree with the findings of Howard (1959) on mixed *Isotricha* species. Under their experimental conditions, H_2, CO_2, acetate, butyrate, lactate and storage polysaccharide (69%) were the major products of carbohydrate fermentation. They were also able to demonstrate the simultaneous breakdown and synthesis of storage amylopectin in the presence of exogenous sugars, below a threshold concentration of 20 mM glucose.

Similar experiments were conducted with suspensions of *Dasytricha ruminantium* (Van Hoven and Prins, 1977). Comparison with the substrates fermented by *Isotricha prostoma* can be summarized as follows: both species ferment glucose, fructose, sucrose, raffinose, pectin and galactose; only *I. prostoma* fermented melibiose; only *D. ruminantium* fermented maltose and cellobiose; and neither species fermented xylose, arabinose or lactose. End-products from glucose fermentation by *D. ruminantium* were H_2, CO_2, acetate, butyrate, lactate and amylopectin. Formate was produced at higher substrate concentrations. The percentage lactate production was much greater in *D. ruminantium*.

Williams and Harfoot (1976) and Williams (1979a), working with preparations of *Dasytricha* isolated from rumen contents by filtration through a sintered glass funnel, studied selectivity in the uptake and metabolism of carbohydrates. *Dasytricha* was not selective in the uptake of available carbohydrates (glucose, sucrose, fructose and galactose) and did not appear to regulate sugar entry by preferential or sequential utilization. The presence of readily fermentable substrates did not preclude the uptake and subsequent effects of the toxic monomers mannose and glucosamine. The data indicate that *Dasytricha*, in the presence of excess substrate, is unable to control the entry of sugars into the cell; however, this excess does not lead to an uncontrolled synthesis of amylopectin as originally thought, but to an intracellular build-up of acidic fermentation products.

In later studies, Williams (1979b) was able to demonstrate exocellular carbohydrase activity, in the absence of cell lysis, in culture fluid of rumen holotrich ciliate suspensions in which bacterial activity was suppressed by antibiotics. Exocellular carbohydrase activity was observed against cellobiose, maltose, isomaltose, maltotriose, sucrose, lactose, raffinose, inulin, amylopectin and pectin. Invertase or sucrase activity was very high and studies conducted with *Dasytricha* preparations indicated that activity increased throughout the fermentation period and was influenced by initial pH, temperature, sucrose concentration and inoculum size.

Based on the results of his studies, Williams (1979a,b) proposed that the absence of selectivity in sugar uptake by *Dasytricha* should enable the protozoan to compete more effectively for substrates in the rumen. It is attracted by chemotaxis to soluble sugars and is able to assimilate them as soon as they become available in the immediate environment.

In 1982, Williams and Yarlett described an improved procedure for isolation of isotrichids from rumen contents. Rumen liquor is strained through a double layer of cheesecloth, diluted two-fold with inorganic salts solution and placed in a separatory funnel under N_2. The protozoa are allowed to sediment for 30-60 minutes and then filtered through defined aperture nylon and polyester textiles. To isolate *Dasytricha*, the protozoal sediment is first pre-filtered though 45 μm aperture cloth to remove large entodiniomorphs and *Isotricha* species. *Dasytricha* were then separated by retention on a 24 or 30 μm filter and recovered by repeated sedimentation and washing or thorough washing on a 15 μm filter. The small entodiniomorph protozoa and bacteria were not retained by this filter. For isotrichs, the large entodiniomorphs were removed by prefiltration within the porosity range of 70-80 µm. The isotrichs were retained on a 45 m filter and the contaminating protozoa and bacteria removed on a 30 µm filter. In both cases, the protozoa isolated were morphologically normal and metabolically active. Contamination by entodiniomorph protozoa was negligible. This procedure allows maintenance of fairly anaerobic conditions and is quite rapid, not requiring a reduced pressure as with previous procedures using sintered glass or stainless steel filters.

Yarlett et al. (1981) reported the presence of microbody-like organelles in the anaerobic ciliate D. ruminantium. These organelles have no typical mitochondrial ultrastructure, but are similar to the hydrogenosomes of the trichomonad protozoa. In subsequent studies, Yarlett et al. (1982) were able to show that D. ruminantium can maintain endogenous respiration under a low O_2 tension (1% v/v), and actually utilize O_2 as a terminal electron acceptor. The organism lacks cytochromes, and their data suggested the operation of flavoprotein-iron-sulphur-mediated electron transport. The hydrogenosomes form H_2 under anaerobic conditions and can act as a respiratory organelle in the presence of O_2 (Lloyd et al., 1982). These particles or microbody like organelles contain a major percentage of the pyruvate synthase and hydrogenase activities and 20% of the lactic dehydrogenase activity. These are the enzymes needed to produce acetate, CO_2 and H_2 from pyruvate, a pathway generally found only in aerotolerant anaerobes (Lloyd et al., 1989). It was discovered that O_2 could act as a terminal electron acceptor during oxidation of pyruvate to acetate plus CO_2 and H_2. Dissolved O_2 levels <1.5 µM causes a reversible inhibition of H_2 production, while higher O_2 levels appeared to irreversibly inactivate the system. On this basis, the authors concluded that the rumen isotrichids are not strictly anaerobic organisms. They apparently possess the ability to inactivate or overcome the damaging affects of low O_2 concentrations (~1 µM). Superoxide dismutase and catalase were not detectable, but a functional NADH oxidase could provide some protection against dioxygen.

Although the rumen is regarded as an anaerobic environment, levels of O_2 ranging from 0.56 to 6.5% by volume have been measured in the head space gas. Sources of O_2 are from food and drinking water, rumination, saliva and diffusion from blood vessels located in the rumen wall. It has been estimated that about 10 liters of O_2 need to be consumed daily by microorganisms and chemical reactions in the rumen (Lloyd et al., 1989). Since the isotrichids are able to utilize low levels of O_2 (< 2 µM) over an extended period of time, they help maintain anaerobiosis in the rumen and stabilize metabolism patterns. A post-feeding increase in rumen O_2 levels was observed in defaunated animals, further establishing the involvement of the protozoa (Lloyd et al., 1989).

Ellis et al. (1989) found that aerotolerant anaerobes exist within both the bacterial and protozoal populations. In addition to the holotrichs, other species of rumen protozoa are somewhat tolerant to low O_2 concentrations and are able to utilize O_2 at low tensions. *Polyplastron multivesiculatum* and *Eudiplodinium maggii*, both rumen entodiniomorphs, and *N. patriciarum*, a rumen fungus, all contain hydrogenosomes (Yarlett et al., 1984, 1986; Paul et al., 1990). These species plus the isotrichids can thus protect the more oxygen sensitive microorganisms, such as the methanogens, by removing

104 Rumen microbiology

O_2 from their environment. The authors estimated that the contribution of the bacterial and protozoal population to O_2 utilization are about equal, with the fungi contributing a much smaller proportion.

Williams (1986) has published a comprehensive review on the rumen isotrichids, with an extensive section on their metabolic activities. Additional information can be found in the monograph, *The Rumen Protozoa,* by Williams and Coleman (1992). In general, *Dasytricha* and *Isotricha* species primarily utilize soluble carbohydrates and non-structural plant storage polysaccharides as energy sources; pentoses, hexuronic acids, polyuronides, cellulose and hemicellulose are not utilized (Table 5.1). To date, intermediary metabolism of the isotrichids has not been studied in great detail.

Table 5.1 PRINCIPAL CARBOHYDRATES UTILILIZED BY *DASYTRICHA RUMINANTIUM* AND MIXED *ISOTRICHA* SPECIES (*INTESTINALIS* AND *PROSTOMA*)[a]

Carbohydrate	Utilized (+ or -)	
	Dasytricha	Isotricha species
Arabinose	-	-
Cellobiose	+	-
Cellulose	-	-
Fructose	+	+
Galactose	+	+
Galacturonic acid	-	-
Glucosamine	-	-
D-Glucose	+	+
Glucuronic acid	-	-
Hemicellulose[b]	±	±
Lactose	-	-
Maltose	+	-
Pectin[bc]	±	±
Polygalacturonic acid	-	-
Starch	-	+
Sucrose	+	+
Xylose	-	-

[a]From Williams and Coleman (1992).
[b]Are able to depolymerize or degrade the polysaccharide, but are unable to utilize the products of degradation.
[c]Pectin contains covalently linked neutral sugars which may be released by glycosidases and subsequently utilized.

Metabolism of the entodiniomorphs

Microscopic observation of the entodiniomorphs revealed quite early in their investigation that they were capable of ingesting plant particles. The only exception appears to be the smaller species of *Entodinium*. However, the small entodinia can be observed to rapidly ingest small starch grains. Most of the early studies with the entodiniomorphs were concerned with the ability of the protozoa to digest cellulose. Hungate (1942, 1943) was able to demonstrate cellulose digestion in cell-free extracts from several species of *Diplodinium*, however, *E. caudatum* extracts could not digest cellulose. His work was criticized on the basis of a large bacterial contamination. Sugden (1953) obtained similar results from longevity studies with cultures of *Metadinium medium* and *Entodinium* spp., cultured with cellulose in the presence of antibiotics. Once again bacterial symbiosis could not be ruled out.

ENTODINIUM

One of the first studies on metabolism in entodiniomorphs was reported by Abou Akkada and Howard (1960). Using defaunation techniques they established sheep containing only *Entodinium* spp., primarily *E. caudatum*. Washed suspensions, almost bacteria-free, were obtained with antibiotic treatment. Protozoal cells in freshly prepared suspensions were filled with starch grains which gradually disappeared with incubation. The principal products produced were acetic and butyric acids, small amounts of propionic and formic acids, CO_2, H_2 and very small amounts of lactic acid. The *E. caudatum* suspensions did not metabolize glucose, maltose, cellobiose, sucrose or soluble starch. Rice starch grains were ingested by the cells and cell-free extracts contained strong maltase and amylase activity. They concluded that *E. caudatum* satisfied its carbohydrate requirements solely by the ingestion of granular starch.

Somewhat contradictory results were subsequently reported by Coleman (1964). Using washed suspensions of *E. caudatum*, to which *E. coli* were added, he found that soluble starch and maltose gave growth comparable to rice starch grains. Cellobiose, glucose or sucrose produced half maximum growth. The *E. coli* cells were rapidly engulfed by the protozoa. Growth of *E. caudatum* in the presence of rice starch was also stimulated by engulfment of *Clostridium welchii* or *Lactobacillus casei*. Coleman (1969b) published results of a rather extensive study on the metabolism of starch, maltose and glucose by washed suspensions of *E. caudatum*. Using ^{14}C he demonstrated uptake of glucose and maltose and their incorporation into protozoal polysaccharide. His data suggested both an active and passive uptake of sugars, but into different compartments of the cell. Evidence is presented which indicates that the protozoal ectoplasm may be freely permeable to sugars in the medium and that a barrier exists between the ectoplasm and endoplasm. The rate of uptake of both sugars was markedly decreased in the presence of penicillin and neomycin.

Abou Akkada and Howard (1962) found that suspensions of *E. caudatum* could rapidly hydrolyze casein, and subsequently demonstrated the presence of a proteinase in cell-free extracts. In later studies, Coleman (1967a,b) observed direct incorporation of free ^{14}C amino acids and ^{14}C labeled amino acids in the cellular protein of *E. coli* into protozoal protein without conversion to any other amino acid.

In a recent study, Fondevila and Dehority (2001b) studied in vitro growth and starch digestion by *Entodinium exiguum*. Using antibiotics to inhibit bacterial growth in their cultures, they found: (1) that protozoal growth was greater in the presence of live bacteria as compared to "no" bacteria or dead bacteria; (2) the initial digestion of autoclaved corn starch was much faster than non-autoclaved; however, the extent of digestion was almost complete for both substrates after 48 h; (3) digestion of rice starch begins approximately 6 - 12 h before the digestion of corn starch; and (4) a synergistic effect was observed between bacteria and protozoa. Figure 5.1 illustrates most of these points quite well.

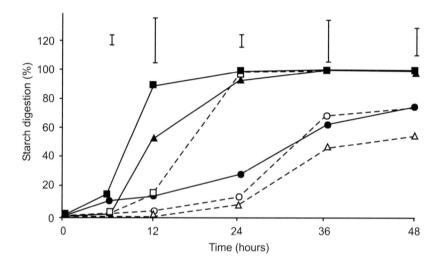

Figure 5.1 In vitro corn (open symbols) and rice (closed symbols) starch digestion by *E. exiguum* without bacteria (O,●), with live bacteria (□,■) and by bacteria alone (△▲). Upper bars show standard error of means (n = 2). From Fondevila and Dehority (2001).

Morgavi *et al.* (1996) have reported the presence of both chitinase and lysozyme activity in homogenates of both mixed rumen protozoa and *Entodinium caudatum*. The mixed protozoa were incubated with antibiotics for 4 h and then washed, to reduce bacterial contamination. *Entodinium caudatum* cultures were washed 10 times prior to use. In general, the mixed and single protozoal preparations both contained chitinase and lysozyme activity which accounts for their ability to degrade bacterial and fungal cell walls.

DIPLODINIINAE

Using defaunation techniques, Abou Akkada *et al.* (1963) established sheep with the sole protozoan species *Polyplastron multivesiculatum*. Cell-free extracts of disintegrated cells hydrolyzed amylose, maltose, cellulose, cellobiose, wheat-flour pentosan, xylobiose, pectin, sucrose, melibiose, raffinose, inulin and lactose. However, it was of interest that extracts of mixed rumen bacteria obtained from ciliate free sheep and prepared in the same manner as the protozoal extracts, did not hydrolyze cellulose.

At about this same time, Bailey and Clarke (1963), working with a clonal culture of *Eudiplodinium bovis*, freed from external bacteria, ruptured the cells and were able to demonstrate hydrolysis of starch, xylans, xylodextrins, cellodextrins, maltose, xylobiose, cellobiose and sucrose. Pectin and cellulose were not attacked.

Naga and el-Shazly (1968) established *Eudiplodinium medium* as the only protozoal species in the rumen of a ciliate-free water buffalo. *E. medium* did not metabolize simple sugars or cellulose, but utilized starch and hemicellulose, the latter quite rapidly. Cell-free extracts showed activities towards carbohydrates similar to those observed with whole cells. *E. medium* appears to differ from many other entodiniomorphs in that formic acid is an end product in addition to acetate and butyrate.

Belzecki and Michalowski (2002), working with sheep containing either *Eudiplodinium maggii* alone or *E. maggii* plus *Entodinium caudatum*, estimated that *E. maggii* contributed from 12 - 76% of the total amylolytic activity occurring in the rumen.

Ellis *et al.* (1991) reported on the influence of rumen O_2 and CO_2 concentrations on metabolic pathways of *P. multivesiculatum*. The normal end products of *P. multivesiculatum* are butyric, acetic, lactic acid, H_2 and CO_2. Increased O_2 concentrations (1-3 µM) depressed acetate, H_2 and CO_2 formation, while higher levels of CO_2 appeared to depress the hydrogenosomal pathway and result in increased production of butyrate. Production of hydrogen by *P. multivesiculatum* is reversibly inhibited by low concentrations of dissolved O_2 (1-3 µM); however, higher concentrations caused complete inactivation. Several other observations of interest were made in this same study. Cytochromes could not be detected in *P. multivesiculatum* and the terminal oxidase in hydrogenosomes is unknown. Presumably the consumption of oxygen is linked to substrate-level phosphorylation as the mechanism of energy generation. Glycerol, identified as a significant metabolite of glucose fermentation by *P. multivesiculatum*, had not been previously identified as a product of this or any other rumen ciliates.

EPIDINIUM

Bailey *et al.* (1962), examined the carbohydrases of *Epidinium ecaudatum*. Extracts prepared under conditions which would not disrupt any associated bacteria, hydrolyzed various plant hemicelluloses and starch. Xylobiose, cellobiose, sucrose, isomaltose, and melibiose were also hydrolyzed, but not cellulose. Previous work by Bailey (1958), and later by Bailey and Howard (1963) demonstrated marked amylase and maltase activity in extracts of *Epidinium ecaudatum*.

Coleman and Laurie (1974), demonstrated that *Epidinium caudatum* could use glucose for synthesis of intracellular polysaccharide and at least 8 amino acids which appeared in protein. Protein was also synthesized from starch grains. Considerable numbers of bacteria were engulfed by the *Epidinium*, as well as taking up a wide range of amino acids.

Clayet *et al*. (1992) studied the different enzymatic activities in cell-free extracts of *Epidinium caudatum* which were fairly well free of bacteria. The cells were ruptured by sonication. The following enzymatic activities were found using gel filtration chromatography: avicellulase, carboxymethylcellulase, laminarinase, xylanase, arabinosidase, cellobiosidase, fucosidase, galactosidase, glucosidase and xylosidase.

OPHRYOSCOLEX

Mah and Hungate (1965) reported on physiological studies with *Ophryoscolex purkynjei* grown in clone culture *in vitro*. The cells were freed from external bacteria by repeated washing. Using ground wheat as a substrate, large amounts of acetate and butyrate were produced, lesser amounts of propionate plus traces of formate and lactate along with CO_2 and H_2. The carbohydrates maltose, glucose, glucose-6-phosphate, cellobiose and sucrose were not fermented. Insoluble cellulose was not ingested by the cells. Pectin was hydrolyzed.

In studies similar to those conducted by Abou-Akkada *et al*. (1963) with *P. multivesiculatum*, Howard (1963) has demonstrated an active cellulase and hemicellulase in extracts of *O. tricoronatus*. Williams *et al*. (1961) observed rapid hydrolysis of pectin, starch and protein by washed suspensions of *O. caudatus*.

Cellulolytic activity of rumen protozoa

Coleman (1985) measured cellulase activity in cell-free extracts of 15 species of entodiniomorphs, using six different assays. The assays included: (1) the production of reducing material, (2) change in viscosity using carboxymethylcellulose (CMC) as a substrate, (3) release of dye from cellulose azure, (4) production of reducing sugars from reprecipitated cellulose or (5) microcrystalline cellulose and (6) measurement of changes in turbidity of a reprecipitated cellulose suspension. The highest activities were found in *Epidinium caudatum, Ostracodinium obtusum dilobum, Eudiplodinium maggii* and *Ophryoscolex caudatus*. Lesser activity was observed in cell free extracts of *Metadinium affine, Eudiplodinium bovis, Polyplastron multivesiculatum,* and *Eudiplodinium dilobum. Diplodinium pentacanthum* extracts contained only a trace of activity. The extent of activity varied considerably between assays, growth conditions and food source and this variability was inconsistent between species. On the other hand, no cellulase activity was found in cell-free extracts of five different *Entodinium* species. Optimum pH values for cellulase activity were 5.0 for microcrystalline cellulose, 5.5 for carboxymethylcellulose and 6.5 for cellulose azure. Bacterial enzymes appeared to have their pH optimum between 5.0 - 6.0. He estimated that in a normal sheep, 62% of the total rumen cellulase activity was present in the protozoal fraction.

Michalowski *et al,* (2001) were able to demonstrate in vitro that *Epidinium ecaudatum* was capable of utilizing microcrystalline cellulose for growth. In contrast, oat spelt xylan had an inhibitory effect, decreasing concentrations of *Epidinium.*

The data on cellulolytic activity of various protozoa has been compiled into Table 5.2. These species apparently are the principal cellulose digestors among the protozoa, although a number of additional Diplodiniinae species do appear to show traces of cellulolytic activity.

Table 5.2 CELLULOLYTIC ACTIVITY OF RUMEN PROTOZOA

Species	*Activity[a]*	*References[f]*
Eudiplodinium maggii	Strong	1,2,3,4,5
Epidinium caudatum[b]	"	3,5,11
Ostracodinium dilobum[c]	"	5
Metadinium affine[d]	Moderate	3,5,10
Eudiplodinium bovis[e]	"	1,2,5
Ophryoscolex caudatus	"	5
Polyplastron multivesiculatum	"	5,6
Diplodinium pentacanthum	Weak	3,5
Enoploplastron triloricatum	?	3
Ophryoscolex tricoronatus	?	7
Entodinium caudatum	Trace	5,8
Ostracodinium gracile	?	9

[a] Activities are based on a relative scale. No quantitative information is available on those species listed as "?"
[b] *Epidinium ecaudatum caudatum* Dogiel 1927
[c] *Ostracodinium obtusum dilobum* Dogiel 1927
[d] *Diploplastron affine* Kofoid and MacLennan 1932
 (*Diplodinium affine* Dogiel and Fedorowa 1925)
[e] *Eremoplastron bovis* Kofoid and MacLennan 1932
 (*Eudiplodinium neglectum* Dogiel 1927)
[f] (1) Hungate, 1942; (2) Hungate, 1943; (3) Coleman *et al.,* 1976; (4) Coleman, 1978; (5) Coleman, 1985; (6) Abou Akkada *et al.,* 1963; (7) Abou Akkada, 1965; (8) Bonhomme-Florentin, 1975; (9) Dehority (unpublished); (10) Wereszka *et al.,* 2002; (11) Michalowski *et al.,* 2001.

In a later study, Coleman (1986) studied the distribution of carboxymethylcellulase activity in various rumen fractions. Activities were determined at three time intervals after feeding in sheep containing no protozoa or one of five different protozoal populations. CMCase activity for the animal without protozoa and the animal containing *Entodinium caudatum* was highest in the bacterial fraction, whereas the protozoal cytoplasm fraction was highest for the other animals. Activities were similar at 1.5, 6.5 and 24 hours after feeding. Low but variable amounts of CMCase activity were associated with plant debris in the rumen, while cell-free rumen fluid was almost devoid of CMCase activity. As might be expected, the amount of CMCase activity associated with the free bacterial fraction was inversely proportional to the amount present in the protozoan cytoplasmic fraction.

Thus, it would appear that almost all of the entodiniomorph species of rumen protozoa are able to ingest plant particles, with the possible exception of some smaller *Entodinium*, and possess the ability to digest some or all of the major polysaccharide components of these plant materials, i.e., cellulose, hemicellulose, starch and pectin. The isotrichid species, on the other hand, appear to primarily utilize soluble sugars as a source of energy. The one exception would be the ingestion of small starch grains by species of *Isotricha*.

Nutritional requirments and cultivation

Over the years it has been assumed that a large portion of the nutritional requirements of the protozoa are satisfied by rumen bacteria, especially with regard to nitrogen. Oxford (1955) reported that the rumen ciliates would not grow in a chemically defined medium; however, a number of investigators have successfully cultured the protozoa in media containing various combinations of such materials as ground alfalfa, ground wheat, rice starch grains, dried grass and protozoa-free fresh rumen fluid.

REQUIREMENT FOR BACTERIA

In studying the *in vitro* culture of *Isotricha*, Gutierrez (1955) observed that this protozoan would not grow if the bacteria were removed from the rumen fluid. Based on the observation that the normal habitat of the protozoa contained millions of bacteria and that they could not be cultured *in vitro* in a bacteria-free environment, it was postulated that the bacteria were required by the protozoa and comprised their nitrogenous food. Appleby *et al.* (1956), on the basis of staining techniques and the culture of crushed and intact ciliates, concluded that the holotrichs were independent of bacteria, while with the entodiniomorphs, the bacterial count increased when the crushed cells were cultured.

Working with cultures of *Dasytricha ruminantium*, Gutierrez and Hungate (1957) microscopically observed that this organism selectively ingested two morphological types of bacteria from a mixed culture of rumen bacteria. A number of bacterial strains were then isolated from rumen contents and their ability to be ingested and support growth of

Dasytricha ruminantium in vitro was determined. Two bacterial strains, one a small coccus, 0.8 µm in diameter, and the other a rod, 1.0 x 1.5 µm, allowed growth of the protozoal cultures for a period of at least two weeks. Parallel control cultures without the added bacteria were dead at 96 hours. In a later study, Gutierrez (1958) worked with cultures of *Isotricha prostoma*, and after allowing the starved protozoa to feed on mixed rumen bacteria, isolated four strains of rod-shaped bacteria from the crushed protozoal cells. In further work, three of the four strains were observed to be ingested by *Isotricha*. In growth studies, one strain gave numerous dividing *I. prostoma* after 48 hours, but the response diminished until all cells were dead at about 6 days. Control cultures showed no division forms and the response to the other three strains alone or in combination with the active strain were no better than the active strain alone.

Using similar procedures, Gutierrez and Davis (1959) extended the observations on bacterial ingestion by holotrichs to a number of species of *Entodinium* and *Diplodinium*. Bacteria isolated from mixed species of *Entodinium* were all strains of gram-positive diplococci, 0.8 x 1.0 - 1.5 µm. These strains were readily ingested by starved cells of two different *Entodinium* species. The isolated strains of gram-positive diplococci were identified as *Streptococcus bovis*. Mah (1964) observed that *Ophryoscolex purkynjei* ingested bacteria and seemed to be selective for a large streptococcus resembling *Peptostreptococcus elsdenii*.

Results of the above studies would suggest that the protozoa utilize bacteria as a source of nutrients for growth and are rather specific as to which species of bacteria they can ingest. Coleman (1962, 1964, 1967a,b), working with cultures of *Entodinium caudatum*, has obtained good evidence for the bacteria requirement of this organism; however, his results do not support the previous data on specificity or selectivity. Almost bacteria-free cultures of *Entodinium caudatum*, containing less than one viable bacterium per ten protozoa, were prepared by aerobic incubation in a medium containing penicillin, streptomycin, dihydrostreptomycin and neomycin in the presence of autoclaved rumen fluid and rice starch grains. These cultures could not be maintained alive for over a period of 3-4 days (Coleman, 1962). Continuation of this work revealed that *Entodinium caudatum* could ingest a variety of different bacterial species and showed no preference for rumen bacteria over bacteria isolated from other habitats (Coleman, 1964). Such diverse species as *Escherichia coli, Clostridium welchii, Serratia marcescems, Lactobacillus casei* and *Streptococcus bovis* were tested. Viability of the engulfed *E. coli* decreased sharply within 30 minutes while other species were much more resistant. Experiments with ^{14}C labeled *E. coli* clearly indicated the ability of the protozoa to digest the bacteria and directly incorporate the amino acids into protozoal protein (Coleman, 1967b).

Free amino acids were also directly incorporated into protozoal protein by *E. caudatum* (Coleman, 1967a). *E. caudatum* does not appear to be able to synthesize amino acids from carbohydrate (starch grains) and NH_3 present in rumen fluid, but probably satisfies its amino acid requirements from the digestion of bacteria. Coleman (1967b) speculates that the inability of *E. caudatum* to biosynthesize or inter-convert amino acids is probably the result of a gradual loss of the necessary cellular enzymes over the period of time when this protozoan first invaded the rumen. The loss of enzymes could have resulted by growth of *E. caudatum* on the microorganisms which probably contain all the low-molecular-weight nitrogenous compounds required by living cells. If the above concept is true, then the observation that growth of the protozoa only occurred when living bacteria were added to the culture is puzzling. No stimulation was obtained from addition of boiled bacteria, although they were engulfed at similar rates to live bacteria. Coleman speculates that the non-specific requirements for living bacteria may be related to the lower oxidation-reduction potential which can be obtained in a medium with viable bacteria; however, the more recent studies by Ellis *et al.*, (1989) would not support this explanation. Coleman also suggested a protozoal requirement for a specific compound or enzyme obtained from the bacteria which was lost or destroyed when the bacteria were boiled. Although the protein or nucleic acids supplied by the bacteria may be important in protozoal nutrition, these components should be supplied by the boiled bacteria.

In a recent study, Fondevila and Dehority (2001a) investigated the requirements of *E. exiguum* and *E. caudatum* for live or dead bacteria when cultured in vitro. They found that these organisms appeared to have a requirement for live bacteria in the culture medium after 48 h for *E. exiguum* and 72 h for *E. caudatum*. Whether this effect is the result of having to use antibiotics in all media without live bacteria could not be determined, since no other procedures are available by which the protozoa can be cultured axenically. However, a slight increase in growth with dead bacteria compared to "no" bacteria suggested a possible nutritional contribution.

CULTIVATION OF *D. RUMINANTIUM*

Clarke and Hungate (1966) reported the successful cultivation of *Dasytricha ruminantium in vitro*. The organisms required anaerobic conditions and had an obligate requirement for rumen fluid and an isotrichid protozoal extract (P.E.). However, the P.E. could be replaced by bovine serum. Dialysis of either of these materials considerably diminished growth of the organism. Sucrose and P.E. were fed to the cultures once daily for 2-4 h and the cells were then transferred to a medium free of these nutrients. The inability of *Dasytricha* to control polysaccharide storage may be the key to previous difficulties encountered in their *in vitro* culture. Division seems to be impaired when the cells are distended with storage material. These observations would, of course, fit with the growth curves obtained *in vivo* for *Dasytricha* which were discussed previously. With animals fed once daily, numbers begin to increase just before or at feeding, peak soon after feeding and then decrease rather markedly and remain low until shortly before the next feeding. The feeding of low concentrations of sucrose for a short time seems to limit deposition of storage polysaccharide, and, in addition, helps to control or limit bacterial growth in the culture.

In contrast, results obtained by Van Hoven and Prins (1977) indicated that *D.*

ruminantium can only store a definite amount of starch per cell, and they suggest that lysis occurs in the presence of additional substrates as a result of the intracellular accumulation of acidic end-products, principally lactic acid.

Although added bacteria were not required for growth in the studies by Clarke and Hungate (1966), considerable numbers of bacteria were present in all their cultures and may have been consumed. Cultures died within 7 days after extensive washing and treatment with antibiotics and showed no division during this period; however, if the washed culture was reinoculated with mixed bacteria from a successful culture, they survived and grew as before washing. The washed and antibiotic treated cultures were not completely bacteria-free, but methane was present in the gas phase of all successful cultures and absent in gas from the washed cultures. The methane bacteria require an extremely low redox potential. One additional point of interest in their study was the fact that they were unable to establish clone cultures of *Dasytricha*. At least 16 ciliates were required to establish a successful culture.

CULTIVATION OF ENTODINIOMORPHS

A number of early studies have been reported on the cultivation of the entodiniomorph protozoa *in vitro*; however, methods have been improved and refined over the years and I will only mention some of the more recent reports. Information on the early studies can be found in Clarke (1963), Coleman (1958, 1960, 1969a), Gutierrez and Davis (1962) and Sugden (1953).

Coleman and Sanford (1980) compared the metabolic activity of spined and spineless forms of *Entodinium caudatum* grown *in vivo*. The spined form engulfed mixed rumen bacteria 3.8 times faster, took up free amino acids 3.1 times and glucose 60 times faster per unit volume of protozoan than the spineless form. When the spineless form was grown both in vitro and *in vivo*, these parameters were 2.5, 0.77 and 10% faster, respectively, *in vitro*. On this basis, they point out the limitations in making generalizations from data obtained only from one form *in vitro*.

The procedure by which Coleman and Sanford (1980) obtained the spined and spineless forms of *Entodinium caudatum* is most interesting. Coleman *et al.* (1977) found that *E. caudatum* cells were required for growth of *Entodinium bursa* (probably a synonym for *E. vorax*) *in vitro*. When spineless *E. caudatum* cells were added in excess, caudal spines developed. This culture of *E. caudatum* had been grown *in vitro* for 17 years as the spineless form. The authors had previously observed that *E. caudatum* always occurs as the spineless form when cultured alone either *in vivo* or *in vitro*. Engulfment of the spined forms by *E. bursa* was very limited, as compared to engulfment of the spineless form. They postulated that when a spined form of *E. caudatum* divides the anterior daughter cell has a slightly shorter spine than present in the original protozoan which becomes part of the posterior daughter cell. If these two daughter cells divide again in the absence of *E. bursa*, because less metabolic energy is required to reproduce the spineless form, it tends to predominate. However, in the presence of *E. bursa*, the spineless forms are engulfed preferentially, thus giving rise to a large population of spined forms.

Onodera and Henderson (1980) published results of a study where they were attempting to develop a procedure for an axenic or bacterial-free culture of *Entodinium caudatum*. Although not completely successful, they did find that growth in the presence of low bacterial numbers could be markedly enhanced by cell-free extracts of rumen bacteria and other soluble nutrients, if these materials were absorbed on insoluble particles (activated charcoal) which are engulfed by the protozoan.

Coleman *et al.* (1972) have reported on the successful cultivation of *Epidinium caudatum* and *Polyplastron multivesiculatum in vitro* in the presence of bacteria. Of particular interest was the observation that live *Epidinium caudatum* cells were required in the culture medium for establishment and growth of *Polyplastron*. The epidinia were engulfed by *P. multivesiculatum* and could not be replaced by dead cells of *Epidinium*, live *Entodinium caudatum*, *E. simplex*, *Diplodinium monocanthum*, or *E. affine*. Live *Eudiplodinium maggii* cells supported growth for a short time, but all the *Polyplastron* cultures were dead after 4 months. The authors were able to eventually grow *P. multivesiculatum* in the absence of epidinia using a sodium-chloride rich medium which had been inoculated the previous day with bacteria from crude rumen fluid or an established protozoal culture. However, no culture was ever maintained over a year in the absence of epidinia. The average size of *Polyplastron* in their host animal was 175 x 127 μm. After 12 months in culture in the presence of epidinia, their mean size was 205 x 123 μm. Those cells grown *in vitro* in the absence of epidinia measured 123 x 98 μm. Under optimum growth conditions each *Polyplastron* engulfed about 10 epidinia per day. The minimum requirement for growth was one epidinia per *Polyplastron* per day.

Coleman *et al.* (1976) found that the species *Enoploplastron triloricatum*, *Eudiplodinium maggii*, *Eudiplodinium affine*, *Epidinium caudatum*, *Diplodinium monocanthum* and *Diplodinium pentacanthum* could be cultured *in vitro* with powdered grass as the only substrate. Extracts of these species digested a ^{14}C-cellulose preparation, liberating soluble ^{14}C-labeled compounds. They concluded that any isolated protozoan which can be grown on dried grass alone will digest cellulose. This was verified in later studies (Coleman, 1985). More detailed studies on nitrogen requirements of *Eudiplodinium maggii* have been reported by Coleman and Sanford (1979).

In another report from Coleman's lab, a culture of *Entodinium caudatum* that had been maintained *in vitro* for 9 3/4 years was used to inoculate a defaunated sheep (Coleman and White, 1970). There were 1×10^7 protozoa cells in the inoculum and after one week the protozoa were visible in rumen fluid and had increased to a concentration of 1.3×10^6 protozoa per ml by four weeks. Thus, the protozoa were still capable of growth in the rumen.

A requirement of *Entodinium caudatum* for choline was discovered by Broad and Dawson (1976). Since the associated bacteria in the *in vitro* culture are also unable to synthesize choline, it was suggested that the normal source of choline was from plant membrane material which the protozoan ingests. This would, of course, substantiate the observation that *E. caudatum* cannot be grown *in vitro* without a small amount of plant material.

GENERATION TIME

Only a few studies have been reported on growth rate or generation time of rumen protozoa *in vivo*. Warner (1962), using division time and percentage of dividing cells as criteria, obtained estimates of generation time for mixed entodinia in sheep ranging from 5.5 h to 58 h, at various times after feeding. Potter and Dehority (1973), using the increase in concentration of total protozoa between 5 and 20 h after feeding, calculated generation times between 13.5 and 37.3 h in sheep. More recently, Williams and Withers (1993) estimated a generation time of 9-10 h for entodinia in sheep during the initial stages of refaunation. Coleman (1979) has estimated mean generation times for eight species of entodiniomorphs, based on measurements taken during logarithmic growth *in vitro*. Values ranged from 6 h for *Entodinium bursa* to 38 h for *E. simplex*.

For any organisms to survive in a continuous system, its generation time must be equal or less than .69 times the fluid turnover time (Hungate 1942, 1966). Assuming the protozoa pass with the liquid phase, which turns over once per 24 h, then an organism must have a generation time of 16.6 h or less to maintain itself. Solids turnover times are much slower; however, it is not clear which of these fractions best estimates protozoal passage. Hungate *et al.* (1971) estimated that 80% of the protozoa move within the liquid fraction which has a turnover time between 10-16 h. Thus, generation times would need to be between 7 and 11 h for protozoa to maintain themselves in the rumen.

Using logarithmic growth from a small inoculum, Coleman *et al.* (1972) reported a generation time of 26 h for *Epidinium caudatum*. Figure 5.2a presents logarithmic growth curves for *Epidinium caudatum* in pure and coculture, measured by Dehority (1998). The coculture contained *Epidinium caudatum* and *Entodinium caudatum*. The generation time in pure culture was 30.8 h (measured between 24-120 h) and in coculture, 19.5 h (0-96 h), which gives a mean of 25.2 h, quite close to the time reported by Coleman *et al.* (1972).

Concentrations of *Epidinium* when the culture was transferred every 1, 2 or 3 days are shown in Fig. 5.3. Figure 5.4 shows concentrations when transfers were made every 4, 6, 8 or 12 h. Graph (a) is the pure culture and (b) is the coculture. At each transfer, half of the culture was transferred to a new tube containing fresh medium. If the transfer interval is shorter than the generation time, the concentration of protozoa should decrease over time. As can be seen, transferring more often than every 12 h resulted in a marked decrease in concentration. Figure 5.5 illustrates the curves to be expected when transferring an organism every 12 h with various theoretical generation times. The actual curve for *Epidinium* in pure culture did not differ from the theoretical curve for a generation time of 12.5 h.

116 Rumen microbiology

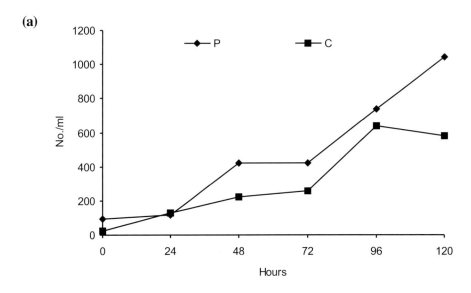

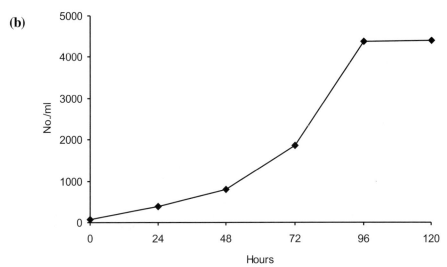

Figure 5.2 (a) Growth curves for *Epidinium caudatum* from a small inoculum, in pure culture (P) or in coculture (C) with *Entodinium caudatum*. (b) Growth curve for *Entodinium caudatum* grown in coculture with *Epidinium caudatum*. Concentrations were measured at 24 h intervals (from Dehority, 1998).

Figure 5.2b is a growth curve of *Entodinium caudatum* from a small inoculum. The generation time from 0 - 96 h was 16.3 h, which is considerably lower than the 23 h reported by Coleman (1979) for this species. Transfer curves, similar to those shown for *Epidinium*, were also determined for *Entodinium caudatum* and suggested a generation time possibly a little longer than 12 h.

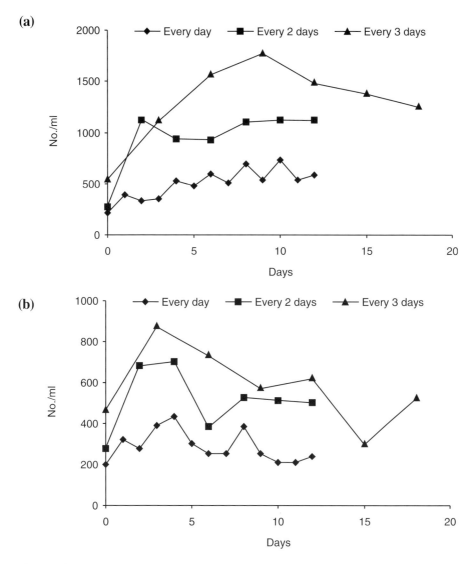

Figure 5.3 *Epidinium caudatum*, alone (a) or in coculture with *Entodinium caudatum* (b), transferred every 1, 2 or 3 d. Protozoal concentrations were determined each time a culture was transferred (from Dehority, 1998).

Mean and median generation times were calculated for both species, considering each transfer to represent a separate growth experiment. Except for the median values calculated from the 24-h growth periods, generation times for both *Epidinium* and *Entodinium* did not differ from 12 h. The probability of a difference between the concentration of cultures transferred every 12 h and concentrations based on the

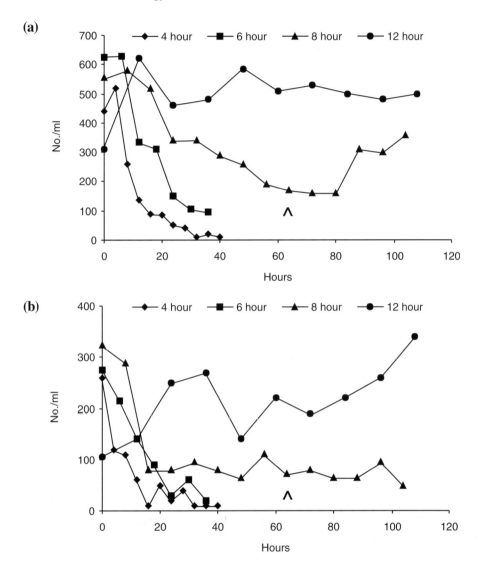

Figure 5.4. *Epidinium caudatum,* alone (a) or in coculture with *Entodinium caudatum* (b), transferred every 4, 6, 8 or 12 h. For the 8-h transfer schedule curves, the arrowheads indicate time at which substrate level was increased. Protozoal concentrations were determined each time a culture was transferred (from Dehority, 1998).

theoretical curves at the generation times shown in Fig. 5.5 was determined.. In pure culture, *Epidinium* did not differ at 12.5 h ($P > 0.41$) and in coculture, at 11.5 and 12 h ($P > 0.34$ and 0.48). For *Entodinium,* only the 13 h theoretical curve did not differ ($P > 0.64$).

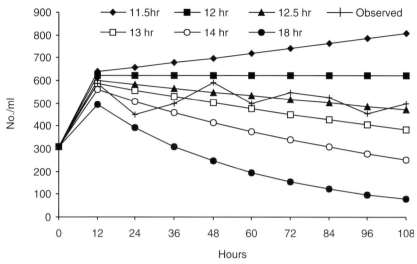

Figure 5.5 Comparison of the concentration changes observed in a culture of *Epidinium caudatum* that was transferred every 12 h with the theoretical changes expected if the organism had a generation time of 11.5, 12, 12.5, 13, 14 or 18 h (from Dehority, 1998).

In summary, both *Epidinium caudatum* and *Entodinium caudatum* appear to be capable of doubling in approximately 12-13 h. These values are lower than most previously reported times and help explain the ability of these organisms to maintain themselves in the rumen.

NUTRIENT REQUIREMENTS

At this time, it would appear that more exacting studies on nutrient requirements of the protozoa are entirely dependent upon improved methods for cultivation. If gnotobiotic cultures could be grown, it would be possible to obtain definitive answers to many questions about which we can only speculate at present. Some progress was made along these lines in the study reported by Jarvis and Hungate (1968) in which they studied the effects of sterilization upon the natural substrates which appear to be required for cultivation of entodiniomorph protozoa (whole meal flour, dried grasses, grains of wheat, etc.). Cultures of *E. simplex* exhibited slow and limited growth when the substrates were autoclaved; however, better growth was obtained when the substrate was sterilized with ethylene oxide vapor. Bacteria were required for the growth of *E. simplex*, either as food for the protozoa or in synergism between the substrate and protozoa. In the studies from Coleman's lab, all attempts to remove bacteria from the protozoal cultures with antibiotics have resulted in death of the protozoa, and they have reached similar conclusions to those of Jarvis and Hungate.

The previously cited study by Fondevila and Dehority (2001) indicated that initiation of both growth and starch digestion *by Entodinium exiguum* were more rapid when corn starch was autoclaved and when rice starch was compared to corn starch. However, there were essentially no differences after 48 h.

Studies by the author on the cultivation of protozoa *in vitro* have indicated that certain *Ostracodinium* species can be grown successfully for several months with sterile purified cellulose as the only energy source added to a sterilized 30% rumen fluid basal medium (unpublished).

EFFECTS OF pH ON VIABILITY AND GROWTH

Cultures of *Entodinium caudatum, Entodinium exiguum, Epidinium caudatum,* and *Ophryoscolex purkynjei* were grown and transferred in poorly buffered media prepared using different concentrations of sodium bicarbonate and a nitrogen gas phase (Dehority, unpublished). By transferring every 12 or 24 h, culture pH was gradually decreased until the protozoa disappeared. The cultures were transferred by placing half of the culture into an equal volume of fresh medium, resulting in pH fluctuations similar to the changes associated with fermentation, eating and saliva production in the rumen (Fig. 5.6). The effect of decreasing the medium pH on concentrations of *Epidinium caudatum* is shown in Fig. 5.7.

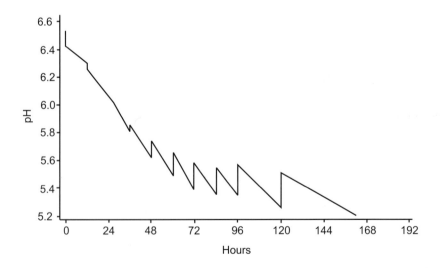

Figure 5.6. Fluctuation and overall decrease in medium pH when half of an *Epidinium caudatum* culture is transferred to an equal volume of fresh poorly buffered medium (Dehority, unpublished).

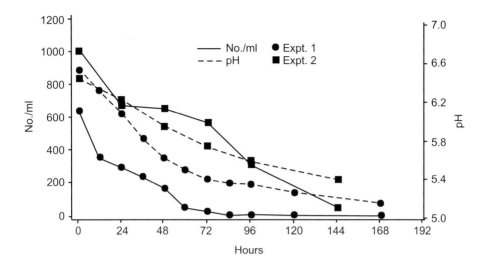

Figure 5.7 Effect of decreasing medium pH on the concentration of *Epidinium caudatum*. Each point represents the pH and concentration at time of transfer (Dehority, unpublished).

In general, all species appeared to maintain their concentrations at pH values at or above 5.8, but numbers began to decrease as pH values fell to 5.6 and below. Minimum pH values were calculated by regressing pH on concentration, and all four species were similar in that they all had a minimum pH value between 5.3 and 5.4. These results are somewhat surprising, since *Entodinium* species have been thought to be more tolerant to low pH than the higher ophryoscolecids. No adaptation to low pH was observed in *Epidinium* cultures after recovery from pH 5.4 medium containing only one or two viable cells.

References

Abou Akkada, A. R. (1965). The metabolism of ciliate protozoa in relation to rumen function. In: *Physiology of Digestion in the Ruminant.* Edited by R. W. Dougherty. Butterworths, Washington, D.C., pp. 335.

Abou Akkada, A. R. and B. H. Howard. (1960). The biochemistry of rumen protozoa. 3. The carbohydrate metabolism of *Entodinium*. *Biochemical Journal*, **76**, 445-451.

Abou Akkada, A. R. and B. H. Howard. (1962). The biochemistry of rumen protozoa. 5. The nitrogen metabolism of *Entodinium*. *Biochemical Journal*, **82**, 313-320.

Abou Akkada, A. R., J. M. Eadie and B. H. Howard. (1963). The biochemistry of rumen protozoa. 7. The carbohydrases of *Polyplastron multivesiculatum*. *Biochemical Journal*, **89**, 268-272.

Appleby, J. C., J. M. Eadie and A. E. Oxford. (1956). Interrelationships between ciliate protozoa and bacteria in the sheep's rumen. *Journal of Applied Bacteriology*, **19**, 166-172.

Bailey, R. W. (1958). Bloat in cattle. X. The carbohydrases of the cattle rumen ciliate *Epidinium ecaudatum* Crawley isolated from cows fed on red clover (*Trifolium pratense* L.). *New Zealand Journal of Agricultural Research*, **1**, 825-833.

Bailey, R. W. and R.T.J. Clarke. (1963). Carbohydrases of the rumen oligotrich *Eremoplastron bovis*. *Nature*, **199**, 1291-1292.

Bailey, R. W. and B. H. Howard. (1963). The biochemistry of rumen protozoa. 6. The maltases of *Dasytricha ruminantium, Epidinium ecaudatum* (Crawley) and *Entodinium caudatum*. *Biochemical Journal*, **86**, 446-452.

Bailey, R. W., R.T.J. Clarke and D. E. Wright. (1962). Carbohydrates of the rumen ciliate *Epidinium ecaudatum* Crawley. Action on plant hemicellulose. *Biochemical Journal*, **83**, 517-523.

Belżecki, G. and T. Michałowski. (2002). The role of the ciliate *Eudiplodinium maggii* in starch digestion in the rumen. *Reproduction Nutrition Development*, **42** (Suppl.1), S78.

Bonhomme-Florentin, A. (1975). Activité cellulolytique des ciliés entodiniomorphs. *Journal of Protozoology*, **22**, 447-451.

Broad, T. E. and R.M.C. Dawson. (1976). Role of choline in the nutrition of the rumen protozoan *Entodinium caudatum*. Journal of General Microbiology, **92**, 391-397.

Clarke, R.T.J. (1963). The cultivation of some oligotrich protozoa. *Journal of General Microbiology*, **33**, 401-408.

Clarke, R.T.J. and R. E. Hungate. (1966). Culture of the rumen holotrich ciliate *Dasytricha ruminantium* Shuberg. *Applied Microbiology*, **14**, 340-345.

Clayet, F., J. Senaud and J. Bohatier. (1992). Chromatographic separation of some cell wall polysaccharide-degrading enzymes of the sheep rumen ciliate *Epidinium caudatum*. *Annales de Zootechnie*, **41**, 81.

Coleman, G. S. (1958). Maintenance of oligotrich protozoa from the sheep rumen *in vitro*. *Nature,* **182**, 1104-1105.

Coleman, G. S. (1960). The cultivation of sheep rumen oligotrich protozoa *in vitro*. *Journal of General Microbiology*, **22**, 555-563.

Coleman, G. S. (1962). The preparation and survival of almost bacteria-free suspensions of *Entodinium caudatum*. *Journal of General Microbiology*, **28**, 271-281.

Coleman, G. S. (1964). The metabolism of *Escherichia coli* and other bacteria by *Entodinium caudatum*. *Journal of General Microbiology*, **37**, 209-223.

Coleman, G. S. (1967a). The metabolism of free amino acids by washed suspensions of the rumen ciliate *Entodinium caudatum*. *Journal of General Microbiology*, **47**, 433-447.

Coleman, G. S. (1967b). The metabolism of the amino acids of *Escherichia coli* and other bacteria by the rumen ciliate *Entodinium caudatum*. *Journal of General*

Microbiology, **47**, 449-464.

Coleman, G. S. (1969a). The cultivation of the rumen ciliate *Entodinium simplex*. *Journal of General Microbiology*, **57**, 81-90.

Coleman, G. S. (1969b). The metabolism of starch, maltose, glucose and some sugars by the rumen ciliate *Entodinium caudatum*. *Journal of General Microbiology*, **57**, 303-332.

Coleman, G. S. (1978). The metabolism of cellulose, glucose and starch by the rumen ciliate protozoon *Eudiplodinium maggii*. *Journal of General Microbiology*, **107**, 359-366.

Coleman, G. S. (1979). Rumen ciliate protozoa. In: *Biochemistry and Physiology of Protozoa*, Vol. 2, 2nd ed. Edited by M. Levondowsky and S. H. Hunter. Academic Press, New York, NY, pp. 381-408.

Coleman, G. S. (1985). The cellulase content of 15 species of entodiniomorphid protozoa, mixed bacteria and plant debris isolated from the ovine rumen. *Journal of Agricultural Science*, **104**, 349-360.

Coleman, G. S. (1986). The distribution of carboxymethylcellulase between fractions taken from the rumens of sheep containing no protozoa or one of five different protozoal populations. *Journal of Agricultural Science*, **106**, 121-127.

Coleman, G. S. and Judith I. Laurie. (1974). The metabolism of starch, glucose, amino acids, purines, pyrimidines and bacteria by three *Epidinium* spp. isolated from the rumen. *Journal of General Microbiology*, **85**, 244-256.

Coleman, G. S. and D. C. Sanford. (1979). The uptake and utilization of bacteria, amino acids and nucleic acid components by the rumen ciliate *Eudiplodinium maggii*. *Journal of Applied Bacteriology*, **47**, 409-419.

Coleman, G. S. and D. C. Sanford. (1980). The uptake and metabolism of bacteria, amino acids, glucose and starch by the spined and spineless forms of the rumen ciliate *Entodinium caudatum*. *Journal of General Microbiology*, **117**, 411-418.

Coleman, G. S. and R. W. White. (1970). Re-establishment of *Entodinium caudatum*, cultured *in vitro* in the rumen of a defaunated sheep. *Journal of General Microbiology*, **62**, 265-266.

Coleman, G. S., Judith I. Davies and Margaret A. Cash. (1972). The cultivation of the rumen ciliates *Epidinium ecaudatum caudatum* and *Polyplastron multivesiculatum* in vitro. *Journal of General Microbiology*, **73**, 509-521.

Coleman, G. S., J. I. Laurie and J. E. Bailey. (1977). The cultivation of the rumen ciliate *Entodinium bursa* in the presence of *Entodinium caudatum*. *Journal of General Microbiology*, **101**, 253-258.

Coleman, G. S., J. I. Laurie, J. E. Bailey and S. A. Holdgate. (1976). The cultivation of cellulolytic protozoa isolated from the rumen. *Journal of General Microbiology*, **95**, 144-150.

Dehority, B. A. (1998). Generation times of *Epidinium caudatum* and *Entodinium caudatum*, determined in vitro by transferring at various time intervals. *Journal of Animal Science*, **76**, 1189-1196.

Ellis, J. E., A. G. Williams and D. Lloyd. (1989). Oxygen consumption by ruminal microorganisms: protozoal and bacterial contributions. *Applied and Environmental Microbiology*, **55**, 2583-2587.

Ellis, J. E., P. S. McIntyre, M. Saleh, A. G. Williams and D. Lloyd. (1991). Influence of CO_2 and low concentrations of O_2 on fermentative metabolism of the ruminal ciliate *Polyplastron multivesiculatum*. *Applied and Environmental Microbiology*, **57**, 1400-1407.

Fondevila, M. and B. A. Dehority. (2001a). Preliminary study on the requirements of *Entodinium exiguum* and *Entodinium caudatum* for live or dead bacteria when cultured in vitro. *Reproduction, Nutrition, Development*, **41**, 41-46.

Fondevila, M. and B. A. Dehority. (2001b). In vitro growth and starch digestion by *Entodinium exiguum* as influenced by the presence or absence of live bacteria. *Journal of Animal Science*, **79**, 2465-2471.

Gutierrez, J. (1955). Experiments on the culture and physiology of holotrichs from the bovine rumen. *Biochemical Journal*, **60**, 516-522.

Gutierrez, J. (1958). Observations on bacterial feeding by the rumen ciliate *Isotricha prostoma*. *Journal of Protozoology*, **5**, 122-126.

Gutierrez, J. and R. E. Davis. (1959). Bacterial ingestion by the rumen ciliates *Entodinium* and *Diplodinium*. *Journal of Protozoology*, **6**, 222-226.

Gutierrez, J. and R. E. Davis. (1962). Culture and metabolism of the rumen ciliate *Epidinium ecaudatum* Crawley. *Applied Microbiology*, **20**, 305-308.

Gutierrez, J. and R. E. Hungate. (1957). Interrelationships between certain bacteria and the rumen ciliate *Dasytricha ruminantium*. *Science*, **126**, 511.

Heald, P. J., A. R. Oxford and B. Sugden. (1952). A convenient method for preparing massive suspensions of virtually bacteria-free ciliate protozoa of the genera *Isotricha* and *Dasytricha* for manometric studies. *Nature*, **169**, 1055-1056.

Howard, B. H. (1959). The biochemistry of rumen protozoa. 1. Carbohydrate fermentation by *Dasytricha* and *Isotricha*. *Biochemical Journal*, **71**, 671-675.

Howard, B. H. (1963). Metabolism of carbohydrates by rumen protozoa. *Biochemical Journal*, **89**, 89P.

Hungate, R. E. (1942). The culture of *Eudiplodinium neglectum* with experiments on the digestion of cellulose. *Biological Bulletin*, **83**, 303-319.

Hungate, R. E. (1943). Further experiments on cellulose digestion by the protozoa in the rumen of cattle. *Biological Bulletin*, **84**,157-163.

Hungate, R. E. (1966). *The Rumen and its Microbes*. Academic Press, New York, NY. USA.

Hungate, R. E., J. Reichl and R. Prins. (1971). Parameters of rumen fermentation in a continuously fed sheep: evidence of a microbial rumination pool. *Applied Microbiology,* **22**,1104-1113.

Jarvis, B.D.W. and R. E. Hungate. (1968). Factors influencing agnotobiotic cultures of

the rumen ciliate *Entodinium simplex*. *Applied Microbiology*, **16**, 1044-1052.
Lloyd, D., J. Williams, N. Yarlett and A. G. Williams. (1982). Oxygen affinities of the hydrogenosome-containing protozoa *Trichomonas foetus* and *Dasytricha ruminantium* and two aerobic protozoa, determined by bacterial bioluminescence. *Journal of General Microbiology*, **128**, 1019-1022.
Lloyd, D., K. Hillman, N. Yarlett and A. G. Williams. (1989). Hydrogen production by rumen holotrich protozoa: Effects of oxygen and implications for metabolic control by *in situ* conditions. *Journal of Protozoology*, **36**, 205-213.
Mah, R. A. (1964). Factors influencing the *in vitro* culture of the rumen ciliate *Ophryoscolex purkynjei* Stein. *Journal of Protozoology*, **11**, 546-552.
Mah, R. A. and R. E. Hungate. (1965). Physiological studies on the rumen ciliate *Ophryoscolex purkynjei* Stein. *Journal of Protozoology*, **12**, 131-136.
Masson, F. M. and A. E. Oxford. (1951). The action of the ciliates of the sheep's rumen upon various water-soluble carbohydrates, including polysaccharides. *Journal of General Microbiology*, **5**, 664-672.
Michałowski, T., K. Rybicka, K. Wereszka and A. Kasperowicz. (2001). Ability of the rumen ciliate *Epidinium ecaudatum* to digest and use crystalline cellulose and xylan for in vitro growth. *Acta Protozoologica*, **40**, 203-211.
Morgavi, D. P., M. Sakurada, Y. Tomita and R. Onodera. (1996). Electrophoretic forms of chitinolytic and lysozyme activities in ruminal protozoa. *Current Microbiology* **32**, 115-118.
Naga, M. A. and K. el-Shazly. (1968). The metabolic characterization of the ciliate protozoan *Eudiplodinium medium* from the rumen of buffalo. *Journal of General Microbiology*, **53**, 305-315.
Onodera, R. and C. Henderson. (1980). Growth factors of bacterial origin for the culture of the rumen oligotrich protozoan, *Entodinium caudatum*. *Journal of Applied Bacteriology*, **48**, 125-133.
Oxford, A. E. (1951). The conversion of certain soluble sugars to a glucosan by holotrich ciliates in the rumen of sheep. *Journal of General Microbiology*, **5**, 83-90.
Oxford, A. E. (1955). The rumen ciliate protozoa: Their chemical composition, metabolism, requirements for maintenance and culture, and physiological significance for the host. *Experimental Parasitology*, **4**, 569-605.
Paul, R. G., A. G. Williams and R. D. Butler. (1990). Hydrogenosomes in the rumen entodiniomorphid ciliate, *Polyplastron multivesiculatum*. *Journal of General Microbiology*, **136**, 1981-1989.
Potter, E. L. and B. A. Dehority. (1973). Effects of changes in feed level, starvation, and level of feed after starvation upon the concentration of rumen protozoa in the ovine. *Applied Microbiology*, **26**, 692-698.
Prins, R. A. and W. Van Hoven. (1977). Carbohydrate fermentation by the rumen ciliate *Isotricha prostoma*. *Protistologica*, **13**, 549-556.
Sugden, B. (1953). The cultivation and metabolism of oligotrich protozoa from the sheep's rumen. *Journal of General Microbiology*, **9**, 44-53.

Sugden, B. and A. E. Oxford. (1952). Some cultural studies with holotrich ciliate protozoa of the sheep's rumen. *Journal of General Microbiology*, **7**, 145-153.

Van Hoven, W. and R. A. Prins. (1977). Carbohydrate fermentation by the rumen ciliate *Dasytricha ruminantium*. *Protistologica*, **13**, 599-606.

Warner, A.C.I. (1962). Some factors influencing the rumen microbial population. *Journal of General Microbiology*, **28**, 129-146.

Wereszka, K., T. Michałowski and A. *Kasperowicz.* (2002). The fibrolytic activity of the rumen ciliate *Diploplastron affine*. *Reproduction Nutrition Development*, **42** (Suppl. 1), S86.

Williams, A. G. (1979a). The selectivity of carbohydrate assimilation by the anaerobic rumen ciliate *Dasytricha ruminantium*. *Journal of Applied Bacteriology*, **47**, 511-520.

Williams, A. G. (1979b). Exocellular carbohydrase formation by rumen holotrich ciliates. *Journal of Protozoology*, **26**, 665-672.

Williams, A. G. (1986). Rumen holotrich ciliate protozoa. *Microbiological Reviews*, **50**, 25-49.

Williams, A. G. and G. S. Coleman. (1992). *The Rumen Protozoa*. Springer-Verlag New York, Inc. New York, N.Y.

Williams, A. G. and C. G. Harfoot. (1976). Factors affecting the uptake and metabolism of soluble carbohydrates by the rumen ciliate *Dasytricha ruminantium* isolated from ovine rumen contents by filtration. *Journal of General Microbiology*, **96**, 125-136.

William, A. G. and S. E. Withers. (1993) Changes in the rumen microbial populations and its activities during the refaunation period after the reintroduction of ciliate protozoa into the rumen of defaunated sheep. *Canadian Journal of Microbiology*, **39**, 61-69.

Williams, A. G. and N. Yarlett. (1982). An improved technique for the isolation of holotrich protozoa from rumen contents by differential filtration with defined aperture textiles. *Journal of Applied Bacteriology*, **52**, 267-270.

Williams, P. P., R. E. Davis, R. N. Doetsch and J. Gutierrez. (1961). Physiological studies of the rumen protozoan *Ophryoscolex caudatus* Eberlein. *Applied Microbiology*, **9**, 405-409.

Yarlett, N., A. C. Hann, D. Lloyd and A. Williams. (1981). Hydrogenosomes in the rumen protozoon *Dasytricha ruminantium* Schuberg. *Biochemical Journal*, **200**, 365-372.

Yarlett, N., D. Lloyd and A. G. Williams. (1982). Respiration of the rumen ciliate *Dasytricha ruminantium* Schuberg. *Biochemical Journal*, **206**, 259-266.

Yarlett, N., G. S. Coleman, A. G. Williams and D. Lloyd. (1984). Hydrogenosomes in known species of rumen entodiniomorphid protozoa. *FEMS Microbiology Letters*, **21**, 15-19.

Yarlett, N., C. G. Orpin, E. A. Munn, N. C. Yarlett and C. A. Greenwood. (1986).

Hydrogenosomes in the rumen fungus *Neocallimastix patriciarum*. *Biochemical Journal*, **236**, 729-739.

CHAPTER 6

DISTRIBUTION, SPECIFICITY AND ROLE OF THE RUMEN PROTOZOA

Distribution

GEOGRAPHIC DISTRIBUTION

Hungate (1966) compiled a list of the genera and species of entodiniomorphs observed in cattle and sheep from Russia, China, New Zealand and Scotland. However, since publication of his book, many reports from various locations around the world have appeared in the literature, and some of the more interesting points in these reports will be discussed.

Clarke (1964) did not observe the genus *Ophryoscolex* in New Zealand cattle and sheep, and although not known for certain, this genus is not mentioned in a number of studies from Australia. A report from Finland (Westerling, 1969), on samples obtained from 24 cattle and 8 sheep does not include the genus *Ophryoscolex*, nor was it observed in sheep from Japan (Nakamura and Kanegasaki, 1969). In those samples which I personally collected from Brazil and Peru, *Ophryoscolex* was not observed in the rumen contents of *Bos indicus, Bos taurus*, sheep, goats, water buffalo or the alpaca. However, this genus was present in several cattle samples obtained from Chile (Dehority, unpublished). These observations are of interest with respect to the studies of Eadie (1962, 1967). She found *Ophryoscolex* was difficult to establish in young sheep and goats, and observed that this species tends to be unstable in older ruminants; completely disappearing in many cases. In addition, there appears to be some antagonism between *Ophryoscolex* and *Epidinium*, in that *Ophryoscolex* slowly disappears when both are present in the fauna.

A very common protozoan in the U.S. and Europe, *Polyplastron multivesiculatum*, was not observed in New Zealand (Clarke, 1964), or in rumen contents of *Bos indicus* (humped cattle) and *Bos gaurus* (gaur) from India and Ceylon (Kofoid and Christenson, 1934; Kofoid and MacLennan, 1932). Occurrence of this species in samples from Brazil was limited to very low numbers in only one animal of *Bos taurus* (Dehority, unpublished). It was also absent from the Peruvian material, but present in Chilean cattle. The dominance of *Polyplastron* by predation over *Epidinium* and many *Eudiplodinium* and *Ostracodinium* species was discussed previously in Chapter 4. On this basis, it seems unusual that *Polyplastron* would be absent from so many geographic areas. However, this may reflect the source of importation of ruminants and their subsequent isolation in certain areas, i.e., New Zealand and Brazil. Obviously, when obtaining samples in a foreign site, one should attempt to sample those animals which are well isolated and not in contact with recently imported ruminants.

In other studies, Abou Akkada and el-Shazly (1964) and Naga *et al.* (1969) observed the protozoal population in both cow and buffalo calves and sheep from various regions in Egypt and have suggested that the genus *Epidinium* is absent from all ruminants in Egyptian territory.

Becker and Talbott (1927) surveyed the protozoa in 26 American cattle. All of the genera were observed; however, marked differences were observed between individual animals. For example, 11 of the 26 animals were devoid of all holotrichs and *Ophryoscolex* occurred in only one. Two species of *Entodinium* and *Epidinium* were present in almost all animals. More recent reports from various locations in the United States and Canada, for both cattle and sheep, have shown that all of the genera except *Elytroplastron* are quite widespread in domestic animals. No particular geographical differences have been noted with regard to the individual species (Abou Akkada *et al.*, 1969; Dehority, 1978; Dogiel, 1927; Ibrahim *et al.*, 1970).

Dehority *et al.* (1983) observed the ciliate *Oligoisotricha bubali* in rumen contents of domestic cattle in two different areas of Tennessee. Concentrations ranged from <1 up to 72% of the total protozoa. It is of interest that the concentration of this species increased when concentrates were fed, which differs markedly from the response shown by the other holotrichs. This species was originally described by Dogiel in 1928, which he observed in rumen contents of two water buffalo from Russia. No additional observation of this species was recorded until 1981, when Imai detected its presence in water buffalo from Taiwan. At this point, any explanation for the occurrence of this species in domestic cattle in two areas of Tennessee is unclear.

Dehority and Orpin (1988) have compiled a listing of protozoa concentrations and number of species per animal in water buffalo, *Bos indicus* (Zebu cattle) and *Bos taurus* (cattle) in various locations around the world (Table 6.1). Although data are limited, protozoan concentrations and number of species appear to be slightly higher in zebu cattle. With the same animal species, higher values were generally observed in animals from Brazil. As can be noted, the number of species in an individual animal varied from 2 to 39. Additional observations on protozoan concentrations from several different geographical areas are listed in Table 6.2. In general, the range of protozoan concentrations ($1.7\text{-}418.7 \times 10^4$/ml) and numbers of species per animal (5-45) are similar to those shown in Table 6.1. An increase in protozoan concentrations in response to feeding concentrates is clearly shown by the data on bison in Table 6.2.

Imai (1985) compared protozoan species composition in water buffalo from a number of different locations. He found that 80.8% of the species were common between Indonesia and Thailand. Similarity was calculated as the number of species in Thailand common to Indonesia divided by the total number of species in Thailand. The percentage of species common between Indonesia and other locations were as follows: Taiwan, 71.4%; Kafkas, 67.9%; India, 50% and Brazil 48.8%. Similarity in protozoa between

Table 6.1 PROTOZOAN CONCENTRATIONS AND NUMBER OF SPECIES PER ANIMAL IN WATER BUFFALO AND CATTLE LOCATED IN DIFFERENT GEOGRAPHICAL AREAS[a]

Host Location	No. of animals	Total protozoa $\times 10^4$/ml	Number of species/ animal	Reference[b]
Water Buffalo				
Indonesia	17	1.5(0.1-31.6)[c]	12.9(8-20)[c]	1
Thailand	10	0.7(0.2-2.0)	9.4(2-17)	2
Taiwan	29	8.9(0.5-316.2)	11.5(3-25)	3
Philippines	2	4.7(1.5-7.8)	8.0(7-9)	4
Brazil	4	22.9(16.6-35.8)	29.0(22-35)	5
Okinawa	5	37.4(27.0-49.5)	9.6[d]	6
Zebu Cattle				
Thailand	46	7.1(0.6-31.6)	26.1(14-39)	2
Philippines	4	15.8(13.2-18.1)	20.0(18-22)	4
Senegal	24	9.0(3.6-31.0)	13.2(8-18)	7
Sri Lanka	20	2.9(0.1-31.6)	18.4(6-29)	8
Brazil	4	26.4(9.0-51.2)	30.2(22-36)	9
Cattle				
Japan	69	13.5(0.5-3981)	10.3(4-25)	10

[a] From Dehority and Orpin, 1988.
[b] References: (1) Imai, 1985; (2) Imai & Ogimoto, 1984; (3) Imai *et al.*, 1981b; (4) Shimizu *et al.*, 1983; (5) Dehority, 1979; (6) Imai *et al.*, 1981a; (7) Bonhomme-Florentin *et al.*, 1978; (8) Imai, 1986; (9) Dehority, 1986c; (10) Imai *et al.*, 1982.
[c] Mean and range.
[d] Range not reported.

Bali cattle and water buffalo in Indonesia was 66.7%. It appears that similar protozoan species tend to occur in a given geographical location, even between different animal species.

EFFECT OF DIET

The data shown in Table 6.3 are taken from a report by Dehority and Mattos (1978) and clearly illustrate the effect of diet upon both protozoan concentration and genera distribution in a single Brazilian cow. Obviously the addition of concentrate increased both concentration and percent *Entodinium*. In general, the percentage *Entodinium* for most domestic ruminants is generally in the range of 80-99%, even on an all forage diet. An average value would be around 88-90% (Ibrahim *et al.*, 1970; Dearth *et al.*, 1974; Dehority, 1978; Imai *et al.*, 1982).

Table 6.2 PROTOZOAN CONCENTRATIONS IN ANIMALS FROM SEVERAL ADDITIONAL GEOGRAPHICAL AREAS

Site Animal	No. of animals	Diet	Total protozoa (10^4/ml)	Number of species/anim.	Reference[a]
Kenya					
SEA cattle (zebu)	14	Varied[b]	10.7(2.5-25.1)	36.6(27-45)	1
Boran cattle (zebu)	13	"	15.1(6.3-39.8)	34.9(28-40)	1
Japan					
Cattle (*Bos taurus*)	71	Varied[b]	53.7(14.5-168.2)	17.2(5-30)	2
Canada					
Cattle (*Bos taurus*)	11	Hay	6.9(2.5-12.6)	20.5(14-24)	3
Sheep	6	Hay	18.6(10-31.6)	13.8(12-16)	3
USA[c]					
Cattle (*Bos taurus*)	40	85% conc.	16(9.7-61.3)[d]	—	4
Bison	21	Forage	27.1(1.7-82.2)	—	5
	45	Forage + conc.	210.1(12.6-407.6)	—	
	15	Conc. type	169.2(42.0-418.7)	—	
Mexico					
Cattle (*Bos taurus*)	14	Varied	9.0(.07-21.9)	—	6
Cattle (*Bos indicus*)	16	Varied	4.2(.07-10.7)	—	
Inner Mongolia, China					
Cattle	6	Varied	31(7-48)	20.8(16-24)	7
Turkey					
Cattle	28	Varied	47.5(16-87.5)	18.7(5-34)	8

[a] References: (1) Imai, 1988; (2) Ito and Imai, 1990; (3) Imai *et al.*, 1989; (4) Towne *et al.*, 1990; (5) Towne *et al.*, 1988; (6) Imai and Kinoshita, 1997; (7) Guirong *et al.*, 2000; (8) Göçmen (unpublished).
[b] Samples obtained either at abattoir or from random sites, with no information given on diets.
[c] Kansas.
[d] Range in mean values from 12 sampling days.

DISTRIBUTION AMONG ANIMAL SPECIES

Clarke (1977), summarized the literature on occurrence of the different genera of entodiniomorphs in both domestic and wild ruminants. In general, the highest number of different genera are found in cattle, sheep, goats and the water buffalo. However, this may possibly be explained by the actual number of studies and animals involved. Most genera are rather widely distributed, except for *Caloscolex, Opisthotrichum* and *Epiplastron*. Williams and Coleman (1988) compiled a similar listing for the holotrichs.

Table 6.3 EFFECT OF DIET ON CONCENTRATION OF TOTAL PROTOZOA AND GENERIC DISTRIBUTION[a]

Ration	Successive days on each ration	Total protozoa (x10³/ml)	Generic distribution (% of total protozoa)				
			Ento-dinium	Diplo-dinium	Isotricha	Dasy-tricha	Charo-nina
Pasture + conc[b]	21	1,236	92.7	4.0	0.5	1.5	1.3
Grass hay[c]	15	96	46.7	6.7	0	7.5	39.1
	16	118	44.3	15.9	0	3.4	36.5
	17	122	55.3	10.7	0.6	4.3	29.0
	20	195	44.4	8.2	1.2	15.7	30.5
	21	141	49.8	13.9	1.6	2.8	32.0
Pasture[d]	17	230	75.7	13.5	0.4	4.5	5.9
Green chop[e]	7	70	55.1	30.7	0	5.1	9.1
	11	60	50.8	19.9	2.0	6.0	21.3
Grass hay + conc[f]	9	344	86.6	7.6	0	5.5	0.3

[a] From Dehority and Mattos, 1978.
[b] Native grass pasture plus 3 kg of concentrate (conc) per day.
[c] Rhodes grass (*Chloris gayana*), 7 kg/day.
[d] Napier grass (*Pennisetum purpurem*).
[e] Napier grass (cut fresh daily and fed in the barn), 60 kg/day.
[f] 5.5 kg of Rhodes grass hay plus 1.5 kg of conc per day.

Isotricha and *Dasytricha* are widely distributed among the different animals species, whereas occurrence of *Buetschlia*, *Charonina* and *Oligoisotricha* is sporadic and limited. Most of the data on wild ruminants represents only one or two observations.

In 1974, Dehority described a new species of *Entodinium* from Alaskan moose. This species, *Entodinium alces*, was subsequently observed in the springbok and giraffe in southern Africa (Kleynhans and van Hoven, 1976; Wilkinson and van Hoven, 1976a,b). In 19 springbok, its concentrations ranged from 0.4 to 21.1%. Also of interest was the occurrence of the species *E. anteronucleatum* in the springbok. This species was first observed in reindeer but has also been observed in other arctic ruminants, i.e., musk-ox and Dall sheep. *E. anteronucleatum* has also been observed in *Bos indicus* located in Dakar, Senegal (Bonhomme-Florentin *et al.*, 1978), thus fairly well establishing its presence on the African continent. *E. alces* averaged 1% of the total ciliates in 8 giraffe, while *E. quadricuspis*, another species previously observed only in reindeer, constituted 2% of the total ciliates. The occurrence of these apparent arctic-type *Entodinium* species in African animals was most unexpected and difficult to explain. It also raises the question as to why they have not been observed in any intermediate locations.

Although the fauna of Brazilian water buffalo differs considerably from that of water buffalo in several other areas of the world (Dehority, 1979; Imai, 1985), it is closely related to the fauna observed in *Bos indicus* and *Bos gaurus* from India and Ceylon (Kofoid and MacLennan, 1930, 1932, 1933; Kofoid and Christenson, 1934). This probably reflects the importation of this species into Brazil from that area of the world. A total of 32 species of protozoa present in the Brazilian water buffalo were previously observed in *B. indicus* and *B. gaurus*. This gives a similarity index of 64% as calculated by the procedure of Imai (1985). Until this time, three of the 32 species had not been observed outside of the original Indian material, and occurrence of several other species was limited. Eight new species were also described from the Brazilian water buffalo. One of these species, *Ostracodinium tiete* was subsequently found in two water buffalo from the Philippines (Shimizu *et al.*, 1983). Another of these new species, *Eudiplodinium bubalus*, was found in four of 69 cattle from Japan (Imai *et al.*, 1982), while a third species, *Entodinium spinonucleatum*, was present in two of five water buffalo sampled in Okinawa (Imai *et al.*, 1981a). The unusual distribution patterns observed for these ciliates is somewhat similar to that observed for the Arctic and African ciliates.

Total numbers and fauna composition have been reported in samples of rumen contents obtained from 13 musk-oxen living on Banks Island, N.W.T., Canada (Dehority, 1985). These animals were quite isolated and their fauna was fairly unusual in that only two species of *Entodinium* were present. In five of the animals, only one species, *E. ovibos* n. sp., was present. *Entodinium* constituted 52.4% of the total ciliates ranging from 45-63%. Although there is no obvious explanation for this distribution, it was suggested that dietary effects, animal isolation or both could be responsible. A somewhat similar situation was observed by van Hoven *et al.* (1979) in the sable antelope in which only a single species of *Entodinium, E. rostratum*, was present in a fairly diverse fauna and constituted about 32% of the total ciliates. A total of 18 protozoan species were identified in the musk-oxen samples from Banks Island. Two of these were new species and six were species which had not previously been observed in this host. This brings the total number of protozoan species observed in musk-oxen to 33. Similarity indexes were 22% with Alaskan musk-oxen and 50% with musk-oxen in two other areas of the N.W.T. of Canada.

Dehority (1990) examined rumen contents of 23 white-tailed deer from east-central Ohio. Samples were obtained during late fall and winter over a 4 year period. Protozoa concentrations averaged 2.96×10^6 per ml and ranged from .002 to 7.25×10^6/ml. The only species present in all 23 animals was *Entodinium dubardi*. Calculation of the volume of an individual *E. dubardi* cell, based on measurements of 100 cells, revealed that 7.25×10^6 cells per ml would actually constitute 10.4% of the rumen contents volume. In a later study on the blue duiker, which also contained only the single species *Entodinium dubardi*, concentrations were considerably higher ranging from 4.5 to 33.7×10^6 per ml. This would constitute between 5.3 to 39.9% of the total volume of rumen contents (Dehority, 1994).

Rumen contents from 5 wild Mongolian gazelles were examined by Imai and Rung (1990a). Concentrations ranged from 12.3 to 67.7 x 10^4 per ml with an average of 24.8 x 10^4. *Entodinium convexum* occurred in all five animals; *E. dubardi* in 3; *and E. nanellum* and *E. exiguum* in 1 animal each. Ito *et al.* (1993) surveyed the rumen ciliate population in 13 adult Ezo deer (*Cervus nippon yesoensis*) from Japan, and found only two species of *Entodinium*, *E. simplex* and *E. dubardi*. Concentrations ranged from 0.31 to 588.2 x 10^4/ml. This "*Entodinium* only condition" has generally been attributed to animals who primarily consume browse and probably have a low rumen pH. In addition to finding an "*Entodinium* only" fauna in both the Ezo deer and Mongolian gazelles, it is of interest that Dehority (1994) subsequently presented information which suggested that *E. simplex*, *E. nanellum*, and *E. convexum* may be variation lines within the species *E. dubardi*. Thus it appears possible that many animals in widely separated areas may actually contain a single species, *E. dubardi*.

In a separate study, Imai and Rung (1990b) obtained samples of stomach contents from four Bactrian camels inhabiting Inner-Mongolia, China. A total of 14 species of ciliates representing 7 genera of protozoa were found, which, except for *Caloscolex*, normally occur in the rumen. Six of the species had not been previously observed in camels. Protozoan concentrations averaged 21.1 x 10^4/ml (7.4-43.7) and mean numbers of species per head was 7.3 (5-10).

Kubesy and Dehority (2002) examined the forestomach contents of 20 dromedary camels from Egypt. As with the bactrian camels, except for the genus *Caloscolex,* the ciliates were rumen ophryoscolecids. Concentrations ranged from 4.9-109.4 x 10^4/ml. Ten genera containing 31 species were identified.

Williams and Coleman (1992) compiled a list of references for the occurrence and in some cases, enumeration and identification, of fauna in both rumen and forestomach contents of over 50 herbivores. Since that time, a number of reports have been published for both ruminant and nonruminant herbivores, some of which have not previously been studied (Table 6.4). A better understanding of both geographical and animal host distribution of rumen protozoa will probably be forthcoming as additional samples are collected around the world.

Specificity

Results of early studies with defaunated animals indicated that the rumen ciliates can only be transmitted by direct contact with other ruminants (Becker & Hsiung, 1929). The genera and species of protozoa found in the rumen appear to be almost unique to that habitat. Except for their occurrence in the first stomach chamber of the pseudo-ruminant camelids, they were not observed in any other locations, including the gastrontestinal tract of other herbivores (Dehority, 1986b). Thus it was concluded that the rumen protozoa are a highly specialized group of organisms which can survive only in the rumen or a very similar environment. In addition, a number of studies would also substantiate the concept that some type of specificity must exist as far as determining the species of protozoa which can live in different animal hosts.

Table 6.4 RECENT REPORTS ON CILIATE PROTOZOAL POPULATIONS IN SEVERAL RUMINANT AND NONRUMINANT SPECIES

Host animal	Location	Conc. ($\times 10^4$/ml)	Reference
Red deer (*Cervus elaphus*)	Australia	15-50.9	Dehority (1997)
Sika deer (*Cervus nippon centralis*)	Japan	0.7-58.1	Imai *et al.* (1993)
Sassaby antelope (*Damaliscus lunatus lunatus*)	Africa	24-45	Ito *et al.* (1997)
Lechwe (*Kobus leche*)	Africa	3.6-67.6	Imai *et al.* (1992)
Elk (*Cervus canadensis*)	USA	47.8-93.0	Dehority (1995)
Pronghorn antelope (*Antiloocapra americana*)	USA	13-29.3	Dehority (1995)
Mule deer (*Odocoileus hemionus*)	USA	11.5-71.8	Dehority (1995)
Yak (*Bos grunniens*)	China	7-29	Guirong *et al.* (2000)
European cattle (*Bos taurus*)	Japan	3.9-172	Ito *et al.* (1994)
Quokka (*Setonix brachyurus*)	Australia	2.2-9.7	Dehority (1996)
Camel (*Camels dromedarius*)	Egypt	4.9-109.4	Selim *et al.* (1996) Kubesy & Dehority (2002)
	Libya	28-75	Selim *et al.* (1999)

On the basis of these observations, two types of specificity might be postulated for the rumen protozoa (Dehority, 1978):

1. Host specificity - the animal itself, by some unknown "physiological factors" would influence the genera and species which could become established in its rumen. Physiological factors might include:

   a. Type and amount of feed consumed
   b. Rate of consumption
   c. Saliva production

   These in turn would influence:

   a. Rumen pH
   b. Rate and type of fermentation
   c. Osmolality
   d. Fluid and particulate matter turnover times.

   Experimental investigation of host specificity would involve attempts to introduce species of protozoa into an animal species where they have never been observed. This would probably require using the more exotic ruminants.

2. Protozoan specificity - This would have to be defined as "races" within a given species; for example, a race of cattle *Polyplastron multivesiculatum* which would differ from a race of sheep *Polyplastron*.

Existence of this type of specificity could be determined by attempting to establish species from one host in the rumen of another host where this species has normally been observed.

HOST SPECIFICITY

Dogiel (1927) considered at least 10 species in reindeer and caribou to be specific for that animal host; however, subsequent studies have shown that all but one of these species, *Eudiplodinium spectabile*, has been observed in one or more additional hosts (Table 6.5). Although occurrence of several of these species in wild African ruminants is quite interesting, no explanation is immediately obvious.

Table 6.5 OCCURRENCE OF PROTOZOAN SPECIES CONSIDERED SPECIFIC TO THE RANGIFER-TYPE FAUNA OF REINDEER AND CARIBOU

	Cattle (1,2,3)[a]	Sheep (2,3)	Red Deer (4,11)	Fallow Deer (4)	Musk-ox (7,9)	Dall Sheep (7)	Moose (7)	Springbok (5)	Giraffe (6)	Sable Antelope (8)	Elk (10)
Entodinium:											
E. anteronucleatum	+[b]				+	+		+			
E. bicornutum					+						+
E. exiguum	+	+			+	+	+			+	+
E. quadricuspis										+	+
Diplodinium:											
D. dogieli			+	+	+					+	
D. rangiferi			+	+					+		
Ostracodinium confluens					+						
O. magnum					+						
Eudiplodinium spectabile											
Epidinium gigas					+						

[a] References: (1) Bonhomme-Florentin *et al.* (1978); (2) Dehority (1978); (3) Westerling (1969); (4) Sládeček (1946); (5) Wilkinson and van Hoven (1976b); (6) Kleynhans and van Hoven (1976); (7) Dehority (1974); (8) van Hoven *et al.* (1979); (9) Tener (1965); (10) Dehority (1995); (11) Dehority (1997).
[b] Observation of the protozoan species in the given animal host.

With the exception of *E. exiguum*, which has a wide distribution, Westerling (1969) found no other species of the rangifer-type fauna in 24 cattle and 8 sheep from the reindeer-raising area of Finland. Dehority (1975) examined rumen contents from domestic sheep grazing the same pastures as wild reindeer on Umnak Island, Alaska, and did not observe any species in the rangifer fauna. Even though each individual species does not appear to be absolutely specific to reindeer and caribou, some degree of specificity is suggested by their joint occurrence in the fauna of reindeer and caribou around the world.

Two genera of Ophryoscolecidae, *Epiplastron* (two species) and *Opisthotrichum* (one species), have only been observed to date in several species of African antelope (Dehority, 1986b). Results of cross inoculating rumen contents from these antelope into defaunated domestic ruminants would be very informative.

Dehority (1986c) reported the presence of several species of ciliates in rumen contents of Brazilian cattle, which were new to the rumen habitat. *Parentodinium africanum*, a member of the family Cycloposthiidae, constituted 4.4, 0.9, < 0.1 and 10% of the total ciliates in four Brazilian cattle. Subsequent unpublished studies have revealed the presence of this species at several widely separated sites in western Brazil. This organism was first observed and described in stomach contents from the African hippopotamus (Thurston and Noirot-Timothée, 1973), and appeared to be unique to that site. *Blepharoconus krugerensis*, previously observed in the intestines of the elephant (Eloff and van Hoven, 1980) and an unknown species of Paraisotrichidae were each observed in a single Brazilian animal. Just recently, Dehority *et al.*(1999) observed *P. africanum* in rumen contents of several domestic cattle in Montana. Concentrations ranged from 1.4 to 130.6 x 10^4 per ml of rumen contents, which comprised 4.6 to 80.3% of the total protozoa. It would thus appear that ciliates in families other than those previously found in the rumen, and which do occur at different sites in the intestinal tract of nonruminant herbivores, can survive and become established in the rumen environment. Although two previous studies were unsuccessful in establishing ciliates (including numerous species of Cycloposthiidae) from the colon of the horse into the rumen (Becker and Hsiung, 1929; Dogiel and Winogradowa-Fedorowa, 1930), this new information might suggest the need for further investigations.

In a somewhat reverse type of experiment, Baker *et al.* (1995) were unsuccessful in establishing ciliate protozoa from the forestomach of the kangaroo into the rumen of defaunated sheep. Although physiological conditions in the two sites are fairly similar, within 12-18 hours following inoculation, kangaroo ciliates could not be found in the rumen contents of seven defaunated sheep.

As mentioned earlier, ciliates in the family Ophryoscolecidae had always been considered unique to the foregut of ruminants and camelids. However, large numbers of rumen ophryoscolecids were recently found in feces samples from two capybara housed in a zoo (Dehority, 1987). Concentrations ranged between 15 and 60 x 10^4 per g of wet feces, which is fairly close to concentrations observed in rumen contents. Obviously the environment and rate of digesta passage in the hindgut of the capybara are compatible for establishment and growth of these rumen ciliates. Fermentation in the hindgut of the capybara occurs primarily in the cecum and the normal fauna is unique to the capybara (Hollande and Batisse, 1959). Faunation of the young, through coprophagy of the mother's feces, apparently did not occur with these two animals. They were housed in the zoo with several llama, a normal foregut host for the rumen ophryoscolecids, which apparently served as the source of their infection. Similar results were obtained in a more recent study from Japan by Imai *et al.* (1997). They examined cecal contents from capybara housed in the Nagasaki Bio-Park zoological garden and observed only rumen ciliate protozoa.

In summary, there is not much experimental evidence to indicate a high degree of specificity between various protozoan species and hosts. Key factors controlling the specific fauna in a given animal would appear to be source of inoculum, type of exposure or inoculation, a suitable rumen environment and diet.

PROTOZOAN SPECIFICITY

One of the first suggestions of protozoan specificity was the report of Dogiel and Winogradowa-Federowa in 1930. They inoculated "almost" ciliate free goats with rumen contents from steers which had been killed in the local slaughterhouse. Although a number of species did become established, some species such as *Epidinium* and *Ophryoscolex* did not survive. More recent studies by Naga *et al.* (1969) on protozoan specificity are quite interesting, though their numbers were limited. Inoculum from adult water buffalo and cows contained *Isotricha, Dasytricha, Entodinium, Diplodinium, Eudiplodinium* and *Ostracodinium*. In the inoculum obtained from sheep, *Ophryoscolex* and *Polyplastron* were also present while *Eudiplodinium* was absent. Cross-inoculation of *Ostracodinium* and *Dasytricha* between buffaloes and cows was unsuccessful. *Ophryoscolex* and *Polyplastron* from sheep were unable to survive in buffalo or cow calves. The newly born buffalo and cows calves were inoculated with about 100 ml of rumen contents and fed on 340 kg of whole milk for 120 days. Chopped sweet Sudan grass was offered from 7 days onward and the animals were kept in individual stalls near faunated animals. No information was given on the ration fed the adult donor animals. In other experiments, repeated inoculation of two fistulated cows and two fistulated buffaloes with sheep rumen contents containing *Ophryoscolex* and *Polyplastron* were unsuccessful in establishing these two genera.

The question of protozoan specificity between cattle and sheep was investigated in more detail by Dehority (1978). Six isolated ciliate-free sheep were inoculated with 300 cc of rumen contents from a steer being fed alfalfa hay. Three of the sheep were fed the same alfalfa hay as the steer, while the other three sheep were fed a concentrate type diet. Rumen samples were taken 3, 7, 15, 30, 50 and 60 days following inoculation. All 24 species in the inoculum were observed in one or more of the sheep at 3 days. By 15 days, all species in the inoculum had become established in the alfalfa fed sheep and persisted throughout the 60 day experimental period. In contrast, two species of *Entodinium* and nine species in the family Diplodiniinae had failed to establish in the concentrate fed sheep after 15 days. *Dasytricha* was no longer present and *Isotricha* was present in only one sheep. Essentially this pattern continued through 60 days, except for the eventual establishment of *Isotricha* in all three concentrate fed sheep. These results suggest that the species of protozoa present in cattle will readily transfer to sheep and does not indicate any particular specificity of the protozoa *per se*. The critical factor appears to be the type of ration consumed both by the original host and the recipient host. At least in this work, all species readily established in the recipient host consuming the same ration as the donor host.

If one now goes back and re-evaluates the work of Dogiel and Winogradowa-Fedorowa (1930), their inoculum was obtained from a slaughter house, and no information is available on the diet of the donor host. In the studies by Naga *et al.* (1969) they attempted to establish species from adult animals into newly born calves primarily receiving a whole milk diet. Thus, in both studies, ration and its subsequent effect on the rumen environment could have been a determining factor in their results.

Imai *et al.* (2002) inoculated two unfaunated Japanese shorthorn calves with rumen contents from a wild sika deer which had previously been held for two months in an enclosure and fed alfalfa hay-cubes and orchard hay. All species established in the two calves which were fed a concentrate type diet, although concentration and percentage composition varied over an 11 week period. The authors concluded that the rumen ciliates of sika deer are not host-specific

Speculation about the origination of individual species and their geographical distribution

Occurrence of a specific protozoal species, *E. alces,* originally described from moose in Alaska and subsequently found in the springbok and giraffe from southern Africa is very intriguing. Similarly, the occurrence of *Parentodinium africanum* in stomach contents of the hippopotamus and subsequent appearance in bovine rumen contents from Brazil and the United States is most unusual. One question which immediately arises is whether this species occurs anywhere else between these two extremes and has just not been observed to date. The data shown in Table 6.6 are four examples of gastrointestinal ciliates found exclusively in different animal species in very widely separated locations in Africa, Turkey, and North and South America.

Table 6.6 UNIQUE GEOGRAPHICAL AND ANIMAL SPECIES DISTRIBUTION OF SEVERAL PROTOZOAL SPECIES

Species	Original observation Site/host (Reference)[a]	Additional observations Site/host (References)[a]
Entodinium alces	Alaska/moose (1)	S. Africa/springbok & giraffe (2,3)
Parentodinium africanum	Africa/hippopotamus (4)	Brazil/Zebu cattle (5)
		USA/cattle (8)
Blepharoconus krugerensis	Africa/elephant (6)	Brazil/Zebu cattle (5)
Entodinium dalli	Alaska/Dall sheep (1)	Turkey/cattle (7)

[a]References: (1) Dehority (1974); (2) Kleynhans and van Hoven (1976); (3) Wilkinson and van Hoven (1976a, b); (4) Thurston and Noirot-Timothee (1973); (5) Dehority (1986c); (6) Eloff and van Hoven (1980); (7) Göçmen and Öktem (1996); (8) Dehority *et al.* (1999).

It is tempting to speculate that this could be explained on the basis of the fact that 200 million years ago all of the continents formed a single land mass called Pangaea. The dinosaurs, many of whom were herbivores, were present at that time and survived for an additional 130 million years. During that time it is theorized that Pangaea broke up into two large land masses, Laurasia and Gondwanaland, which both subsequently split into our present continents and drifted to their present locations at a speed of about 1 inch per year. About 65 million years ago, plant eating mammals began to appear and the herbivorous reptiles died out. Did the dinosaurs pass protozoa on to the plant eating mammals?

Protozoal passage

Leng *et al.* (1984, 1986) have studied the turnover time of rumen protozoa and factors which affect this parameter. They concluded that the holotrich protozoa are extensively retained in the rumen; only a small proportion flowing out with the digesta. They further estimated that the rate of lysis was approximately 85% of the turnover rate in the rumen. A previous study on other protozoal species had suggested that as many as 65% of the protozoa could die and lyse in the rumen (Leng, 1982). The data of Ankrah *et al.* (1990), discussed previously, indicated that this value may be nearer to 50%. Michalowski *et al.* (1986), estimated that under normal feeding conditions the rumen residence time for individual species of protozoa is about 2.55 days. This is about four to six times longer than the residence time of soluble markers as well as the generation times for protozoa determined both in vivo and in vitro.

If the protozoa do lyse in the rumen, the enzymes released could be of possible importance in the breakdown of structural carbohydrates. Coleman (1985) found that washed suspensions of rumen protozoa were killed either by freezing or by heating at 49°C for 5 min before normal incubation at 39°C. This latter treatment, along with aeration during incubation or incubation in hypotonic salt solution (30% of normal) resulted in death of the protozoa. Subsequent incubation of the protozoal cells resulted in a progressive release of cellulase, amylase and probably other enzymes from the cell. Coleman (1985) did not believe it likely that the protozoa would die of starvation very rapidly in animals fed once a day and proposed that death resulted from physiological trauma such as exposure to oxygen and the hypotonic conditions which occur immediately after feeding and drinking Exposure of the protozoa to these treatments for as little as 2 minutes resulted in death of a number of the cells suggesting a high probability for achieving these conditions in vivo. Since the released enzymes appeared to be fairly stable for 1½ h in the presence of rumen bacteria, they could potentially contribute to overall rumen metabolism.

Role of the protozoa

Since the first observations on the occurrence of ciliate protozoa in the rumen, about the middle 1800's, two questions have been of extreme interest. The first concerns the specificity of these ciliates for this habitat and second, are the protozoa essential for the host. In essence, both questions were eventually answered by using the same experimental technique, that of working with defaunated or protozoa-free animals.

Several procedures have been used to remove the rumen protozoa; however, most of them are fairly drastic and in addition to causing a major upset to the animal, their effect on the bacterial population is uncertain. Animals have reportedly been defaunated by adding HCl to the rumen, starving for 6-7 days without feed or water, feeding milk, and starving for 3 days and adding a 2% solution of copper sulfate for two consecutive days to the rumen (Hungate, 1966). Eadie and Oxford (1957) developed a procedure in which the rumen contents are entirely removed and the inside of the rumen is washed repeatedly with H_2O and physiological saline. A portion of the rumen contents are heated to 50°C for 15 min, which kills only the protozoa, and the contents are placed back in the animal. Appetite was soon regained by the animals. Although the animals were kept isolated, in many instances, entodiniomorphs reappeared after several weeks. In 1968, Abou Akkada et al. reported a procedure for defaunation using dioctyl sodium sulfosuccinate. The compound, a surfactant, is given just prior to feeding on two consecutive days and supposedly does not affect intake, etc., of the animals.

Orpin (1977) investigated defaunation procedures using dioctyl sodium sulfosuccinate (DSS) and found that the quantity of DSS required to remove protozoa from the rumen of sheep was about 30 times the lethal concentration *in vitro* (1000-2000 µg/ml vs 33.5 µg/ml). Subsequent studies indicated that this discrepancy resulted from an interaction of DSS with rumen particulate matter and only after the particulate matter was saturated with DSS were the protozoa killed. Starvation for 24 h prior to treatment markedly improved protozoa removal, probably because of the reduction in particulate matter.

Towne and Nagaraja (1990) sampled rumen and omasal contents at slaughter from 54 cattle, 15 bison and 40 sheep. Total protozoa concentrations, % generic distribution, dry matter and pH were determined. Concentrations of omasal protozoa were about 10% of those in the rumen for cattle and 17-18% from bison and sheep. Omasal DM was approximately double rumen DM (30% compared to 15%), and pH was not different. Weight of omasal digesta contents multiplied by protozoan concentrations would give total numbers in the omasum of approximately 2.4×10^8, 8.0×10^8 and 0.3×10^8 in cattle, bison and sheep, respectively. These numbers would be 10% or less of the total numbers which normally occur in the rumen of cattle, 20 to 550×10^8 (Puch, H.,1977, M.S. Thesis, The Ohio State University, Columbus, OH), and sheep, $14.4 - 22.5 \times 10^8$ (Dehority, 1978). Towne and Nagaraja suggested that the difficulty encountered in defaunating cattle compared to sheep results from the fact that the omasum in cattle is much larger and the contents are not saturated with the defaunating agent. Omasal backflow can then reinoculate the rumen. They evacuated the rumen, flushed out the omasum several times with a water hose, removing all fluid from the rumen after each flushing, and finally sprayed the rumen walls with a defaunating agent. However, despite isolation of their animal, protozoa were observed in the rumen one day after treatment. This would be a most intriguing area for further study.

Perhaps the best procedure, and one which has been employed successfully by the author, is isolation of the animals at birth. However, this is time consuming, requires special facilities and feeding practices, and in addition, is not applicable to adult ruminants.

To return to our first question, are the rumen ciliate protozoa specific for this habitat? The early workers had thought that the rumen protozoa were the same as could be seen with hay infusions (hay soaked in H_2O at room or incubator temperatures), and that they were simply transmitted as cysts in the hay, infecting the animal when hay was consumed. However, work with defaunated animals in the early 1930's clearly demonstrated that the rumen ciliates are transmitted only by direct contact (Becker and Hsiung, 1929; Hungate, 1966). Isolation of a defaunated animal kept the animal ciliate-free, even though normal hay and grasses were used as feeds. Thus, it has been concluded that the rumen protozoa are a highly specialized group of organisms which can only survive in the rumen or closely related habitat.

The second question, the essentialness of the ciliate protozoa for the host, has been studied extensively. Beginning with the early studies of Becker *et al*. (1930) and Pounden and Hibbs (1950), up to the more recent studies of Eadie and Gill (1971) and Veira *et al*. (1983), it is quite obvious that the rumen protozoa are not essential for viability and growth of the host animal or digestibility of fibrous roughages in the rumen. Several recent reviews, Williams and Coleman (1988) and Hobson and Jouany (1988), have summarized the different areas in which the rumen protozoa appear to influence or affect the ruminant animal. Animal responses can be positive, negative or essentially unchanged as a result of removing the ciliate protozoa. Williams and Coleman (1988) compiled a list of the reported effects of the absence of rumen ciliate protozoa upon ruminants. This survey was used as a source for the information presented in Table 6.7, which is essentially an attempt to document the major changes and the number and consistency of those responses. The major changes observed in the absence of protozoa appear to be an increase in rumen bacterial numbers, a slight decrease in rumen digestibility and little, if any, change in animal growth. Presumably the increased numbers of bacteria quantitatively take over the metabolic activities of the protozoa (Hobson and Jouany, 1988). Overall diet digestibility remains about the same because of an increase in hindgut digestion (Coleman, 1988), which in turn results in little, if any, change in growth parameters (Veira, 1986).

Over the years many investigators have attempted to establish and define a role for the rumen ciliates. One of the most popular suggestions was based on the premise that although bacterial and protozoal protein are of similar biological value, digestibility of the protozoal protein is significantly greater (McNaught *et al*., 1954; Bergen *et al*., 1968). However, a number of studies have strongly suggested that passage of the rumen protozoa down the digestive tract is extremely limited (Potter and Dehority, 1973; Weller and Pilgrim, 1974; Leng, 1982; Leng *et al*., 1986; Michalowski *et al*., 1986). Studies by Ankrah *et al*. (1990) indicated that about 50% of the normal decrease in protozoan

Table 6.7 MAJOR CHANGES OBSERVED IN ANIMALS WITHOUT RUMEN CILIATE PROTOZOA AND OCCURRENCE OF THESE OBSERVATIONS[a]

	Number of references reporting this effect in animals without ciliate protozoa		
	Increase	*Decrease*	*No change*
Rumen parameters:			
Bacterial numbers	13	0	0
Ammonia concentration	0	29	0
VFA concentration	5	19	0
Acetic acid (molar proportion)	5	10	0
Propionic acid (molar proportion)	15	12	0
Butyric acid (molar proportion)	10	14	0
Lactic acid concentration	8	1	0
pH	2	6	0
Rumen digestibility:			
Organic matter	1	15	0
ADF	0	7	0
Cellulose	0	7	2
Starch	0	6	0
Nitrogen	0	0	4
Proteolytic activity	0	3	1
Methanogenesis	0	5	0
Efficiency of bacterial protein synthesis	10	0	0
Nitrogen flow to duodenum	14	0	0
Plasma levels of:			
Urea	2	3	0
Amino acids	3	2	0
Glucose	5	1	0
Animal responses:			
Food conversion efficiency	5	2	0
Live weight gain	7	7	3

[a] From Williams and Coleman, 1988.

concentrations after feeding can be attributed to passage down the tract and 50% to lysis. Essentially all of the concentration decrease occurred with the ophryoscolecid protozoa. This compares fairly well with the estimates of 65% lysis of small ophryoscolecids determined by Leng (1982) using radioactive carbon labeled protozoa. A later study by Leng *et al.* (1986) indicated that the percentage lysis of the larger protozoa may be even higher.

Coleman (1975) proposed that the increased rumen ammonia in faunated animals resulted from extensive digestion of rumen bacteria by the protozoa. The protozoa engulf large quantities of bacteria, as much as 1% of the total per minute in high concentrate fed animals. Digestion products of the bacteria are principally amino acids, half of which are retained by the cell and the other half are released into the medium. These are then fermented to VFA and ammonia. Although this decreases the flow of bacterial amino acids to the host animal, the higher digestibility of the protozoal protein would balance this loss. However, if the protozoa themselves have a very limited extent of passage, then this advantage is also lost. In truth, it would appear that the rumen protozoa add another link to the food chain of the ruminant animal without having any unique or offsetting advantages.

As one reviews the relatively large number of studies concerning differences between faunated and ciliate-free ruminants, it becomes obvious that the protozoa contribute to or influence the overall rumen fermentation (Viera, 1986, Hobson and Jouany, 1988, Williams and Coleman, 1988). Many of their direct and subsequent effects (growth, feed intake, etc.) can readily be measured. However, many factors seem to influence the effect of the protozoa on rumen function and determine whether their presence is advantageous, detrimental or neutral. These are summarized in Table 6.8. As one reviews this list, potential reasons for the reported discrepancies about the effects of protozoa become a little more obvious.

Some recent observations reported in relation to the role of the protozoa in the rumen are:

(1)   Nagaraja *et al.* (1992) found that high-grain fed protozoa-free steers had lower ruminal pH values than faunated cattle (pH 5.97 as compared to pH 6.45), about four-fold higher bacterial concentrations and higher VFA concentrations. The authors suggest that the protozoa moderate the rumen fermentation in the high-grain fed steers through reduction of bacterial numbers.

(2)   Chaudhary *et al.* (1995) measured digestibility of forage structural carbohydrates in water buffalo fed wheat straw to appetite plus a concentrate mixture. They concluded that defaunation decreased the digestibility of structural carbohydrates, both in the rumen and total gastrointestinal tract.

(3)   Takenaka and Itabashi (1995) established five groups of calves with specific populations of protozoa: PF = protozoa-free, Epi = *Epidinium ecaudatum* - mono-faunated, Eud = *Eudiplodinium maggli* - mono-faunated; Ent = *Entodinium spp.* - mono-faunated, Mix = Mixed ophryoscolecids. They observed the following differences: (a)Total viable bacteria in rumen - lower in the Epi, Eud and Mix than PF; (b) Amylolytic bacteria - lower in Epi than PF; (c) Pectinolytic bacteria - higher in Ent than other faunated; and (d) Methanogenic bacteria - higher in Ent, Eud, and Mix than PF. Epi lower than all other faunated.

(4)   The importance of the methanogenic bacteria associated with ciliate protozoa was investigated by Newbold *et al.* (1995). They measured the amount of methane

Table 6.8 FACTORS WHICH CAN INFLUENCE THE EFFECT OF CILIATE PROTOZOA ON RUMINAL FUNCTION AND SUBSEQUENT NUTRITION OF THE HOST ANIMAL

Factor	Effect	References[a]
Diet	Protozoan numbers increase with concentrate level	1,2,3,4
	Both pH and protozoan numbers decrease at very high energy levels	
	Protozoa can have leveling effect on starch and protein fermentation in the rumen	
Frequency of feeding	Protozoan concentrations are more stable as number of feedings increase	1,6,7
Level of intake	Protozoan numbers decrease at low or very high intake levels	8,9,10
Age of animal	Growing animals have different nutritional requirements	3,4
	Microbial ecosystem may differ in young and older ruminants	
Animal host	Variation in protozoan concentrations and occurrence of species	1,4,11
Protozoan species and concentration	Bacterial numbers and rumen digestibility both change	12,13,14
Defaunation method	Chemical methods can eliminate or change proportions of certain bacteria or fungi	3,14,15
	Chemicals cause changes in digestive tract physiology	
	Isolation of young animals can cause partial shift in digestion to hindgut	

[a](1) Dehority and Orpin, 1988; (2) Coleman, 1980; (3) Coleman, 1988; (4) Veira, 1986; (5) Bird and Leng, 1978; (6) Moir and Somers, 1956; (7) Bragg et al., 1986; (8) Warner, 1962; (9) Potter and Dehority, 1973; (10) Dearth et al., 1974; (11) Jouany and Sevaud, 1979; (12) Williams and Coleman, 1988; (13) Fonty et al., 1983; (14) Hobson and Jouany, 1988; (15) Lovelock et al., 1982.

produced by strained rumen fluid, centrifuged rumen fluid and protozoa. The authors estimated that approximately 9 to 25% of the methane produced in whole rumen fluid was by endosymbiotic methanogens associated with protozoa. Ushida and Jouany (1996) studied the effects of inhibiting the methanogens associated with rumen protozoa upon dry matter digestion. They estimated that the daily production of methane from the methanogens associated with a single protozoal cell ranged from a trace to 2 nmol. In addition, methanogenisis increased dry matter disappearance, possibly as a result of interspecies hydrogen transfer.

Those microorganisms which live in the digestive tract of the ruminant are an excellent example of mutualism, i.e., a symbiotic relationship exists which is advantageous to all organisms involved. An environmentally suitable niche is provided by the animals with a continuous supply of food and removal of end products. The microbes (bacteria, protozoa and fungi) digest a large portion of these feedstuffs, making energy available to the host animal which would not be available through its own digestive processes (Hungate, 1966); Orpin and Joblin, 1988; Stewart and Bryant, 1988; Williams and Coleman, 1988). Becker et al. (1930) suggested that the rumen protozoa were mere commensals. Presumably this meant that they were of little or no value to the host and the protozoan was neither benefitted or harmed. However, the protozoa would appear to be benefited, since they have rather specific requirements for their growth and multiplication. These requirements include a specific range of temperature and pH, food, low redox potential and apparently live bacteria (Coleman, 1980; Williams and Coleman, 1988). Under these circumstances, the rumen protozoa must be considered as symbionts, depending upon the animal host and other rumen microbes for their survival. The fact that similar metabolic activities can be carried out by the rumen bacteria and possibly fungi should not affect this classification.

References

Abou Akkada, A. R. and K. el-Shazly. (1964). Effect of absence of ciliate protozoa from the rumen on microbial activity and growth of lambs. *Applied Microbiology*, **12**, 384-390.

Abou Akkada, A. R., E. E. Bartley and L. R. Fina. (1969). Ciliate protozoa in the rumen of the lactating cow. *Journal of Dairy Science*, **52**, 1088-1091.

Abou Akkada, A. R., E. E. Bartley, R. Berube, L. R. Fina, R. M. Meyer, D. Henricks and F. Julius. (1968). Simple method to remove completely ciliate protozoa of adult ruminants. *Applied Microbiology*, **16**, 1475-1477.

Ankrah, P., S. C. Loerch and B. A. Dehority. (1990). Sequestration, migration and lysis of protozoa in the rumen. *Journal of General Microbiology*, **136**, 1869-1875.

Baker, S. K., B. A. Dehority, N. L. Chamberlain and D. B. Purser. (1995). Inability of protozoa from the kangaroo forestomach to establish in the rumen of sheep.

Annales de Zootechnie, **44**, 143.

Becker, E. R. and T. S. Hsiung. (1929). The method by which ruminants acquire their fauna of infusoria, and remarks concerning experiments on the host-specificity of these protozoa. *Proceedings of the National Academy of Science*, **15**, 684-690.

Becker, E. R. and M. Talbot. (1927). The protozoa fauna of the rumen and reticulum of American cattle. *Iowa State College Journal of Science*, **1**, 345-373.

Becker, E. R., J. A. Schulz and M. A. Emmerson. (1930). Experiments on the physiological relationships between the stomach infusoria of ruminants and their hosts, with a bibliography. *Iowa State College Journal of Science*, **4**, 215-251.

Bergen, W. G., D. B. Purser and J. H. Cline. (1968). Determination of limiting amino acids of rumen isolated microbial proteins fed to rats. *Journal of Dairy Science*, **51**, 1698-1700.

Bird, S. H. and R. A. Leng. (1978). The effects of defaunation of the rumen on the growth of cattle on low-protein high-energy diets. *British Journal of Nutrition*, **40**, 163-167.

Bonhomme-Florentin, A., J. Blancou and B. Latteur. (1978). Étude des variations saisonnières de la microfaune du rumen de zebus. *Protistologica*, **14**, 283-289.

Bragg, D. St. A., M.R. Murphy and C.L. Davis. (1986). Effect of source of carbohydrate and frequency of feeding on rumen parameters in dairy steers. *Journal of Dairy Science*, **69**, 392-402.

Chandhary, L. C., A. Srivastava and K. K. Singh. (1995). Rumen fermentation pattern and digestion of structural carbohydrates in buffalo *(Bubalus bubalis)* calves as affected by ciliate protozoa. *Animal Feed Science and Technology*, **56**, 111-117.

Clarke, R.T.J. (1964). Ciliates of the rumen of domestic cattle (*Bos taurus* L.). *New Zealand Journal of Agricultural Research*, **7**, 248-257.

Clarke, R.T.J. (1977). Protozoa in the rumen ecosystem. From *Microbial Ecology of the Gut*. Edited by R.T.J. Clarke and T. Bauchop. Academic Press, New York, N.Y., pp 251-275.

Coleman, G. S. (1975). The interrelationship between rumen ciliate protozoa and bacteria. From *Digestion and Metabolism in the Ruminant*. Edited by I. W. McDonald and A.C.I. Warner. University of New England Publishing Unit, Armidale, Australia. pp 149-164.

Coleman, G. S. (1980). Rumen ciliate protozoa. In: *Advances in Parasitology*. Edited by W.H.R. Lumsden, R. Muller, and J. R. Baker. Academic Press, New York, pp. 121-173.

Coleman, G. S. (1985). Possible cause of the high death rate of ciliated protozoa in the rumen. *Journal of Agricultural Science*, **105**, 39-43.

Coleman, G. S. (1988). The importance of rumen ciliate protozoa in the growth and metabolism of the host ruminant. *International Journal of Animal Science*, **3**, 75-95.

Dearth, R. N., B. A. Dehority, and E. L. Potter. (1974). Rumen microbial numbers in lambs as affected by level of feed intake and dietary diethylstilbesterol. *Journal of Animal Science*, **38**, 991-996.

Dehority, B. A. (1974). Rumen ciliate fauna of Alaskan moose (*Alces americana*), musk-ox (*Ovibos moschatus*) and Dall mountain sheep (*Ovis dalli*). *Journal of Protozoology*, **21**, 26-32.

Dehority, B. A. (1975). Rumen ciliate protozoa of Alaskan reindeer and caribou (*Rangifer tarandus* L.). In: *Proceedings of the 1st International Reindeer and Caribou Symposium*, Special Report Number 1, Biological Sciences Publication #18, University of Alaska, Fairbanks, pp 241-250.

Dehority, B. A. (1978). Specificity of rumen ciliate protozoa in cattle and sheep. *Journal of Protozoology*, **25**, 509-513.

Dehority, B. A. (1979). Ciliate protozoa in the rumen of Brazilian water buffalo, *Bubalus bubalis* Linnaeus. *Journal of Protozoology*, **26**, 536-544.

Dehority, B. A. (1985). Rumen ciliates of musk-oxen (*Ovibos moschatus* Z.) from the Canadian Arctic. *Journal of Protozoology*, **32**, 246-250.

Dehority, B. A. (1986a). Microbes in the foregut of arctic ruminants. In: *Control of Digestion and Metabolism in Ruminants*. Edited by L. P. Milligan, W. L. Grovum, and A. Dobson. Reston Publishing Company, Inc., Reston, Virginia, pp. 307-325.

Dehority, B. A. (1986b). Protozoa of the digestive tract of herbivorous mammals. *Insect Science and its Application*, **7**, 279-296.

Dehority, B. A. (1986c). Rumen ciliate fauna of some Brazilian cattle: occurrence of several ciliates new to the rumen, including the cycloposthid *Parentodinium africanum*. *Journal of Protozoology*, **33**, 416-421.

Dehority, B. A. (1987). Rumen ophryoscolecid protozoa in the hindgut of the capybara (*Hydrochoerus hydrochaeris*). *Journal of Protozoology*, **34**, 143-145.

Dehority, B. A. (1990). Rumen ciliate protozoa in Ohio white-tailed deer (*Odocoileus virginianus*). *Journal of Protozoology*, **37**, 473-475.

Dehority, B. A. (1994). Rumen ciliate protozoa of the blue duiker (*Cephalophus monticola*), with observations on morphological variation lines within the species *Entodinium dubardi*. *Journal of Eukaryotic Microbiology*, **41**, 103-111.

Dehority, B. A. (1995). Rumen ciliates of the pronghorn antelope (*Antilocapra americana*), mule deer (*Odocoileus hemionus*), white-tailed deer (*Odocoileus virginianus*) and elk (*Cervus canadensis*) in the northwestern United States. *Archiv für Protistenkunde*, **146**, 29-36.

Dehority, B. A. (1996). A new family of entodiniomorph protozoa from the marsupial forestomach, with a description of a new genus and five new species. *Journal of Eukaryotic Microbiology*, **43**, 285-295.

Dehority, B. A. (1997). Rumen ciliate protozoa in Australian red deer (*Cervus elaphus* L.). *Archiv für Protistenkunde*, **148**, 157-165.

Dehority, B. A. and W.R.S. Mattos. (1978). Diurnal changes and effect of ration on concentrations of the rumen ciliate *Charon ventriculi*. *Applied and Environmental Microbiology*, **36**, 953-958.

Dehority, B. A. and C. G. Orpin. (1988). Development of, and natural fluctuations in, rumen microbial populations. In: *The Rumen Microbial Ecosystem*. Edited by P. N. Hobson. Elsevier Applied Science, London, pp. 151-183.

Dehority, B. A., W. S. Damron and J. B. McLaren. (1983). Occurrence of the rumen ciliate *Oligoisotricha bubali* in domestic cattle (*Bos taurus*). *Applied and Environmental Microbiology*, **45**, 1394-1397.

Dehority, B. A., E. E. Grings and R. E. Short. (1999). Effects of cross-inoculation from elk and feeding pine needles on the protozoan fauna of pregnant cows: occurrence of *Parentodinium africanum* in domestic U. S. Cattle (*Bos taurus*). *Journal of Eukaryotic Microbiology*, **46**, 632-636.

Dogiel, V. A. (1927). Monographie der familie Ophryoscolecidae. *Archiv für Protistenkunde*, **59**, 1-288.

Dogiel, V. A. (1928). La faune d'infusoires habitant l'estomac du buffle et du dromadaire. *Annales de Parasitologie*, **6**, 323-338.

Dogiel, V. A. and T. Winogradowa-Fedorowa. (1930). Experimentelle Unte suchungen zur Biologie der Infusorien des Wiederkäuermagens. Wissenschaftliche Arhiv für Landwirtschaftlichen. *Abt. B, Archive für Tierernährung und Tierzuecht*, **3**, 172-188.

Eadie, J. M. (1962). Interrelationships between certain rumen ciliate protozoa. *Journal of General Microbiology*, **29**, 579-588.

Eadic, J. M. (1967). Studies on the ecology of certain rumen ciliate protozoa. *Journal of General Microbiology*, **49**, 175-194.

Eadie, J. M. and J. C. Gill. (1971). The effect of the absence of rumen ciliate protozoa on growing lambs fed on a roughage-concentrate diet. *British Journal of Nutrition*, **26**, 155-167.

Eadie, J. M. and A. E. Oxford. (1957). A simple and safe procedure for the removal of holotrich ciliates from the rumen of an adult fistulated sheep. *Nature*, **179**, 485.

Eloff, A. K. and W. van Hoven. (1980). Intestinal protozoa of the African elephant *Loxodonta africana* (Blumenbach). *South African Journal of Zoology*, **15**, 83-90.

Fonty, G., Ph. Garrett, J. P. Jouany and J. Senaud. (1983). Ecological factors determining establishment of cellulolytic bacteria and protozoa in the rumens of meroxenic lambs. *Journal of General Microbiology*, **129**, 213-223.

Göçmen, B., and N. Öktem. (1996). New rumen ciliates from Turkish domestic cattle (*Bos taurus* L.) I. The presence of *Entodinium dalli* Dehority, 1974 with a new forma, *E. dalli rudidorsospinatum* n. f. and comparisons with *Entodinium williamsi* n. sp. *European Journal of Protistology*, **32**, 513-522.

Guirong, N.-R. Su, Z. X. Hua, S. Zhu and S. Imai. (2000). Rumen ciliated protozooan fauna of the yak (*Bos grunniens*) in China with the description of *Entodinium monuo* n. sp. *Journal of Eukaryotic Microbiology*, **47**, 178-182.

Hobson, P. N. and J.-P. Jouany. (1988). Models, mathematical and biological, of the rumen function. In: *The Rumen Microbial Ecosystem*. Edited by P. N. Hobson. Elsevier Applied Sciences, London, pp. 461-511.

Hollande, A. and A. Batisse. (1959). Contribution à l'étude des infusoires parasites du coecum de l'hydrocheire (*Hydrocheirus capybara* L.). 1. La famille des *Cycloposthiidae*. *Memórias do Instituto Oswaldo-Cruz*, **57**, 1-16.

Hungate, R. E. (1966). *The Rumen and Its Microbes*. Academic Press, New York.

Ibrahim, E. A., J. R. Ingalls and N. E. Stanger. (1970). Effect of dietary diethylstilbestrol on populations and concentrations of ciliate protozoa in dairy cattle. *Canadian Journal of Animal Science*, **50**, 101-106.

Imai, S. (1981). Four new rumen ciliates, *Entodinium ogimotoi* sp.n., *E. bubalum* sp.n., *E. fujitai* sp.n. and *E. tsunodai* sp.n. and *Oligoisotricha bubali* (Dogiel, 1928) n. comb. *Japanese Journal of Veterinary Science*, **43**, 201-209.

Imai, S. (1985). Rumen ciliate protozoal faunae of Bali cattle (*Bos javanicus domesticus*) and water buffalo (*Bubalus bubalis*) in Indonesia, with the description of a new species, *Entodinium javanicum* sp. nov. *Zoological Science*, Tokyo, **2**, 591-600

Imai, S. (1986). Rumen ciliate protozoal fauna of zebu cattle (*Bos taurus indicus*) in Sri Lanka, with the description of a new species, *Diplodinium sinhalicum* sp. nov. *Zoological Science*, Tokyo, **3**, 699-706.

Imai, S. (1988). Ciliate protozoa in the rumen of Kenyan Zebu cattle, *Bos taurus indicus*, with the description of four new species. *Journal of Protozoology*, **35**, 130-136.

Imai, S. and M. Kinoshita. (1997). Comparison of rumen ciliate compositions among Hereford, Holstein and Zebu cattle in Mexico. *Revista Sociedad Mexicana de Historia Natural,* **47**, 85-91.

Imai, S. and K. Ogimoto. (1984). Rumen ciliate protozoal fauna and bacterial flora of the zebu cattle (*Bos indicus*) and the water buffalo (*Bubalus bubalis*) in Thailand. *Japanese Journal of Zootechnical Science*, **55**, 576-583.

Imai, S. and G. Rung. (1990a). Rumen ciliates from the Mongolian Gazelle, *Procapra gutturosa*. *Japanese Journal of Veterinary Science*, **52**, 1063-1067.

Imai, S. and G. Rung. (1990b). Ciliate protozoa in the forestomach of the Bactrian camel in Inner-Mongolia, China. *Japanese Journal of Veterinary Science*, **52**, 1069-1075.

Imai, S., K. Ogimoto and J. Fujita. (1981a). Rumen ciliate protozoal fauna of water buffalo, *Bubalus bubalis* (Linnaeus) in Okinawa, Japan. *Bulletin of the Nippon Veterinary and Zootechnical College*, **29**, 82-85.

Imai, S., S. S. Han, K.-J. Cheng and H. Kudo. (1989). Composition of the rumen ciliate population in experimental herds of cattle and sheep in Lethbridge, Alberta, Western Canada. *Canadian Journal of Microbiology*, **35**, 686-690.

Imai, S., M. Matsumoto, A. Watanabe and H. Sato. (1993). Rumen ciliate protozoa in Japanese sika deer (*Cervus nippon centralis*). *Animal Science and Technology,*

64, 578-583.

Imai, S., M. Matsumoto, A. Watanabe and H. Sato. (2002). Establishment of a spinated type of *diplodinium rangiferi* by transfaunation of the rumen ciliates of Japanese sika deer (*Cervus nippon centralis*) to the rumen of two Japanese shorthorn calves (*Bos taurus taurus*). *Journal of Eukaryotic Microbiology*, **49**, 38-41.

Imai, S., Y. Tsutsumi, S. Yumura and A. Mulenga. (1992). Ciliate protozoa in the rumen of Kafue lechwe, *Kobus leche kafuensis*, in Zambia, with the description of four new species. *Journal of Protozoology*, **39**, 564-572.

Imai, S., C.-H. Chang, J.-S. Wang, K. Ogimoto and J. Fujita. (1981b). Rumen ciliate protozoal fauna of the water buffalo (*Bubalus bubalis*) in Taiwan. *Bulletin of the Nippon Veterinary and Zootechnical College*, **29**, 77-81.

Imai, S., A. Ito, T. Ichikawa, T. Morita and Y. Kimura. (1997). Ciliate protozoa composition found from the hindgut of capybara, *Hydrochoerus hydrochaeris*. Programme and Abstracts of 10th International Congress of Protozoology, p 109.

Imai, S., M. Shimizu, M. Kinoshita, M. Toguchi, T. Ishii and J. Fujita. (1982). Rumen ciliate protozoal fauna and composition of the cattle in Japan. *Bulletin of the Nippon Veterinary and Zootechnical College*, **31**, 70-74.

Ito, A. and S. Imai. (1990). Ciliated protozoa in the rumen of Holstein-Friesian cattle (*Bos taurus taurus*) in Hokkaido, Japan, with the description of two new species. *Zoological Science*, **7**, 449-458.

Ito, A., S. Imai and K. Ogimoto. (1993). Rumen ciliates of Ezo deer (*Cervus nippon yesoensis*) with the morphological comparison with those of cattle. *Journal of Veterinary Medical Science*, **55**, 93 98.

Ito, A., S. Imai and K. Ogimoto. (1994). Rumen ciliate composition and diversity of Japanese beef black cattle in comparison with those of Holstein-Friesian cattle. *Journal of Veterinary Medical Science*, **56**, 707-714.

Ito, A., N. Arai, Y. Tsutsumi and S. Imai. (1997). Ciliate protozoa in the rumen of sassaby antelope, *Damaliscus lunatus lunatus*, including the description of a new species and form. *The Journal of Eukaryotic Microbiology* **44**, 586-591.

Jouany, J. P. and J. Senaud. (1979). Role of rumen protozoa in the digestion of food cellulosic materials. *Annales de Recherches Veterinaires*, **10**, 261-263.

Kleynhans, C. J. and W. van Hoven. (1976). Rumen protozoa of the giraffe with a description of two new species. *East African Wildlife Journal*, **14**, 203-214.

Kofoid, C. A. and J. F. Christenson. (1934). Ciliates from *Bos gaurus* H. Smith. *University of California Publications in Zoology*, **30**, 341-391.

Kofoid, C. A. and R. F. MacLennan. (1930). Ciliates from *Bos indicus* Linn., I. The genus *Entodinium* Stein. *University of California Publications in Zoology*, **33**, 471-544.

Kofoid, C. A. and R. F. MacLennan. (1932). Ciliates from *Bos indicus* Linn., II. A revision of *Diplodinium* Schuberg. *University of California Publications in Zoology*, **37**, 53-152.

Kofoid, C. A. and R. F. MacLennan. (1933). Ciliates from *Bos indicus* Linn., III. *Epidinium* Crawley, *Epiplastron* gen. nov. and *Ophryoscolex* Stein. *University of California Publications in Zoology*, **39**, 1-34.

Kubesy, A. A. and B. A. Dehority. (2002). Forestomach ciliate protozoa in Egyptian dromedary camels (*Camelus dromedarius*). *Zootaxa*, **51**, 1-12.

Leng, R. A. (1982). Dynamics of protozoa in the rumen of sheep. *British Journal of Nutrition*, **48**, 399-415.

Leng, R. A., D. Dellow and G. Waghorn. (1986). Dynamics of large ciliate protozoa in the rumen of cattle fed on diets of freshly cut grass. *British Journal of Nutrition*, **56**, 455-462.

Leng, R. A., J. V. Nolan, G. Cumming, S. R. Edwards and C. A. Graham. (1984). The effects of monensin on the pool size and turnover rate of protozoa in the rumen of sheep. *Journal of Agricultural Science*, **102**, 609-613.

Lovelock, L.K.A., J. G. Buchanan-Smith and C. W. Forsberg. (1982). Difficulties in defaunation of the ovine rumen. *Canadian Journal of Animal Science*, **62**, 299-303.

McNaught, Mary L., E. C. Owen, Kathleen M. Henry and S. K. Kon. (1954). The utilization of non-protein nitrogen in the bovine rumen 8. The nutritive value of the proteins of preparations of dried rumen bacteria, rumen protozoa and brewer's yeast for rats. *Biochemical Journal*, **56**, 151-156.

Michalowski, T., J. Harmeyer and G. Breves. (1986). The passage of protozoa from the reticulo-rumen through the omasum of sheep. *British Journal of Nutrition*, **56**, 625-634.

Moir, R. J. and M. Somers. (1956). A factor influencing the protozoal population in sheep. *Nature*, **178**, 1472.

Naga, M. A., A. R. Abou Akkada and K. el-Shazly. (1969). Establishment of rumen ciliate protozoa in cow and water buffalo (*Bos bubalus* L.) calves under late and early weaning systems. *Journal of Dairy Science*, **52**, 110-112.

Nagaraja, T. G., G. Towne and A. A. Beharka. (1992). Moderation of ruminal fermentation by ciliated protozoa in cattle fed a high-grain diet. *Applied and Environmental Microbiology*, **58**, 2410-2414.

Nakamura, K. and S. Kanegasaki. (1969). Densities of ruminal protozoa of sheep established under different dietary conditions. *Journal of Dairy Science*, **52**, 250-255.

Newbold, C. J., B. Lassalas and J. P. Jouany. (1995). The importance of methanogens associated with ciliate protozoa in ruminal methane production in vitro. *Letters in Applied Microbiology*, **21**, 230-234.

Orpin, C. G. (1977). Studies on the defaunation of the ovine rumen using dioctyl sodium sulphosuccinate. *Journal of Applied Bacteriology*, **43**, 309-318.

Orpin, C. G. and K. N. Joblin. (1988). The rumen anaerobic fungi. In: *The Rumen Microbial Ecosystem*. Edited by P. N. Hobson. Elsevier Applied Science, London. pp. 129-150.

Potter, E. L. and B. A. Dehority. (1973). Effects of changes in feed level, starvation, and level of feed after starvation upon the concentration of rumen protozoa in the ovine. *Applied Microbiology*, **26**, 692-698.

Pounden, W. D. and J. W. Hibbs. (1950). The development of calves raised without protozoa and certain other characteristic rumen microorganisms. *Journal of Dairy Science*, **33**, 639-644.

Selim, H. M., S. Imai, O. Yamato, E. Miyagawa and Y. Maede. (1996). Ciliate protozoa in the forestomach of the dromedary camel (*Camelus dromedarius*), in Egypt, with description of a new species. *Journal of Veterinary Medical Science*, **58**, 833-837.

Selim, H. M., S. Imai, A. K. El Sheik, H. Attia, E. Okamoto, E. Miyagawa and Y. Maede. (1999). Rumen ciliate protozoal fauna of native sheep, friesian cattle and dromedary camel in Libya. *Journal of Veterinary Medical Science*, **61**, 303-305.

Shimizu, M., M. Kinoshita, J. Fujita and S. Imai. (1983). Rumen ciliate protozoal fauna and composition of the zebu cattle, *Bos indicus*, and water buffalo, *Bubalus bubalis*, in Philippines. *Bulletin of the Nippon Veterinary and Zootechnical College*, **32**, 83-88.

Sládeček, F. (1946). Ophryoscolecidae from the stomach of *Cervus elephus* L., *Dama dama* L., and *Capreolus capreolus* L. *Vestnik Ceskoslovenske Zoologicke Spolecnosti*, **10**, 201-231. (in Czech, English summary).

Stewart, C. S. and M. P. Bryant. (1988). The rumen bacteria. In: *The Rumen Microbial Ecosystem*. Edited by P. N. Hobson. Elsevier Applied Science, London, pp. 21-75.

Takenaka, A. and H. Itabashi. (1995). Changes in the population of some functional groups of rumen bacteria including methanogenic bacteria by changing the rumen ciliates in calves. *Journal of General and Applied Microbiology*, **41**, 377-387.

Tener, J. S. (1965). *Muskoxen in Canada*. Canadian Wildlife Service, Queen's Printer, Ottawa, Canada.

Thurston, J. P. and C. Noirot-Timothée. (1973). Entodiniomorph ciliates from the stomach of *Hippopotamus amphibius* with descriptions of two new genera and three new species. *Journal of Protozoology*, **20**, 562-565.

Towne, G. and T. G. Nagaraja. (1990). Omasal ciliated protozoa in cattle, bison and sheep. *Applied and Environmental Microbiology*, **56**, 409-412.

Towne, G., T. G. Nagaraja and K. K. Kemp. (1988). Ruminal ciliated protozoa in bison. *Applied and Environmental Microbiology*, **54**, 2733-2736.

Towne, G., T. G. Nagaraja, R. T. Brandt, Jr. and K. E. Kemp. (1990). Dynamics of ruminal ciliated protozoa in feedlot cattle. *Applied and Environmental Microbiology*, **56**, 3174-3178.

Ushida, K. and J. P. Jouany. (1996). Methane production associated with rumen ciliated protozoa and its effect on protozoan activity. *Letters in Applied Microbiology*,

23, 129-132.

van Hoven, W., V. L. Hamilton-Attwell and J. H. Grobler. (1979). Rumen ciliate protozoa of the sable antelope *Hippotragus niger*. *South African Journal of Zoology*, **14**, 37-42.

Veira, D. M. (1986). The role of ciliate protozoa in nutrition of the ruminant. *Journal of Animal Science*, **63**, 1547-1560.

Veira, D. M., M. Ivan and P. Y. Jui. (1983). Rumen ciliate protozoa: Effects on digestion in the stomach of sheep. *Journal of Dairy Science*, **66**, 1015-1022.

Warner, A.C.I. (1962). Some factors influencing the rumen microbial population. *Journal of General Microbiology*, **28**, 129-146.

Weller, R. A. and A. F. Pilgrim. (1974). Passage of protozoa and volatile fatty acids from the rumen of the sheep and from a continuous in vitro fermentation system. *British Journal of Nutrition*, **32**, 341-351.

Westerling, B. (1969). Våmciliatfaunan has tamboskap i finska Lappland, med Speciell hånsyn til arter anaedda som specifika för ren. *Nordisk Veterinaermedicin*, **21**, 14-19.

Wilkinson, R. C. and W. van Hoven. (1976a). Geographical distribution and population structure of springbok *Antidorcas marsupialis* rumen protozoa in southern Africa. *Koedoe*, **19**, 17-26.

Wilkinson, R. C. and W. van Hoven. (1976b). Rumen ciliate fauna of the springbok (*Antidorcas marsupialis*) in southern Africa. *Zoological Africana*, **11**, 1-22.

Williams, A. G. and G. S. Coleman. (1988). The rumen protozoa. In: *The Rumen Microbial Ecosystem*. Edited by P. N. Hobson. Elsevier Applied Sciences, London, pp. 77-128.

Williams, A. G. and G. S. Coleman. (1992). *The Rumen Protozoa*. Springer-Verlag, New York, NY, pp 305-306.

CHAPTER 7

RUMEN BACTERIA — HISTORY, METHODS OF *IN VITRO* CULTIVATION, AND DISCUSSION OF MIXED CULTURE FERMENTATIONS

Early observations and experiments which led to the establishment of the role played by the bacterial flora in digestion of feedstuffs in the rumen are discussed in the Introduction to *The Rumen and Its Microbes* by Hungate (1966). In general, from the first experiments by von Tappeiner in 1884, little progress was made until the late 1940's. Baker and Harriss (1947), using direct microscopic observations concluded that the cocci forms of bacteria were primarily responsible for degradation of cellulose in the rumen. Also, in 1947, Hungate published a report on the isolation in pure culture of several types of cellulolytic bacteria from the rumen of cattle. A more detailed account of his technique was published in 1950. Quite independently, Sijpesteijn (1948, 1951), working in Holland, succeeded in growing enrichment cultures of rumen cellulolytic bacteria and eventually obtained one pure strain. At this same time Marston (1948), working in England, reported on *in vitro* studies with mixed cultures of rumen bacteria. From this point onward, rather rapid advances were made in the field of rumen bacteriology. Hungate and his students modified and improved the anaerobic culture techniques and applied them to the problems of estimating total viable numbers, determining the types of anaerobic bacteria which occurred in relatively large numbers in the rumen, and isolation of pure cultures (Hungate, 1950; Bryant and Burkey, 1953a,b). Concurrently, the *in vitro* mixed culture fermentation method was used by a number of investigators and has yielded much valuable information on the overall rumen fermentation.

Methods of *in vitro* cultivation

As outlined in the first chapter, the rumen has an anaerobic environment, a temperature of 39-40°C and a pH range of 5.5-7.0. Food is continuously supplied to the microorganisms and fermentation products are removed by the host animal. Bacterial concentrations far exceed those of the protozoa and fungi, and most of the fermentative activity in the rumen is generally ascribed to this large bacterial population.

The methods available for studying the rumen bacteria can be divided into three general categories: pure cultures, *in vitro* mixed culture fermentations and *in vivo - in vitro* techniques.

PURE CULTURES

This method involves isolation of a single strain of bacteria and its subsequent characterization. The procedure is quite involved and time consuming and, in addition, only provides detailed information on one organism. Since the overall rumen fermentation is a synergistic and symbiotic system involving many species of bacteria, the data obtained from pure cultures can be difficult to interpret with regard to understanding total rumen activity.

IN VITRO MIXED CULTURE FERMENTATIONS

These studies are essentially conducted by incubating either whole rumen contents, or more commonly, strained rumen fluid, with specific substrates. Effects of adding various compounds or changing environmental conditions can be measured. Two general approaches have been used, the first is simply incubating rumen contents in a static or closed system, while the second is a continuous culture system where an attempt is made to maintain steady state conditions. Obviously the static system suffers from such drawbacks as the accumulation of end-products, disappearance of substrate and possible flora shifts, depending on length of the fermentation period. The continuous culture system is an attempt to overcome these difficulties and simulate actual *in vivo* conditions.

Washed suspensions of rumen bacteria have been used to study metabolism of specific carbohydrates, utilization of various nitrogen sources, unknown growth factor requirements, and overall metabolic pathways. The primary objection to this approach is that when the bacteria are separated from their normal environment, washed and subsequently grown in a semi-purified medium, marked population changes can occur. Some quite valid data might be obtained for the proliferating type; however, this is hard to relate to the rumen fermentation itself. Washed resting-cell suspensions can provide information on occurrence of specific enzymatic activity, metabolic pathways, etc.

IN VIVO — *IN VITRO* METHODS

The "so—called" vivar technique (Fina *et al.*, 1958; Fina *et al.*, 1962), developed by Fina and co-workers at Kansas State, has only been used by a few investigators and although quite sound in theory has not lived up to previous expectations. It involves placing a container inside the rumen, which is permeable to all materials except bacteria and protozoa. Thus, supposedly, all *in vivo* conditions would be met. Samples can be withdrawn or materials added through a rigid tube. The main difficulty with this procedure has been equilibration across the permeable portion of the container. The membrane type filters require about 48 h for equilibration of VFA, while stainless steel, ceramic and porous vycor glass filters reach only about 50% equilibration in that time. Despite these drawbacks the method was very useful for the studies on protozoan antagonism conducted by Eadie (1967), since the protozoa survived well in this apparatus.

The nylon or dacron bag technique (Hopson *et al*., 1963; Johnson, 1966) would also fit under this general heading. This procedure is sometimes referred to as the "*in situ*" or "*in sacco*" technique (Nocek, 1988). Small bags made of an indigestible synthetic fiber material such as nylon or dacron are filled with feed, usually a forage, tied tightly and then placed in the rumen. Two factors appear to be of importance with this technique. First, the bags must be suspended in such a manner that they do not become lodged in the bottom of the rumen or some pocket, and second, that the pore size of the bag material is of fine enough mesh to prevent wash-out of undegraded forage particles but still allow influx of the rumen microbes. Bags can be removed at varying time intervals and digestion curves for a forage determined. Using this procedure, Hopson *et al*. (1963) obtained digestion curves quite similar to those found with *in vitro* fermentations. These authors also noted an effect of the animals ration on digestibility of the forage in the nylon bags.

In a study reported by Trabalza Marinucci *et al*. (1992), some possible drawbacks to the synthetic fiber bag procedure were uncovered. The authors simultaneously measured dry matter and cellulose disappearance *in vitro* from alfalfa incubated inside and outside of synthetic fiber bags. In general, dry matter digestion (DMD), cellulose digestion (CD) and pH were all markedly reduced inside of the bags, compared to outside. Subsequent studies indicated that the bags became expanded with gas and there was little or no liquid exchange inside of the bag, with a subsequent decrease in pH and decrease in DMD and CD. By intermittently creating a vacuum in the flask, the bags deflated and liquid exchange was increased. This resulted in a significant increase in all three parameters inside the bags. When bags were incubated *in vivo*, free or inside a perforated rigid container, DMD and pH values were higher in the free bags. Apparently the physical action of the rumen contents promotes exchange of fluid. Bacterial concentrations were also higher on fiber inside of free bags as compared to those bags in containers. These results were later confirmed by Nozièrs and Michalet-Doreau (1996).

Although there are shortcomings with both the synthetic fiber bag and "vivar" techniques, they do offer a procedure in which one can compare digestibility between diets in the rumen. Obviously, some caution is needed in accepting such data as absolute values. These procedures might also be useful in providing information on relative rates of digestion in the rumen itself.

Pure cultures

Descriptions of isolated species of rumen bacteria will be presented in subsequent Chapters, according to the major plant substrates which they digest, i.e., cellulolytic, amylolytic, proteolytic, etc. Isolation of pure cultures was originally accomplished by picking individual colonies from anaerobic roll tubes as described by Hungate (1969) and Bryant (1972). More recently, Petri plates have been used in anaerobic glove boxes

(Leedle and Hespell, 1980). An additional advantage of being able to use Petri plates is it allows use of replicate plating techniques to screen for many different activities, i.e., substrates fermented, antibiotic sensitivity, etc.

The anaerobic technique used in culturing rumen microorganisms was primarily developed by Hungate (1950). It involves carrying out all the standard bacteriological procedures under a stream of O_2 free CO_2. Flasks and culture tubes are closed or sealed with rubber stoppers. Modifications to improve the procedure have been added by Bryant and Robinson (1961), Dehority (1969) and Bryant (1972).

Many early workers had attempted to isolate the cellulolytic bacteria from rumen contents, however, in general they were unsuccessful. In 1947, Hungate succeeded in isolating a number of pure cultures by using methodology which met the rigid anaerobiosis requirements and a habitat-simulating medium. The medium contained 40% rumen fluid, minerals, resazurin (oxidation-reduction indicator), cysteine as a reducing agent and $NaHCO_3$, all under a gaseous phase of carbon dioxide. He also used an acid-treated ball-milled cellulose as a substrate, which was more readily attacked by the cellulolytic bacteria, and allowed growth of visible colonies which could then be isolated. After isolation and study of the bacteria, their requirement for complex organic nutrients not present in most bacteriological media were discovered. This, in addition to their requirement for strict anaerobiosis, might explain the difficulties experienced by previous workers.

Sijpesteijn (1948, 1951), working with enrichment cultures and a strip of filter paper as substrate, noted that the bacteria appeared to "attach" themselves to the fibers and dissolve the filter paper. She continually found spore-forming anaerobes in her initial studies, but when she added rumen fluid and a reducing agent, ascorbic acid, a coccoid cellulose digesting bacteria proliferated as colonies visible on the surface of the filter paper Her cultures were incubated in an anaerobic jar under H_2. By incorporating agar into her medium, she could remove the agar plug, separate the filter paper out and pick from an isolated colony. Using these techniques she successfully isolated a cellulolytic coccus. Hungate's procedure was obviously much simpler and could be adapted to study many types of rumen bacteria by simply changing the substrate in the basal medium.

In vitro fermentations

Marked emphasis on the mixed culture or *in vitro* fermentation also began in the late 1940's. Two excellent reviews on this topic have been published by Johnson (1963, 1966).

Burroughs and co-workers in 1950 developed an *in vitro* system using 500 ml flasks which contained filter paper, mineral solution, rumen fluid and distilled water. The flasks were placed in a water bath at 39°C and bubbled with CO_2. After 36 hours, half of the contents were transferred to a second flask. They found that cellulose digestion by the bacteria decreased markedly after the second transfer; however, when certain additions such as the ash of alfalfa extract, autoclaved rumen fluid or an autoclaved water extract of manure were added, cellulose digestion was markedly increased. Using this procedure they established that cellulose digestion in good quality forages was much higher than in poor quality forages, but marked improvement in the digestibility of poor quality roughage could be obtained by adding available nitrogen, complex minerals and manure extract. These investigators also found that the cellulolytic rumen bacteria did not require proteins or amino acids, but could utilize ammonia or urea as the sole added nitrogen source.

Bentley and co-workers (1954a) separated the bacteria from rumen fluid by centrifugation and investigated cellulose digestion in a purified medium. After a considerable number of studies, they found that the so-called "cellulolytic" factor in rumen fluid was steam volatile and eventually identified the active material as valeric acid (Bentley *et al.*, 1954b, 1955). They also found that biotin and PABA had to be included in their basal medium. It is of interest that shortly after publication of this information, Bryant and Doetsch (1955), working with pure cultures, reported that the cellulolytic species, *B. succinogenes*, had an absolute requirement for several volatile fatty acids. Both studies were conducted completely independent of each other.

A non-volatile "cellulolytic" factor activity was also observed in autolyzed yeast, alfalfa meal and casein hydrolysate by Bentley *et al.* (1954a). Using a washed suspension of rumen bacteria as an inoculum, along with a purified medium, Dehority *et al.* (1957), found that the amino acids valine, proline and the leucines were the active compounds in these complex natural materials. Subsequent studies with radioactive valine and proline revealed that these amino acids were degraded by the mixed culture to isobutyric and valeric acids, respectively (Dehority *et al.*, 1958). This would, of course, account for their activity in enhancing cellulose digestion.

Some preliminary work was also done at this time on inoculum preparation and the effects of VFA concentrations in the basal medium (Johnson *et al.*, 1958). Discarding the liquid portion of the rumen ingesta and extracting the solids with buffer gave a more consistent and active cellulolytic inoculum. When acetic, propionic and butyric acids were added to the medium at levels normally found near the end of the *in vitro* fermentation, little if any, inhibition was observed. However, inhibition was observed at higher levels (300, 300 and 30 mg/100 ml, respectively), indicating that this factor must be considered in *in vitro* studies.

Particle size of a purified cellulose substrate was found to affect digestion rate by mixed cultures of rumen bacteria (Dehority, 1961). Total digestibility did not appear to be affected and it was concluded that true or maximum digestion rate was not changed. However, the lag phase was reduced as particle size decreased. It was suggested that surface area or available sites for attachment were responsible for these differences in lag phase.

The *in vitro* fermentation method has been used for a number of other studies. For example, Dehority and Johnson (1961) were able to draw the following conclusions from their study on the effect of particle size on cellulose digestion from intact forages: (1) the percent cellulose digested by rumen bacteria was found to decrease with increasing maturity and lignification of the plant (Table 7.1); (2) the total amount of cellulose in a forage available for digestion by rumen bacteria was almost completely utilized after 30 h of fermentation *in vitro* (Figures 7.1a and 7.1b); (3) physical reduction of the forage particle size by ball-milling increased the amount of cellulose which could be digested *in vitro* and this increase was directly related to the length of ball-milling, at least up to 72 h (Figures 7.1c and 7.1d); (4) the increase in *in vitro* cellulose digestibility due to ball-milling became larger as the forage matured (Figures 7.1a and 7.1b); (5) there appeared to be a basic difference in grasses and legumes in regard to the amount of cellulose which could be digested per given amount of lignin in the plant; and (6) simple physical solubility of forage cellulose in cupriethylene diamine (a cellulose solvent) decreased with maturity and was markedly increased after ball-milling (Table 7.2). These conclusions support the theory that decreased cellulose digestibility of mature forages is caused by a physical barrier of lignin or other forage components between the bacteria and the cellulose, and not solely upon the total concentration of lignin. Clark (1938) has postulated that the cell wall is a continuous interpenetrating system of cellulose and lignin similar to reinforced concrete. The iron rods would represent the cellulose framework while lignin and other constituents, the concrete. This model may best fit the actual spatial relationship between cellulose and lignin in the mature plant.

Table 7.1. EFFECT OF PLANT MATURITY AND LIGNIFICATION UPON CELLULOSE DIGESTION[a]

Forage	Cellulose digested (%)	Lignin (%)
Timothy, 1st stage[b]	83.0±2.8[c]	8.5
Timothy, 2nd stage	75.7±1.9	11.9
Timothy, 3rd stage	62.4±0.8	15.3
Alfalfa, 1st stage[d]	67.8±2.5	8.0
Alfalfa, 2nd stage	58.1±2.7	11.8
Alfalfa, 3rd stage	54.8±1.5	13.8

[a] Data from Dehority and Johnson (1961).
[b] 1st, 2nd and 3rd stages are vegetative, heading and headed, respectively.
[c] Mean and standard deviation.
[d] 1st, 2nd and 3rd stages are early bloom, late bloom and seed stage, respectively.

Table 7.2. SOLUBILITY OF FORAGE CELLULOSE IN CUPRIETHYLENE DIAMINE[a]

Timothy forage[b]	Cellulose dissolved (%)	
	Ground[c]	Ball-milled[d]
1st stage	78.2±2.2[e]	86.0±1.5
2nd stage	72.9±1.6	87.2±1.0
3rd stage	61.7±1.7	82.8±1.6
4th stage	49.7±1.9	79.4±0.8

[a] Data from Dehority and Johnson (1961).
[b] Maturity stages, 1st through 4th, are vegetative, heading, headed and seed ripe, respectively.
[c] Ground through a 40-mesh screen.
[d] Ball-milled for 72 hours.
[e] Mean and standard deviation.

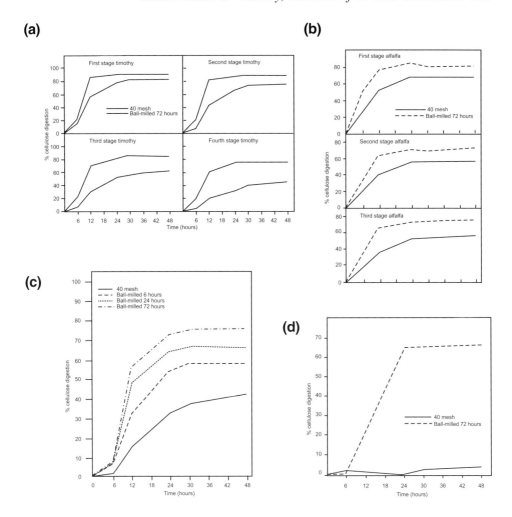

Figure 7.1. (a) Time curves of *in vitro* cellulose digestion in four maturity stages of timothy as affected by particle size; (b) time curves of *in vitro* cellulose digestion in three maturity stages of alfalfa as affected by particle size; (c) Effect of ball-milling time upon rate and extent of *in vitro* cellulose digestion in mature timothy; (d) Effect of physically reducing particle size on the availability of cellulose in the residue from a 48 h *in vitro* fermentation of mature timothy. From Dehority and Johnson (1961).

Surprisingly, as shown in Figure 7.2, very similar results were obtained on the effect of plant species, maturity and lignification upon hemicellulose and pectin digestibility (Dehority et al., 1962). Some very interesting results have also been obtained with regard to the differential effect lignin concentration appears to have on grasses and legumes (Tomlin et al., 1965). In general, 12 h *in vitro* cellulose digestibility values decreased from approximately 75% to 5% in grasses and 62% to 28% in legumes as lignin concentration increased from 3% to 14%.

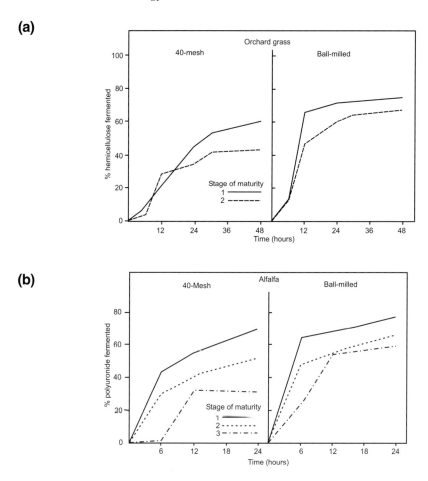

Figure 7.2. Time curves of: (a) hemicellulose digestion by rumen bacteria, using two maturity stages of orchardgrass (1, early bloom; 2, early seed), ground through a 40-mesh screen or ball-milled 72 h; (b) pectin digestion by rumen bacteria using three maturity stages of alfalfa (1, early bloom; 2, late bloom; 3, seeded), ground through a 40-mesh screen or ball-milled 72 h. From Dehority *et al.* (1962).

The other major area where the *in vitro* fermentation has had considerable application has been that of laboratory forage evaluation. Barnes (1967) served as coordinator in a 17 laboratory collaborative study to evaluate methodology between labs for determining *in vitro* digestibility of forage cellulose and dry matter. Three forages were analyzed in duplicate in three runs at fermentation times of 6-, 12-. 24- and 48-hours. Considerable variation was observed in digestibility values between laboratories and it was concluded that a standard *in vitro* procedure would be necessary for valid comparisons. Table 7.3 presents a compilation of studies conducted by Johnson and Dehority (1968), and illustrates the type of information which can be obtained with these procedures.

Table 7.3 CORRELATIONS BETWEEN *IN VIVO* DRY MATTER DIGESTIBILITY, RELATIVE INTAKE, AND NUTRITIVE VALUE INDEX AND SEVERAL INDEXES DETERMINED *IN VITRO*[a,b]

Item[c]	IVCD X DMS[d]	CED X DMS	2-stage IVDMD
Grasses (22)			
DMD	0.88	0.89	0.93
RI	0.83	0.64	0.67
NVI	0.92	0.78	0.82
Legumes (25)			
DMD	0.61	0.82	0.87
RI	0.48	0.42	0.41
NVI	0.87	0.79	0.83
Mixed forages (30)			
DMD	0.82	0.87	0.92
RI	0.40	0.40	0.28
NVI	0.73	0.75	0.68
All forages (77)			
DMD	0.70	0.82	0.90
RI	0.62	0.39	0.08
NVI	0.85	0.69	0.46

[a] Data from Johnson and Dehority (1968).
[b] Abbreviations used: IVCD, 12-h *in vitro* cellulose digestibility; DMS, dry matter solubility; CED, cellulose solubility in cupriethylenediamine; IVDMD, *in vitro* dry matter disappearance.
[c] Numbers in parenthesis indicates number of forages in each group. Abbreviations: DMD (dry matter digestibility); RI (relative intake) = observed intake x 100 ÷ 80 (W kg$^{.75}$); NVI (nutritive value index) = RI x energy digestibility (*in vivo*).
[d] Correlation coefficients required for significance at the 5% and 1% level, respectively, are: n=22, 0.41 and 0.53; n=25, 0.38 and 0.49; n=30, 0.35 and 0.45; n=80(77), 0.22 and 0.28.

In general, the mixed culture or *in vitro* fermentation methods can be of considerable use in rumen microbiological research. One has to be well aware of their limitations and consider these when attempting to evaluate the results. Warner (1956), published a list of criteria for establishing the "so-called" validity of the *in vitro* fermentation. These criteria, also proposed somewhat later by Davey *et al*. (1960) are as follows:

(1) The maintenance of normal numbers, appearance and proportions of the bacteria, selenomonads and protozoa.
(2) The maintenance of normal rates of digestion of cellulose, starch and protein and the normal interaction between these.
(3) The ability to predict quantitative results *in vivo*.

Using a semipermeable membrane system and substrates similar to that fed the animal, Warner (1956) estimated that most of the criteria could be met for periods of up to 8 hours. After that many changes began to occur. The question becomes one of whether you are trying to actually duplicate the rumen fermentation *in vitro*, as might be desirable in studies on rates and amount of VFA production and/or specific substrate utilization rates, or estimate criteria like the availability of forage nutrients or nitrogen sources to the bacteria, study nutritional requirements of certain types of bacteria, check for specific types of activity which might occur in rumen contents, or study inhibition of the fermentation.

Fermentations by a mixed culture of rumen bacteria would tend to imply that one is actually measuring an activity or parameter as it might occur in the rumen. However, this is rarely true, especially in the case of a closed vessel type of *in vitro* fermentation. First, either the protozoa are removed in preparation of the inoculum, or die out very early in the fermentation; and second, if a purified or single substrate is used, one would expect a rapid proliferation of those species capable of using that particular energy source with a concomitant shift in numbers and types. Another factor to be considered is the possible effects of end-product accumulation. These criticisms become especially important when fermentations are carried out over long periods. The work of el-Shazly *et al.* (1961) suggested that one or two types of bacteria proliferated in an all-glass *in vitro* fermentation with purified cellulose as the substrate. Dehority (1963) subsequently isolated those species which proliferated after a 24 h *in vitro* mixed culture fermentation on purified cellulose, and found that these organisms were the major cellulolytic species which occur in the rumen, i.e., *Fibrobacter succinogenes* (formerly *Bacteroides succinogenes*) and *Ruminococcus flavefaciens*. Their nutritional requirements in pure culture were quite similar to those observed previously by the mixed culture techniques.

Leedle and Hespell (1982) investigated possible changes which might occur in carbohydrate-specific bacterial groups during preparation of a mixed rumen bacterial inoculum. In addition, this same criteria was evaluated with regard to population shifts during short incubations. In general they found that: (a) viable cell counts were similar after two washings with no change in the proportions of major carbohydrate-specific groups; (b) if strict anaerobiosis was not maintained during washing, a decrease was noted in the cellulolytic and amylolytic bacterial groups; (c) a mixture of urea and acid hydrolyzed casein was found to be the best nitrogen source for maintaining normal proportions of specific carbohydrate-fermenting bacterial groups and appeared to enhance growth of the cellulolytic and xylanolytic groups; (d) when individual carbohydrates were added as the only substrate, glucose, cellobiose and starch fermentations were predominated by *Strep. bovis*-like bacteria within 3 h and the cellulolytic bacteria disappeared; (e) using pectin or xylan plus xylose as substrates gave no marked population shifts in 6 h and enhanced growth of cellulolytic and xylanolytic groups. Obviously these are factors which need to be considered when using mixed rumen bacteria as an inoculum for *in vitro* fermentations.

In further studies, Leedle and Hespell (1983) studied the effects of washing the mixed inoculum upon *in vitro* fermentations. Bacterial composition remained fairly similar for both the washed and the unwashed inoculum when the substrate was primarily forage. However, when readily fermentable substrates were used the population shifted to starch and glucose fermenting groups.

Numerous investigations have been conducted with the *in vitro* technique and have shed considerable light on the metabolic activities of the rumen bacteria. Some examples of the different types of studies conducted would include:

1. Biohydrogenation of unsaturated fatty acids (Wilde and Dawson, 1966; Van Nevel and Demeyer, 1996; Mosley *et al.*, 2002).
2. Metabolism of citric acid (Wright, 1971).
3. Hydrolysis of biuret (Bauriedel, 1971; Bauriedel *et al.*, 1971).
4. Effect of cellulose crystallinity on digestibility (Baker *et al.*, 1959).
5. Degradation and effects of oxalate (James *et al.*, 1967).
6. Toxicity of various insecticides, antibiotics, etc. (Williams *et al.*, 1968).
7. Nitrogen fixation in the rumen (Jones and Thomas, 1974).
8. Effect of fat on fiber digestibility (Jenkins and Palmquist, 1982).
9. Fermentation of forage organic acids (Callaway and Martin, 1997).
10. Degradation of various lignin type compounds and other plant toxins (Chen et al., 1985; Fukushima *et al.*, 1991; Weimer, 1998).
11. Degradation of protein (Luchini *et al.*, 1996; Depardon *et al.*, 1996).
12. Degradation of biogenic amines (Van Os *et al.*, 1995).
13. Stability of feed enzymes (Morgavi *et al.*, 2001).
14. Degradation of pectic polysaccharides (Hatfield and Weimer, 1995).
15. Inoculation of mixed culture fermentations with organisms having specific activities (Kung and Hession, 1995).

A rather interesting variation of the *in vitro* fermentation technique was developed by el-Shazly and Hungate (1965), in which they used the fermentation capacity of whole rumen contents to estimate net growth of rumen microorganisms. A sample of whole rumen contents is brought into the lab and placed in a flask in a water bath. A portion of the contents are added to a second flask containing buffer, minerals and substrate (similar to that being fed the animal is preferable). Gas production is measured for 1 h and calculated as µliters/g rumen contents/min. Meanwhile, the original sample of rumen contents has been allowed to ferment anaerobically for the same hour period. A second sample, after 1 h incubation, is taken from the whole rumen contents and treated as the first, again measuring gas production. Based on preliminary work, conditions are such that maximum rate of gas production is being estimated. The % difference between rates before and after the 1 h incubation is then said to be equal to % net growth of the rumen microorganisms. The lowest net growth, some values were even negative, was obtained in samples taken just before feeding, while maximum values were obtained about 6 h after feeding in animals fed once daily. The amount of gas produced in the first maximal rate fermentation should be a relative estimate of the size of the rumen population. This value times the % net growth would allow comparison of cells produced per hour by different animals on different rations. In a later study (el-Shazly and Hungate, 1966), these same authors used diaminopimelic acid concentration to estimate bacterial growth and obtained good agreement with their growth rates established from fermentation capacity. Another point of interest, the average relative growth rate from their data was about 8% per hour or 192% per day or 1.92 turnovers per day. This would be in close agreement with values for liquid turnover rates which mostly fall between 1 and 2 turnovers per day.

Zaki-el Din and el-Shazly (1969a,b) found that values for net growth rate, as determined by fermentation capacity, were significantly correlated with changes in numbers of viable rumen bacteria or total ciliate protozoa. These results would strongly support the conclusion that bacteria and protozoa grow in the rumen at the same rate. If true, then substrate limitation in the rumen must be the primary factor controlling microbial growth. The time at which the rumen sample is obtained with relation to feeding would be important in comparing different animals and rations by this method.

An automated continuous culture-type system would obviously be the most desirable for duplicating the total rumen fermentation. Numerous procedures and techniques have been devised and tested. These are described in the review articles mentioned earlier (Johnson, 1963, 1966). Slyter and Putnam (1967) have described a system, where they followed both bacteria and protozoa numbers for a period of 14 days. They also isolated and presumptively identified large numbers of bacteria from the continuous culture and the donor animals. Protozoa numbers were markedly lower and bacterial numbers higher *in vitro*; however, the same bacterial groups were predominant in both. They do point out that their pH was lower and fatty acid concentration and osmolality higher *in vitro* than *in vivo*, indicating improvement in methodology might be beneficial. Abe and Kumeno (1973) investigated the effects of dilution rate with a continuous *in vitro* fermentation system and found that the fermentation patterns resembled those *in vivo* when a low dilution rate was used with a semi-permeable vessel. Entodiniomorph, but not isotrichid populations were maintained over the four day period. However, % distribution of VFA and DNA content indicated shifts in the microbial population.

Nakamura and Kurihara (1978) included a dialyzing system in their continuous-flow apparatus and found that the concentration of ciliate protozoa, pH, VFA concentrations and NH_3 concentrations could be maintained within normal rumen limits for more than 145 days by appropriate choice of mechanical agitation rate, amount of substrate and the physical way in which substrate was added. Their results suggested that no major shifts in the bacterial population had occurred.

One of the more widely used continuous-flow type of *in vitro* fermentation systems is the rumen simulation technique (Rusitec). It was designed to provide three of the four compartments found *in vivo* and to use natural fibrous feeds as substrates (Czerkawski and Breckenridge, 1977). The microbial population in the rumen can be described as occurring in four different compartments:

Compartment 1 - Strained rumen contents, lowest of the microbial concentrations, largest volume, relies on soluble substrates, markedly influenced by dilution rate and supply of soluble food.

Compartment 2 - Intermediate between compartments 1 and 3, microorganisms are loosely attached to feed particles and are removed by gentle agitation such as rumination, functions to transfer microbial matter, nutrients and end-products between 1 and 3.

Compartment 3 - Microorganisms are firmly bound to particulate matter, break down fibrous feeds, probably invade the fibers and attack from within, large proportion are cellulolytic bacteria.

Compartment 4 - Microbial population close to or attached to the rumen wall, less than 1% of total microbes, carries out proteolytic digestion and recycling of the protein of sloughed epithelial cells, produces urease.

The Rusitec apparatus is shown diagrammatically in Figure 7.3. The fermentation is started by placing solid rumen digesta in a coarse nylon bag (3a) and the animal feed to be used in a second nylon bag (3b). These two bags are placed inside a perforated cage (2) which is agitated at an amplitude of 5-6 cm at about 8 cycles/min. The reaction vessel (1) is filled with strained diluted rumen contents. Artificial saliva enters into the

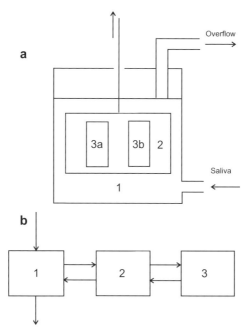

Figure 7.3. Diagrammatic sketch of the RUSITEC apparatus. (a) Compartment 1 is the free bacteria, compartment 2 represents the bacteria loosely associated with the solids and compartments 3a and 3b are the bacteria firmly attached to the solids fraction. (b) Schematic diagram as to the movement of bacteria through these three compartments (redrawn from Czerkawski and Cheng, 1988).

170 *Rumen microbiology*

bottom of the vessel (1) and is forced out through an overflow by a slight positive pressure. These three compartments represent the first three compartments in the rumen. After 24 hours the inoculum bag is removed and replaced with a new bag of food. Removal of the oldest bag (48 hours) and adding a new bag is repeated each day. After removal, the bag is allowed to drain, placed in a plastic bag and washed twice with artificial saliva by gentle squeezing. The washings are added back to the reaction vessel and the washed solids are dried and analyzed. Movement of the microbial population through these three compartments is shown schematically in Fig. 7.3b. The bacteria move from compartments 1 to 2 to 3, and after the food particles are essentially all digested, the bacteria move back out to compartment 1. In essence, the Rusitec is a rumen without a rumen wall. The activity of the bacteria associated with the rumen wall is missing and removal of substances is only by overflow and manually removing undigested solids in the nylon bags. However, the fermentation patterns and product yield per unit mass of food digested are similar to those parameters in sheep kept on the same diet (Czerkawski and Breckenridge, 1977, 1979a,b).

Figure 7.4 illustrates how rumen bacteria move through those three compartments in the rumen. Theoretically, any remaining energy substrates in the feed particle will be utilized either by the enzymatic activity in the animal's digestive tract or by further microbial fermentation in the hindgut. The bacteria themselves are a source of protein to the host animal.

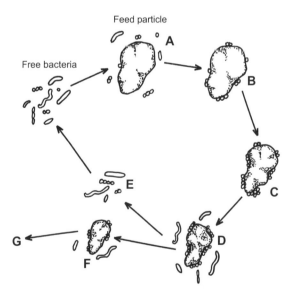

Figure 7.4. Schematic diagram of bacterial movement through the three compartments in the rumen as feed particles are digested. The free bacteria in compartment 1 move into compartment 2, that area near the feed particles (A). The colonizing bacteria attach to the feed particle and establish compartment 3 (B). The attached bacteria begin to grow and digest the feed particle which increases the microbial mass in compartment 3 (C). Release of end-products or soluble substrates from the feed particle attracts other bacteria from compartment 2 and markedly increases microbial mass (D). As the feed particle is digested and substrate may become limiting, some of the bacteria dissociate and return to compartment 1 (E) while the bacteria still firmly attached to the remaining portion of the feed particle (F) pass on down the digestive tract (G) (redrawn from McAllister *et al.*, 1994).

In summary, much useful information can be obtained from mixed culture fermentations *in vitro*; however, one has to be aware of the limitations of the method. The use of natural type substrates, relatively short fermentation times and whole rumen contents as inoculum are the most desirable conditions, in that large population shifts can probably be avoided. Particular care should be taken not to draw unwarranted conclusions from mixed culture fermentations, i.e. make sure the methods and experimental design allow a valid comparison of the treatments under investigation.

References

Abe, M. and Kumeno, F. (1973). *In vitro* simulation of rumen fermentation: apparatus and effects of dilution rate and continuous dialysis on fermentation and protozoal population. *Journal of Animal Science*, **36**, 941-948.

Baker, F. and S. T. Harris. (1947). The role of the microflora of the alimentary tract of herbivora with special reference to ruminants. 2. Microbial digestion in the rumen (and caecum) with special reference to the decomposition of structural cellulose. *Nutrition Abstracts and Reviews*, **18**, 3-12.

Baker, T. I., G. V. Quicke, O. G. Bentley, R. R. Johnson and A. L. Moxon. (1959). The influence of certain physical properties of purified celluloses and forage celluloses or their digestibility by rumen microorganisms *in vitro*. *Journal of Animal Science*, **18**, 655-662.

Barnes, R. F. (1967). Collaborative *in vitro* rumen fermentation studies on forage substrates. *Journal of Animal Science*, **26**, 1120-1130.

Bauriedel, W. R. (1971). Hydrolysis of ^{14}C-biuret by *in vitro* rumen fermentation and crude biuretase preparations. *Journal of Animal Science*, **32**, 704-710.

Bauriedel, W. R., L. F. Craig, J. C. Ramsky and E. O. Camehl. (1971). Hydrolysis of ^{15}N-biuret by *in vitro* rumen fermentation and ruminal biuretase. *Journal of Animal Science*, **32**, 711-715.

Bentley, O. G., R. R. Johnson, S. Vanecko and C. H. Hunt. (1954a). Studies on factors needed by rumen microorganisms for cellulose digestion *in vitro*. Journal of Animal Science, **13**, 711-715.

Bentley, O. G., A. Lehmkuhl, R. R. Johnson, T. V. Hershberger and A. L. Moxon. (1954b). The "cellulolytic factor" activity of certain short-chained fatty acids. *Journal of American Chemical Society*, **76**, 5000-5001.

Bentley, O. G., R. R. Johnson, T. V. Hershberger, J. H. Cline and A. L. Moxon. (1955). Cellulolytic-factor activity of certain short-chain fatty acids for rumen microorganisms *in vitro*. *Journal of Nutrition*, **57**, 389-400.

Bryant, M. P. (1972). Commentary on the Hungate technique for culture of anaerobic bacteria. *The American Journal of Clinical Nutrition*, **25**, 1324-1328.

Bryant, M. P. and L. A. Burkey. (1953a). Cultural methods and some characteristics of some of the more numerous groups of bacteria in the bovine rumen. *Journal of Dairy Science*, **36**, 205-217.

Bryant, M. P. and L. A. Burkey. (1953b). Numbers and some predominant groups of bacteria in the rumen of cows fed different rations. *Journal of Dairy Science*, **36**, 218-224.

Bryant, M. P. and R. N Doetsch. (1955). Factors necessary for the growth of *Bacteroides succinogenes* in the volatile acid fraction of rumen fluid. *Journal of Dairy Science*, **38**, 340-350.

Bryant, M. P. and I. M. Robinson. (1961). An improved nonselective culture medium for ruminal bacteria and its use in determining diurnal variation in numbers of bacteria in the rumen. *Journal of Dairy Science*, **44**, 1446-1456.

Burroughs, W., N. A. Franks, P. Gerlaugh and R. M. Bethke. (1950). Preliminary observations upon factors influencing cellulose digestion by rumen microorganisms. *Journal of Nutrition*, **40**, 9-24.

Callaway, T. R. and S. A. Martin. (1997). Effects of cellobiose and monensin on *in vitro* fermentation of organic acids by mixed ruminal bacteria. *Journal of Dairy Science*, **80**, 1126-1135.

Chen, W., K. Ohmiya, S. Shimizu and H. Kawakami. (1985). Degradation of dehydrodivanillin by anaerobic bacteria from cow rumen fluid. *Applied and Environmental Microbiology*, **49**, 211-216.

Clark, S. H. (1938). Fine structure of the plant cell wall. *Nature*, **142**, 899.

Czerkawski, J. W. and G. Breckenridge. (1977). Design and development of a long-term rumen simulation technique (Rusitec). *British Journal of Nutrition*, **38**, 371-384.

Czerkawski, J. W. and G. Breckenridge. (1979a). Experiments with the long-term rumen simulation technique (Rusitec); response to supplementation of the rations. *British Journal of Nutrition*, **42**, 217-228.

Czerkawski, J. W. and G. Breckenridge. (1979b). Experiments with the long-term rumen simulation technique (Rusitec); use of soluble food and an inert solid matrix. *British Journal of Nutrition*, **42**, 229-245.

Czerkawski, J. W. and K.-J. Cheng. (1988). Compartmentation in the rumen. In: *The Rumen Microbial Ecosystem*. p. 361. Edited by P. N. Hobson. Elsevier Applied Science, London. pp. 361-386.

Davey, L. A., G. C. Cheeseman and C.A.E. Briggs. (1960). Evaluation of an improved artificial rumen designed for continuous control during prolonged operation. *Journal of Agricultural Science*, **55**, 155-163.

Dehority, B. A. (1961). Effect of particle size on the digestion rate of purified cellulose by rumen cellulolytic bacteria *in vitro*. *Journal of Dairy Science*, **44**, 687-692.

Dehority, B. A. (1963). Isolation and characterization of several cellulolytic bacteria from *in vitro* rumen fermentations. *Journal of Dairy Science*, **46**, 217-222.

Dehority, B. A. (1969). Pectin-fermenting bacteria isolated from the bovine rumen. *Journal of Bacteriology*, **99**, 189-196.

Dehority, B. A. and R. R. Johnson. (1961). Effect of particle size upon the *in vitro* cellulose digestibility of forages by rumen bacteria. *Journal of Dairy Science*, **44**, 2242-2249.

Dehority, B. A., R. R. Johnson and H. R. Conrad. (1962). Digestibility of forage hemicellulose and pectin by rumen bacteria *in vitro* and the effect of lignification thereon. *Journal of Dairy Science,* **45**, 508-512.

Dehority, B. A., O. G. Bentley, R. R. Johnson and A. L. Moxon. (1957). Isolation and identification of compounds from autolyzed yeast, alfalfa meal and casein hydrolysate with cellulolytic factor activity for rumen microorganisms *in vitro*. *Journal of Animal Science*, **16**, 502-514.

Dehority, B. A., R. R. Johnson, O. G. Bentley and A. L. Moxon. (1958). Studies on the metabolism of valine, proline, leucine and isoleucine by rumen microorganisms *in vitro*. *Archives of Biochemistry and Biophysics*, **78**, 15-27.

Depardon, N., D. Debroas and G. Blanchart. (1996). Breakdown of peptides from a casein hydrolysate by rumen bacteria. Simultaneous study of enzyme activities and physicochemical paaarameters. *Reproduction Nutrition Development*, **36**, 457-466.

el-Shazly, K. and R. E. Hungate. (1965). Fermentation capacity as a measure of net growth of rumen microorganisms. *Applied Microbiology*, **13**, 62-69.

el-Shazly, K. and R. E. Hungate. (1966). Method for measuring diaminopmelic acid in total rumen contents and its application to the estimation of bacterial growth. *Applied Microbiology*, **14**, 27-30.

el-Shazly, K., R. R. Johnson, B. A. Dehority and A. L. Moxon. (1961). Biochemical and microscopic comparison of *in vivo* and *in vitro* rumen fermentations. *Journal of Animal Science*, **20**, 839-843.

Eadie, J. M. (1967). Studies on the ecology of certain rumen ciliate protozoa. *Journal of General Microbiology*, **49**, 175-194.

Fina, L. R., G. W. Teresa and E. E. Bartley. (1958). An artificial rumen technique for studying rumen digestion *in vivo*. *Journal of Animal Science*, **17**, 667-674.

Fina, L. R., C. L. Keith, E. E. Bartley, P. A. Hartman and N. L. Jacobson. (1962). Modified *in vivo* artificial rumen (vivar) techniques. *Journal of Animal Science*, **21**, 930-934.

Fukushima, R. S., B. A. Dehority and S. C. Loerch. (1991). Modification of a colorimetric analysis for lignin and its use in studying the inhibitory effects of lignin on forage digestion by ruminal microorganisms. *Journal of Animal Science*, **69**, 295-304.

Hatfield, R. D. and P. J. Weimer. (1995). Degradation characteristics of isolated and *in situ* cell wall lucerne pectic polysaccharides by mixed ruminal microbes. *Journal of the Science of Food and Agriculture*, **69**, 185-196.

Hopson, J. D., R. R. Johnson and B. A. Dehority. (1963). Evaluations of the dacron bag technique as a method for measuring cellulose digestibility and rate of forage digestion. *Journal of Animal Science*, **22**, 448-453.

Hungate, R. E. (1947). Studies on cellulose fermentation. III. The culture and isolation of cellulose-decomposing bacteria from the rumen of cattle. *Journal of Bacteriology*, **53**, 631-645.

Hungate, R. E. (1950). The anaerobic mesophilic cellulolytic bacteria. *Bacteriological Reviews*, **14**, 1-49.

Hungate, R. E. (1966). *The Rumen and Its Microbes*. Academic Press, NY, NY.

Hungate, R. E. (1969). A roll tube method for cultivation of strict anaerobes. In: *Methods in Microbiology*. Edited by J. R. Norris and D. W. Ribbons. Academic Press, New York, USA. pp. 117-132.

James, L. F., J. C. Street and J. E. Butcher. (1967). In vitro degradation of oxalate and of cellulose by rumen ingesta from sheep fed *Halogeton Glomeratus*. *Journal of Animal Science*, **26**, 1438-1444.

Jenkins, T. C. and D. L. Palmquist. (1982). Effect of added fat and calcium on *in vitro* formation of insoluble fatty acid soaps and cell wall digestibility. *Journal of Animal Science*, **55**, 957-963.

Johnson, R. R. (1963). Symposium on microbial digestion in ruminants: *in vitro* rumen fermentation techniques. *Journal of Animal Science*, **22**, 792-800.

Johnson, R. R. (1966). Techniques and procedures for *in vitro* and *in vivo* rumen studies. *Journal of Animal Science*, **25**, 855-875.

Johnson, R. R. and B. A. Dehority. (1968). A comparison of several laboratory techniques to predict digestibility and intake of forages. *Journal of Animal Science*, **27**, 1738-1742.

Johnson, R. R., B. A. Dehority and O. G. Bentley. (1958). Studies on the *in vitro* rumen procedure: improved inoculum preparation and the effects of volatile fatty acids on cellulose digestion. *Journal of Animal Science*, **17**, 841-850.

Jones, K. and J. G. Thomas. (1974). Nitrogen fixation by the rumen contents of sheep. *Journal of General Microbiology*, **85**, 97-101.

Kung, L. Jr. and A. O. Hession. (1995). Preventing *in vitro* lactate accumulation in ruminal fermentations by inoculaton with *Megasphaera elsdenii*. *Journal of Animal Science*, **73**, 250-256.

Leedle, J.A.Z. and R. B. Hespell. (1980). Differential carbohydrate media and anaerobic replica plating techniques in delineating carbohydrate-utilizing subgroups in rumen bacterial populations. *Applied and Environmental Microbiology*, **39**, 709-719.

Leedle, J.A.Z. and R. B. Hespell. (1982). Brief incubations of mixed ruminal bacteria: Effects of anaerobiosis and sources of nitrogen and carbon. *Journal of Dairy Science*, **66**, 1003-1014.

Leedle, J.A.Z. and R. B. Hespell. (1983). Changes of bacterial numbers and carbohydrate fermenting groups during *in vitro* rumen incubations with feedstuff materials. *Journal of Dairy Science*, **67**, 808-816.

Luchini, N. D., G. A. Broderick and D. K. Combs. (1996). Characterization of the proteolytic activity of commercial proteases and strained ruminal fluid. *Journal of Animal Science*, **74**, 685-692.

Marston, H. R. (1948). The fermentation of cellulose *in vitro* by organisms from the rumen of sheep. *Biochemistry Journal*, **42**, 564-574.

McAllister, T. A., H. D. Bae, G. A. Jones, and K.-J. Cheng. (1994). Microbial attachment and feed digestion in the rumen. *Journal of Animal Science*, **72**, 3004-3018.

Morgavi, D. P., K. A. Beauchemin, V. L. Nsereko, L. M. Rode, T. A. McAllister, A. D. Iwaasa, Y. Wang and W. Z. Yang. (2001). Resistance of feed enzymes to proteolytic inactivation by rumen microorganisms and gastrointestinal proteases. *Journal of Animal Science*, **79**, 1621-1630.

Mosley, E. E., G. L. Powell, M. B. Riley, and T. C. Jenkins. (2002). Microbial biohydrogenation of oleic acid to *trans* isomers *in vitro*. *Journal of Lipid Research*, **43**, 290-296.

Nakamura, F. and Y. Kurihara. (1978). Maintenance of a certain rumen protozoal population in a continuous *in vitro* fermentation system. *Applied and Environmental Microbiology*, **35**, 500-506.

Nocek, J. E. (1988). In situ and other methods to estimate ruminal protein and energy digestibility: A Review. *Journal of Dairy Science*, **71**, 2051-2069.

Nozière, P. and B. Michalet-Doreau. (1996). Validation of in sacco method: influence of sampling site, nylon bag or rumen contents, on fibrolytic activity of solid associated microorganisms. *Animal Feed Science and Technology*, **57**, 203-210.

Sijpesteijn, A. K. (1948). Cellulose decomposing bacteria from the rumen of cattle. Ph.D. Thesis, Leiden.

Sijpesteijn, A. K. (1951). On *Ruminococcus flavefaciens*, a cellulose-decomposing bacterium from the rumen of sheep and cattle. *Journal of General Microbiology*, **5**, 869- 879.

Slyter, L. L. and P. A. Putnam. (1967). *In vivo* vs *in vitro* continuous culture of ruminal microbial populations. *Journal of Animal Science*, **26**, 1421-1427.

Tomlin, D. C., R. R. Johnson and B. A. Dehority. (1965). Relationship of lignification to *in vitro* cellulose digestibility of grasses and legumes. *Journal of Animal Science*, **24**, 161-165.

Trabalza Marinucci, M., B. A. Dehority and S. C. Loerch. (1992). *In vitro* and *in vivo* studies of factors affecting digestion of feeds in synthetic fiber bags. *Journal of Animal Science*, **70,** 296-307.

Van Nevel, C. J. and D. I. Demeyer. (1996). Influence of pH on lipolysis and biohydrogenation of soybean oil by rumen contents *in vitro*. *Reproduction Nutrition Development*, **36**, 53-63.

Van Os, M., B. Lassalas, S. Toillon and J. P. Jouany. (1995). *In vitro* degradation of amines by rumen micro-organisms. *Journal of Agricultural Science*, ***125,*** 299-305.

von Tappeiner, H. (1884). Untersuchungen über die gärung der cellulose insbesondere über deren lösung in darmkanale. *Zeitschrift für Biologie*, **20**, 52-134.

Warner, A.C.I. (1956). Criteria for establishing the validity of *in vitro* studies with rumen micro-organisms in so-called artificial rumen systems. *Journal of General Microbiology*, **14**, 733-748.

Weimer, P.J. (1998). Manipulating ruminal fermentation: A microbial ecological perspective. *Journal of Animal Science*, **76**, 3114-3122.

Wilde, P. F. and R.M.C. Dawson. (1966). The biohydrogenation of α-linolenic acid and oleic acid by rumen micro-organisms. *Biochemical Journal*, **98**, 469-475.

Williams, P. P., K. L. Davison and E. J. Thacker. (1968). *In vitro* and *in vivo* rumen microbiological studies with 2-chloro-4, 6-bis (isopropylamino)-α-triazine (propazine). *Journal of Animal Science*, **27**, 1472-1476.

Wright, D. E. (1971). Citric acid metabolism in the bovine rumen. *Applied Microbiology*, **21**, 165-168.

Zaki el-Din, M. and K. el-Shazly. (1969a). Evaluation of a method of measuring fermentation rates and net growth of rumen microorganisms. *Applied Microbiology*, **17**, 801-804.

Zaki el-Din, M. and K. el-Shazly. (1969b). Some factors affecting fermentation capacity and net growth of rumen microorganisms. *Applied Microbiology,* **18**, 313-317.

CHAPTER 8

CELLULOSE DIGESTING RUMEN BACTERIA

Before discussing the individual species of cellulolytic rumen bacteria, it would seem worthwhile to discuss the criteria for determining whether or not a species is an authentic rumen bacteria or a transient organism taken in with the food. Bryant (1959) has suggested that the most important criteria which can be used are that the organism be shown to grow in the rumen and that it have a metabolism compatible with the reactions occurring and the environment present in the rumen. The numbers of a given species which occur in the rumen in relation to its numbers in the feed and water consumed would also be of considerable value in establishing its significance. The organism should be able to attack substrates present in the rumen, either those present in the feed (cellulose, hemicellulose, pectin, starch, protein, etc.), hydrolytic products of these feed constituents or fermentation end products of other microbes, such as organic acids and hydrogen. Fermentation products of an organism should be compatible with those present or readily metabolized in the rumen. Cultural characteristics such as pH, Eh, temperature range and nutritional requirements should be compatible with the rumen environment. If an organism is isolated from 1×10^{-8} or higher dilutions of rumen contents (this would be 100 million cells per ml) and meets a majority of the criteria listed above, most workers would probably consider the particular organism to have some significance in the total rumen fermentation. Repeated isolation of a particular species over a period of time, from different host animals at various locations, would be further evidence for its authenticity as a true ruminal bacteria.

Most readers will be familiar with the names of several bacteria, for example *Escherichia coli*. *Escherichia* refers to the genus in which the organism is classified and *coli* is the species. In much of the material to be presented, it will be noted that given bacterial cultures are designated as strains. Classification by strain primarily refers to the physical isolation of an organism. If on a given day, two cultures of the same species were isolated, both from separate colonies, these would be different strains. If this same species was isolated from the same source at a later date, this is again a separate strain. In other words, strain designation refers to a pure culture isolated from a single cell, and thus no two identical strains can possibly exist. Strain differences are generally obvious even in the limited number of physiological and biochemical characteristics normally measured; however, it is possible for two strains to be almost identical with regards to the characteristics tested and still differ from each other in unmeasured criteria.

Cellulolytic species

Based on their relative numbers in the rumen of domestic animals, plus their ability in pure culture to hydrolyze purified and intact forage cellulose, the principal or most important species of cellulolytic bacteria in the rumen appear to be *Ruminococcus flavefaciens, Ruminococcus albus* and *Fibrobacter succinogenes* (formerly *Bacteroides succinogenes*). Many strains of *Butyrivibrio fibrisolvens*, which occurs in high numbers on widely differing rations, are also cellulolytic, but only weakly so. Another species, *Eubacterium* (formerly *Cillobacterium*) *cellulosolvens*, first isolated in low numbers by Bryant *et al.* in 1958 has been observed in much higher numbers in the Netherlands and South Africa (Van Gylswyk and Hoffman, 1970; Prins *et al.*, 1972). Several cellulolytic species in the genus *Clostridium*, anaerobic spore formers, have also been found on occasion; however, they usually occur in quite low numbers (Hungate, 1957; Shane *et al.*, 1969).

FIBROBACTER (FORMERLY *BACTEROIDES*) *SUCCINOGENES* HUNGATE

In 1947, Hungate succeeded in isolating what appeared to be one of the major cellulolytic bacteria in the rumen. He called the organism an actively cellulolytic rod and isolated it from roll tubes with a cellulose-agar medium. After subsequent characterization studies he placed it in the genus *Bacteroides* and established the species *succinogenes* (Hungate, 1950). In 1953, Bryant and Burkey isolated 56 presumptively identified strains of this species in a medium containing the soluble sugars, cellobiose and glucose, as the only added energy source. Eight of these strains were described and characterized in a later publication (Bryant and Doetsch, 1954). Dehority (1963), using glucose and cellobiose as substrates, subsequently isolated two strains of *B. succinogenes* from 24 h *in vitro* mixed culture fermentations with purified cellulose as the only substrate.

Strains of cellulolytic rumen bacteria classified as *Bacteroides succinogenes* appeared to differ in composition from most other strains in that genus. Specifically, they did not contain sphingolipids or large amounts of branched long-chain fatty acids. With the newer techniques, it became possible to determine phylogenetic relatedness among various bacterial strains, without having to rely on phenotypic characteristics for classification purposes. Using 16S ribosomal ribonucleic acid sequences, Montgomery *et al.* (1988), found that strains of bacteria classified as *Bacteroides succinogenes* were not closely related to other species of *Bacteroides*, including the type species, *B. fragilis*. On this basis, they proposed a new genus *Fibrobacter*, and established two species within the new genus, *F. succinogenes* and *F. intestinalis*. *F. succinogenes* differs from *F. intestinalis* by its requirement for biotin and the site of isolation, i.e. rumen versus the cecum of nonruminant animals. The type strain for *F. succinogenes* is S85.

Fibrobacter succinogenes is an anaerobic, nonsporeforming, gram-negative rod, generally varying in diameter from 0.3 to 0.5 µm and in length from 1-2 µm. This species tends to be quite pleomorphic, exhibiting some variation in the shape of cells even in young cultures. As cultures age, many swollen forms and rounded bodies are observed. Table 8.1 lists the physiological characteristics for several strains of this species. Table 8.2 lists the carbohydrates fermented and end-products produced from cellulose fermentation by this species. Aside from a few exceptions, *F. succinogenes* ferments only cellulose, glucose and cellobiose and its primary end-products are acetic and succinic acids.

Table 8.1. CHARACTERISTICS OF SEVERAL STRAINS OF *FIBROBACTER SUCCINOGENES*

		Strain				
	Type species[a]	S85[b]	S111[b]	A3c[c]	B21a[c]	BL2[d]
Isolation medium	Cellulose agar	RGCA[e]	RGCA	RGCA	RGCA	Cellobiose agar
Size, µm						
Length	1-2	1-2	0.5-0.6	1-2	0.5-1.5	0.9-1.9
Width	0.3-0.4	1-1.2		0.5	0.5	0.5-0.8
Gram stain	-	-	-	-	-	-
Motility	-	-	-	-	-	-
Anaerobic	+	+	+	+	+	+
H_2S production				-	-	
Indole production		-	-	-	-	
Catalase				-	-	
Nitrate reduction		-	-	-	-	
Gelatin liquefaction		-	-	-	-	
Casein digestion		+	+			
Cellulose digestion	+	+	+	+	+	+
Starch digestion	+	-	-	-	-	-
CO_2 requirement		+	+	+	+	+
NH_3 requirement		+		+	+	+
VFA requirement[f]				+	+	
Replacement of rumen fluid by trypticase and YE[g]		-	-	-	-	
Final pH-lowly buffered glucose or cellobiose broth		5.5		5.2	5.1	

[a] Hungate (1950)
[b] Bryant and Doetsch (1954)
[c] Dehority (1963)
[d] Stewart *et al.* (1981)
[e] Rumen fluid-glucose-cellobiose-agar medium (Bryant and Burkey, 1953).
[f] VFA = volatile fatty acid
[g] YE = yeast extract

Table 8.2. CARBOHYDRATES FERMENTED AND END-PRODUCTS PRODUCED BY *FIBROBACTER SUCCINOGENES*

			Strain			
	Type species[a]	S85[b]	S111[b]	A3c[c]	B21a[c]	BL2[d]
Acid from:						
Glucose	+	+	+	+	+	+
Cellobiose	+	+	+	+	+	+
Maltose	+	-	+	-	-	-
Lactose	-	±	-	-	-	-
Dextrin	+	-	-	-	-	
Trehalose	+	-	-	-	-	-
Pectin	-	+	+	-	-	
Products in rumen fluid cellulose medium:						
Formic acid	0[e]	0.28[f]	0.23[f]	0.17[g]	0.15[g]	0.24[h]
Acetic acid	0.208	1.00	0.86	1.14	0.98	0.31
Propionic acid	0.026	0.01	0	0	0	0
Butyric acid	0	-0.03	0	0	0	0
Lactic acid	0	0	0	0	0	0
Succinic acid	0.424	2.46	0.89	3.07	2.80	0.39
Ethanol	0	0	0	0	0	
Reducing sugars	0	0	0	0	0	

[a] Hungate (1950)
[b] Bryant and Doetsch (1954)
[c] Dehority, (1963)
[d] Stewart et al. (1981)
[e] millimoles
[f] millimoles/150 ml medium
[g] millimoles/100 ml medium
[h] millimoles/millimole glucose utilized.

In general, bacterial colonies isolated from cellulose agar roll tubes are predominantly ruminococci along with lesser numbers of *Butyrivibrio*. The ruminococci will rapidly digest cellulose in broth culture, while the *Butyrivibrio* strains have limited, if any, ability to degrade cellulose in liquid medium (Dehority, 1966). *F. succinogenes* appears to be one of the most active rumen cellulolytics, digesting appreciable amounts of both purified and forage cellulose (Halliwell and Bryant, 1963; Dehority and Scott, 1967); however, it is rarely isolated from cellulose agar roll tubes. Stewart *et al.* (1981) were able to isolate numerous strains of *F. succinogenes* by growing enrichment cultures on cotton fibers and then isolating bacteria from the enrichment cultures in cellobiose roll tubes. They isolated 11 strains of *F. succinogenes*, all of which digested cellulose in broth culture but would not form clear zones in cellulose agar. Hungate (1947, 1950) obtained the original isolates of this species from roll tubes containing ball-milled cotton as the only substrate; however, based on later studies he proposed that some strains, although not motile, were able to migrate through the agar to the cellulose particles, whereas other strains could not (Hungate, 1966). This explanation was supported by the observations of Macy *et al.* (1982), who found that lowering the agar concentration from 2.0% to 0.5% allowed *F. succinogenes* to form clear zones in cellulose agar.

Huang and Forsberg (1990) studied several parameters concerned with growth and cellulase activity of *F. succinogenes*. *F. succinogenes* grew as rapidly on amorphous cellulose (acid-swollen cellulose) as on glucose or cellobiose. On the other hand, the rate of growth on crystalline cellulose was about three times slower. It would appear that solubilization or disruption of the crystalline structure, not hydrolysis of the polysaccharide chain, is the limiting factor. They also concluded that the cellulase enzymes of *F. succinogenes* were constitutive, which agrees with the previous observation of Hiltner and Dehority (1983). However, the two studies disagree in that Huang and Forsberg found that glucose or cellobiose was used preferentially to cellulose while Hiltner and Dehority observed a simultaneous disappearance of both cellobiose and cellulose. Although concentrations of the soluble carbohydrates were considerably higher in the study by Huang and Forsberg, it is somewhat difficult to explain the observed differences.

THE CELLULOLYTIC COCCI

Based on the morphology and characteristics of a cellulolytic coccus isolated from bovine rumen contents, Sijpesteijn proposed a new genus, *Ruminococcus* in 1948 and expanded the description in 1951 as follows: Spherical cells; gram-positive; generally in chains or pairs; non-motile; no endospores. Cellulose and other carbohydrates fermented with production of large amounts of succinic acid. Anaerobic. Type species is *Ruminococcus flavefaciens*.

Hungate (1957) studied 10 strains of cellulolytic cocci, 7 isolated from cattle and 3 from sheep. In order to accommodate all of his strains, plus some additional strains isolated by other workers, he redefined the genus *Ruminococcus*: spherical cells, somewhat elongated prior to division; single, in twos or in chains, never in tetrads or cubical packets. Non-motile, non-sporeforming. Gram-positive, gram-negative or gram-variable. Anaerobic. Ferments carbohydrates to form acetic acid, at least traces of H_2 and various combinations of ethanol, formic acid, lactic acid and succinic acid. Type species *Ruminococcus flavefaciens* Sijpesteijn.

Description of the type species *Ruminococcus flavefaciens* Sijpesteijn is: cells almost spherical, diameter 0.8 - 0.9 µm; generally in chains; a yellow pigment is produced by many strains on cellulose; utilizable carbon sources: cellulose and cellobiose, glucose used by some strains; maltose, lactose, xylose and starch not used. Principle end-products are acetic, formic and succinic acids, traces of H_2 and lactate. Catalase negative. Obligate anaerobe, mesophilic.

Since several of Hungate's cocci differed from this description (1957), he established a new species, *Ruminococcus albus*: cells usually single or in twos; often slightly elongated prior to division; 0.8 to 2.0 µm in diameter; produce little or no yellow pigment. Gram-negative to gram-variable. Capsule often formed. Ferments cellulose and cellobiose, but usually does not ferment glucose and other sugars. Hydrogen, CO_2, ethanol, acetic acid, formic acid and lactic acid are produced in various combinations and proportions, but no succinic acid. Usually not iodophilic, strain 69 is type strain.

Bryant *et al.* (1958) published the characteristics of twelve strains of cellulolytic ruminococci isolated from cattle which they were able to place in the two described species. However, they suggested that the description of *Ruminococcus albus* be amended to include organisms that produce small amounts of succinic acid. On the basis of this work and subsequent studies by numerous other workers (Dehority, 1963; Kistner and Gouws, 1964; Jarvis and Annison, 1967; Shane *et al.*, 1969; Van Gylswyk and Roche, 1970) the most useful criteria for differentiating these two species would be the general lack of gas and ethanol production by *R. flavefaciens*, and little or no succinate production by *R. albus*. Chain formation by *R. flavefaciens* is also considered by many workers to be an important characteristic.

Other general characteristics of *Ruminococcus* are an obligate requirement for CO_2 and NH_3 and presence of reducing sugars in the medium when grown on an excess of cellulose. All strains ferment cellulose and cellobiose. The number of additional carbohydrates fermented is quite limited for most strains, although occasional strains do ferment a large number of carbohydrates. Characteristics and fermentation end-products for many different strains of *Ruminococcus flavefaciens* and *Ruminococcus albus* can be found in the references listed in the previous paragraph. In 1972, Moore *et al.* amended the genus description of *Ruminococcus* Sijpesteijn, based on the isolation of 124 strains of a gram-positive, anaerobic, strongly amylolytic coccus from the feces of humans and hogs. The emended description allows species which do not ferment cellulose and do hydrolyze starch to be included in the genus. They proposed a new species, *Ruminococcus bromii* sp. n. be established and included all 124 strains in this species. In more recent work from the same laboratory, five additional species of *Ruminococcus* have been described (Holdeman and Moore, 1974; Moore *et al.*, 1976). All of the organisms were isolated from human intestinal contents or feces. As far as can be determined from the descriptions of these species, none are cellulolytic.

Dehority (1977), isolated five strains of anaerobic, gram-variable cellulolytic cocci from cecal contents of the guinea pig. They were classified as belonging to the genus *Ruminococcus*, but differed from most previously described strains of the two recognized cellulolytic species of this genus as follows: (a) Lactate was the major fermentation product. Lesser amounts of formate and ethanol along with a trace of succinate were also produced. No gas production was observed and an uptake of acetate occurred; (b) No growth occurred at 30°C; however, good growth was observed at 38°C and 45°C;

(c) Xylose, arabinose, sucrose and lactose were fermented by all strains. Rumen fluid was required for growth in a complete medium containing all nutrients previously found to be required by species in this genus.

Ten strains of cellulolytic cocci, eight isolated from rumen contents of Alaskan reindeer and two isolated from musk-oxen, were characterized by Dehority (1986). The two musk-oxen strains were identified as *R. albus* and one reindeer strain as *R. flavefaciens*; however, the seven remaining strains differed from the two described species in that the major end-products were approximately equimolar amounts of ethanol, formic acid and lactic acid, with lesser amounts of acetic acid and only a trace of hydrogen. The magnitude of difference between these seven strains and the two described species is no larger than that observed between strains isolated from other animal species and habitats. Without further information, these cultures can be classified as *Ruminococcus* species, possibly a biotype of *R. flavefaciens* or *R. albus*. Other than cellobiose, the seven strains utilized only polysaccharides as energy sources, i.e., cellulose, xylan and pectin. This may reflect an adaptation or selection of *Ruminococcus* which has occurred in arctic ruminants where plants contain relatively low concentrations of soluble sugars.

BUTYRIVIBRIO FIBRISOLVENS

The first isolation of *Butyrivibrio fibrisolvens* was reported by Hungate in 1950. He termed his isolate (strain W) a less actively cellulolytic rod. Although the species was isolated in cellulose medium, he noted that the cellulose was not completely digested around the colony. Bryant and Small (1956) established the species on the basis of a study of 48 strains which had been isolated in 40% rumen fluid-glucose-cellobiose-agar (RGCA) medium. It was of extreme interest that only three of their 48 strains were cellulolytic. Hungate (1966) reported that over several years, a large number of *Butyrivibrio* species were isolated in his laboratory, and in general, those isolated in cellulose medium were cellulolytic, whereas only a few cellulolytic strains were isolated on soluble sugar medium. Dehority (1966) isolated five strains of *B. fibrisolvens* with a selective xylan medium. Quantitative measurement of cellulose digestion for these isolates, with 0.75% cellulose substrate, gave digestibilities of 0, 5.6, 10.0, 9.8 and 23.2%. Under these same conditions, *F. succinogenes, R. albus* and *R. flavefaciens* digest about 90-100% of the cellulose.

Although *Butyrivibrio fibrisolvens* occurs in fairly large numbers in most animals, its slow and limited ability to digest cellulose with respect to *F. succinogenes* and the cellulolytic cocci, would suggest that it does not play a very important role *in vivo* as far as cellulose digestion is concerned. On the other hand, workers in South Africa have found *B. fibrisolvens* to be the most abundant cellulose digesting organism occurring in the rumen of sheep fed low-protein Teff hay (Shane *et al.*, 1969; Gilchrist and Kistner, 1972).

Butyrivibrio fibrisolvens is an anaerobic, nonsporeforming, gram-negative, motile, slightly curved rod. Dimensions usually vary between 0.4 and 0.8 µm in width and 1.0 - 3.0 µm in length. In general, CO_2, rumen fluid, and NH_3, are not required for growth. H_2S and indole are not produced, nitrate is not reduced, and gelatin is not liquified. Starch is hydrolyzed. A fairly large number of carbohydrates are fermented with considerable differences occurring between strains. End-products of fermentation are H_2, CO_2, formic, butyric and lactic acids and ethanol. Slight production or an uptake of acetic acid is generally also observed. Although *Butyrivibrio* consistently gives a gram-negative reaction with standard staining procedures, electron microscopy studies indicated that its cell wall is characteristic of a gram-positive organism (Cheng and Costerton, 1977). However, the cell wall is extremely thin which may account for its gram-negative staining. Characteristics of a number of *B. fibrisolvens* strains can be found in publications by Hungate (1966), Dehority (1966), Shane *et al*. (1969) and Dehority and Grubb (1977). Attempts to separate the genus *Butyrivibrio* into more than one species, based on phenotypic characteristics have been unsuccessful.

Moore *et al*. amended the genus description for *Butyrivibrio* in 1976 as follows: curved rods which occur singly or in chains or filaments and which may or may not be helical; cells are motile, monotrichous or lophotrichous, (tuft of flagella on one end), with polar or subpolar flagella; nonmotile variants may occur. No resting stages are known. Cells are gram-negative. Metabolism is fermentative, carbohydrates being the main fermentable substrates, with the production of butyrate as one of the important products. Strains are strictly anaerobic. Type species, *B. fibrisolvens*. These authors then describe *Butyrivibrio crossotus* sp. nov. which they isolated from human feces. The amended genus description which includes lophotrichous flagellation allows this classification. They felt that the properties of this species were close enough to those of the genus *Butyrivibrio* that it would be better to amend the genus than to create a new genus.

Margherita and Hungate (1963) have reported some very interesting data on the serological analysis of rumen *Butyrivibrio* strains isolated from different areas. Some cross-reactivity was noted for all strains; however, much serological heterogeneity was observed. The greatest degree of agglutinating cross-reactivity was observed between a Pullman, Washington strain and an isolate from an African zebu, and two strains isolated simultaneously from two African zebu in the same herd. In a second study (Margherita *et al*., 1964), serological relationships were tested between five *Butyrivibrio* strains isolated from a single animal. The strains were serologically monospecific, even those very closely related biochemically. Two years later fluorescein-conjugated antisera against three of these strains was tested against rumen contents of the same animal. No homologous cell types were found. It would thus appear that a great deal of variability exists between the serological characteristics of morphologically and biochemically similar strains within this species.

Mannarelli (1988) examined 39 strains of *B. fibrisolvens* for DNA relatedness, using guanine plus cytosine base contents and DNA hybridization studies. His results indicated that the 39 strains comprised a genetically heterogenous group and probably represent a number of separate species and even possibly several genera. Data suggested that 20 strains could probably be grouped into 5 separate species, while the remaining 19 strains were not closely related to any other strain. The highest number of strains which could be grouped into one species was six.

An interesting study was reported by Teather (1982) in which he was able to show that plasmids are a common feature of *B. fibrisolvens*. Plasmids are extracellular bodies which contain DNA and are capable of transmitting genetic information from one cell to another. The similarity of the plasmids in all strains of *B. fibrisolvens* examined suggested to the authors that they carried information which was essential for survival of the host cell under the growth conditions used. The considerable variation observed in the fermentative patterns for different strains suggests that these may be plasmid-determined traits.

EUBACTERIUM CELLULOSOLVENS (FORMERLY *CILLOBACTERIUM CELLULOSOLVENS*)

In 1958, Bryant *et al.* isolated a single strain of a new species of cellulose digesting bacteria from the bovine rumen. It was an anaerobic, gram-positive, peritrichous rod with pointed ends that produced primarily lactic acid in rumen fluid-cellobiose medium. They classified the organism as *Cillobacterium cellulosolvens*, and based on its low numbers judged it to be relatively unimportant in the rumen.

Van Glyswyk and Hoffman reported the isolation and characterization of nine strains of cellulolytic *Cillobacterium* from the ovine rumen in 1970. They estimated that the organism occurred at numbers of 10^6 in rumen contents. Since end-products of their strains differed from that of the type strain, they broadened the species description and classified the organisms as *Cillobacterium cellulosolvens*.

Subsequently, Prins *et al.* (1972) isolated seven strains of cellulolytic, gram-positive, motile rods. One strain was isolated from a heifer at Davis, California and the remaining six from cows in the Netherlands. They were identified as *Cillobacterium cellulosolvens*, now named *Eubacterium cellulosolvens*. The organisms were isolated from 10^{-8} dilutions of rumen contents and counts in three cows were 3.2, 6.1 and 7.1 x 10^8/ml rumen fluid. The authors concluded that despite the high numbers observed and the high rate of cellulose digestion observed *in vitro*, their importance as cellulolytic bacteria in the rumen may be doubtful since so many soluble carbohydrates are fermented. They suggested its importance in cellulose digestion in the rumen to possibly be similar to that of *B. fibrisolvens*. However, very few strains of *B. fibrisolvens* appear to be as strongly cellulolytic in vitro. The authors described their strains morphologically as gram-positive in young cultures, showing long chains with a zig-zag pattern. In older cultures, cells became gram-negative and the chains broke up into pairs and singles. The bacteria were actively motile by means of peritrichous flagella, present in low numbers up to many per cell (peritrichous means flagella located completely around the cell). Cells measured 0.7 to 3.0 µm in length (typically 1-2 µm) by 0.5 to 1.2 µm in width (typically 0.6 to 0.8 µm). Cells appeared coccoid to rod-shaped.

CELLULOLYTIC *CLOSTRIDIUM* SP.

Until 1987, only four species of cellulolytic, anaerobic spore-forming *Clostridium* had been isolated and identified from the rumen: *C. cellobioparus, C. locheadii, C. longisporum* and *C. polysaccharolyticum* (Hungate, 1944; Hungate, 1957; van Gylswyk *et al.*, 1980). In general they are gram-positive, anaerobic, sporeforming, non-motile rods, which digest cellulose rapidly producing CO_2, H_2, acetic, formic, butyric acids and ethanol. Based on their sporadic occurrence in relatively low numbers it has been suggested that they are of limited importance. Shane *et al.* (1969) isolated two anaerobic spore formers from the rumen of sheep in South Africa, which were classified as belonging to the genus *Clostridium*. They differed from all other species, but were not described and named.

Kelly *et al.* (1987) were trying to isolate bacteriophage from rumen contents by treating the contents with 1% chloroform, and repeatedly grew bacteria which produced clear zones on cellulose agar plates prepared and incubated in a CO_2 glove box. Most of the colonies were orange and occurred in numbers ranging between 2×10^4 and 3×10^6 cells/ml. They repeated their studies over a year's time, and the bacterium persisted for that period. Based on morphology and biochemical characteristics, the organism was designated as a new species, *C. chartatabidum*. It most closely resembles *C. longisporum*, but differs in not producing formate, producing butyrate and not fermenting galactose. The organism was observed to bind very tightly to cellulose; however, it does not ferment xylan. The authors enumerated cellulolytic ruminococci in their animals and found numbers ranging from $0.3 - 6.3 \times 10^8$/ml. Thus, *C. chartatabidum* would occur in numbers of 10% or less of the more common rumen cellulolytics. However, its persistence over time would suggest it is probably a true rumen microorganism.

ADDITIONAL SPECIES OF CELLULOLYTIC BACTERIA IN THE RUMEN

Several additional species of cellulolytic bacteria have been isolated from rumen contents. Leatherwood and Sharma (1972) isolated an unusual bacterium which ferments cellulose and produces butyric acid. It grows in long twisted chains and often forms a double-helical pattern. The organism is an obligate anaerobe, gram-negative rod, $0.3 \times 1\text{-}3 \, \mu m$, and non-motile. Maluszynska and Janota-Bassalik (1974) isolated a cellulolytic *Micromonospora* from the rumen of a sheep, similar, but not identical with the cellulolytic actinomycete isolated by Hungate (1946) from the alimentary tract of a termite. Neither of these organisms is considered to be important in the rumen because of low numbers and such sporadic occurrence.

In 1980, Van Gylswyk isolated a gram-negative nonsporeforming rod from sheep rumen contents which fermented both cellulose and starch. The organism, *Fusobacterium polysaccharolyticum* n. sp. was isolated from several different animals and occurred at concentrations of at least 10^6 per g ingesta. The principal end products from cellulose fermentation were formate and butyrate while acetate was utilized. These characteristics are similar to those of *B. fibrisolvens*; however, *F. polysaccharolyticum* is peritrichous with numerous flagella.

Nutrient requirements of cellulolytic species

In 1955, Bryant and Doetsch reported that the factors in rumen fluid necessary for the growth of *F. succinogenes* were in the volatile acid fraction of rumen fluid. Subsequent investigation revealed that this species required a combination of a branched-chain acid (isobutyric, isovaleric, or 2-methylbutyric) and a straight chain acid (C_5 to C_8). The minimum concentrations for good growth with strain S85 were 0.3 and 0.15 µM/ml of medium for valeric and isovaleric acids, respectively. Allison *et al.*, in 1958, reported that a number of strains of ruminococci require branched-chain volatile fatty acids for growth. This requirement could be satisfied by isovaleric acid. Bryant and Robinson confirmed these observations with additional strains in 1961.

Dehority *et al.* (1967) investigated the volatile fatty acid (VFA) requirements of the cellulolytic rumen bacteria. Using gas chromatography, they found that most commercial samples of isovaleric acid were contaminated with 2-methylbutyric acid. However, they were able to obtain pure samples of the various acids and their results on VFA requirements of the cellulolytic bacteria are presented in Table 8.3. Strains of *F. succinogenes* required a combination of valeric plus either isobutyric or 2-methylbutyric acid. Isovaleric acid was completely inactive. Either isobutyric or 2-methylbutyric acid was required for the growth of *R. albus* 7. Strain C-94 of *R. flavefaciens* grew slowly in the presence of any one of the three branched-chain acids, but later studies indicated that a combination of isobutyric and 2-methylbutyric acids appeared to satisfy this organism's growth requirements. None of the individual acids or mixtures of straight- and branched-chain acids allowed growth of *R. flavefaciens* strain C1a which would approach the response obtained from the total mixture of acids. Further work indicated that all three branched-chain acids were required for optimal growth by this strain, although isovaleric acid only appeared to influence the rate of growth. Either 2-methylbutyric or isovaleric acid allowed growth of nearly the same magnitude as that of the positive control for *R. flavefaciens* B34b. Determination of the quantitative fatty acid requirements for the three *F. succinogenes* strains indicated that 0.1 µmole of valeric per ml and 0.05 µmole of 2-methylbutyric per ml permitted maximal growth. However, with isobutyric acid as the branched-chain component, strains A3c and B21a required 0.1 µmole/ml in contrast to S85 which exhibited optimal growth at the 0.05 µmole/ml level. By use of mixtures of isobutyric and 2-methylbutyric acids, good growth of C94 was obtained at concentrations of 0.1 and 0.01 µmole/ml, respectively. About 0.3 µmole/ml of each acid was required for satisfactory growth of C1a.

Table 8.3. GROWTH RESPONSE OF CELLULOLYTIC RUMEN BACTERIA TO THE ADDITION OF VARIOUS VOLATILE FATTY ACIDS[a]

	Maximum optical density						
	Bacteriodes succinogenes			Ruminococcus flavefaciens			
Acids added	A3c	S-85	B21a	C-94	C1a	B34b	R. albus 7
None	0	0	0	0	0	0.27	0
	(62)[b]	(62)	(62)	(62)	(67)	(118)	(54)
All	1.53	1.4	1.37	0.85	0.68	0.69	0.75
	(26)	(20)	(21)	(26)	(17)	(28)	(25)
Valeric	0	0.05	0	0	0.03	0.49	0
	(62)	(40)	(60)	(64)	(73)	(92)	(54)
Isobutyric	0.74	0.60	0.06	0.75	0.27	0.22	0.72
	(59)	(64)	(45)	(63)	(135)	(67)	(30)
2-Methylbutyric	0.04	0	0.03	0.57	0.04	0.69	0.78
	(51)	(62)	(45)	(150)	(75)	(31)	(27)
Isovaleric	0	0	0	0.54	0.08	0.62	0
	(62)	(62)	(60)	(100)	(103)	(36)	(54)
Valeric + isobutyric	1.47	1.38	1.38	0.76	0.37	0.38	0.86
	(26)	(19)	(24)	(59)	(91)	(51)	(22)
Valeric + 2-methylbutyric	1.50	1.38	1.34	0.57	0.05	0.60	0.82
	(28)	(19)	(18)	(151)	(83)	(35)	(25)
Valeric + isovaleric	0	0.13	0	0.54	0.15	0.62	0
	(62)	(47)	(60)	(112)	(115)	(39)	(54)

[a] Data from Dehority et al. (1967).
[b] The figure in parentheses indicates the hours of incubation required.

Wegner and Foster (1963) have shown that the VFA's required by *F. succinogenes* are used as precursors for the synthesis of long-chain fatty acids and fatty aldehydes, which in turn were used in the synthesis of phospholipid. Allison and Bryant (1963) have also shown that these acids are used as carbon skeletons in the biosyntheis of the amino acids valine, leucine and isoleucine.

Vitamin requirements of the cellulolytic species have been studied by Bryant et al. (1959), Bryant and Robinson (1961a) and Scott and Dehority (1965). A total of seven strains of *F. succinogenes* have been studied and all except one have an absolute requirement for biotin. Growth of the one strain not having an absolute requirement was markedly stimulated. A stimulation of two strains was observed with PABA. The remaining B-vitamins were without effect on the growth of *F. succinogenes*. The vitamin requirements of *R. albus* and *R. flavefaciens* are a bit more complex. All twelve strains studied had an absolute requirement for biotin. Other B-vitamins which were essential or stimulatory for some of the individual strains were PABA, pyridoxine, folic acid, riboflavin and thiamine. One strain of *R. flavefaciens* was shown by Scott and Dehority (1965) to have an absolute requirement for B_{12} in the absence of methionine.

Considerable variation appears to exist between individual strains. Gill and King (1958), studied one strain of *B. fibrisolvens* and found biotin, folic acid and pyridoxal to be required.

With regard to mineral requirements, Bryant *et al.* (1959) found $PO_4^=$, NH_4^+, Mg^{++}, Ca^{++}, K^+ and Na^+ to be essential for the growth of one strain of *F. succinogenes*. Caldwell and Hudson (1974) found sodium to be an obligate growth requirement for almost all the predominant species of rumen bacteria, including the cellulolytics. One of their conclusions was extremely interesting, "the rumen appears analogous to an inland sea, and appears to be the first terrestrial environment studied in which the majority of the predominant bacteria required Na^+". They suggest that a growth requirement for Na^+ appears to be more frequent among non-marine bacteria than had been previously believed.

For *F. succinogenes* and the ruminococci, NH_3 is essential and is utilized as the sole source of nitrogen by most strains. *B. fibrisolvens* strains are divided into two groups, NH_3 is essential for good growth in one, and the other utilized either NH_3 or mixtures of amino acids.

All species of cellulolytic rumen bacteria appear to have an absolute requirement for CO_2 based on detailed studies conducted by Dehority (1971). *F. succinogenes* and *R. flavefaciens* require at least 0.05% CO_2 in the medium for optimal growth. These two species produce succinic acid as one of their major end-products and CO_2 must be fixed in the pathway to succinate production. Thus without CO_2, these species are unable to obtain energy for growth. *R. albus* and *B. fibrisolvens* require much lower concentrations of CO_2, probably for biosynthetic purposes involved in cell growth and multiplication.

Many strains of *Ruminococcus* and at least one known strain of *B. fibrisolvens* have requirements for still unknown nutrients present in rumen fluid (Bryant and Robinson, 1961; Dehority, 1963, 1966; Jarvis and Annison, 1967; Slyter and Weaver, 1969). These strains cannot be cultured in a medium containing casein hydrolysate, cellobiose, VFA, B-vitamins, minerals, CO_2 and cysteine. Addition of 10% clarified rumen fluid to the above medium will generally support maximal growth of most of the *Ruminococcus* strains.

Studies on the requirement of several *Ruminococcus albus* strains for rumen fluid revealed that phenylpropanoic acid (PPA) accounted for at least part of the stimulatory effect of rumen fluid on the rate of growth and of cellulose digestion by *R. albus* 8 grown on chemically defined medium (Hungate and Stack, 1982). Subsequent work by Stack *et al.*, (1983) showed that the rate of cellulose digestion in defined medium with PPA could be increased further by adding at least 6.6% (v/v) of rumen fluid. Eventually they identified phenylacetic acid (PAA) as the active component. Later, Stack and Hungate (1984) reported that PPA-grown cells of *R. albus* 8 produced substantial quantities of cell-bound cellulase as well as a very high-molecular-weight extracellular cellulase and lesser quantities of two low-molecular weight cellulases. In contrast, PPA-deprived bacteria produced greater quantities of total cellulase but all of it in the soluble, low-molecular-weight forms. *R. albus* cells grown in the presence of PPA produced an extensively lobed capsule which contained cellulase activity. Stack and Cotta (1986) found that the addition of PPA increased the rate of cellulose utilization by two different strains of *R. albus*; however, it had little effect on the rate of growth when cellobiose was the substrate. Rates of growth for two strains of *R. flavefaciens* and three strains of *B. fibrisolvens* were not affected by PPA, regardless of energy source. These same authors suggested that the enhancement of cellulose digestion in *R. albus* by PPA may have use in differentiating between species of ruminococci. More recently, Odenyo *et al*. (1991) found that the addition of PPA and PAA significantly increased degradation of alkaline hydrogen peroxide-treated wheat straw in a defined medium by *R. albus* 8, but not by *R. flavefaciens* FD-1. No stimulation of *R. albus* 8 was observed in a complex medium. Their data also suggested that *R. flavefaciens* FD-1 had no preference in digesting cellulose or hemicellulose, whereas *R. albus* 8 appeared to prefer hemicellulose over cellulose. In other studies, Morrison *et al*. (1990) found that PPA, but not PAA, markedly increased the extent of purified cellulose hydrolysis in continuous culture by a strain of *R. albus* isolated in South Africa. From their studies, they concluded that adherence of *R. albus* to the insoluble substrate appears to be improved in the presence of PPA.

EFFECT OF SOLUBLE CARBOHYDRATES ON CELLULOSE DIGESTION

The effects of soluble carbohydrates on the rate and extent of cellulose digestion by *F. succinogenes, R. albus* and *R. flavefaciens* were studied by Hiltner and Dehority (1983). Experiments on rate of cellulose digestion were run comparing a standard inoculum, a large inoculum (5x), simulating possible rapid increase in numbers of bacteria from utilization of a soluble sugar, and standard inoculum plus 0.15% cellobiose. Data for *F. succinogenes* are shown in Figure 8.1a. Rates of cellulose digestion were similar between 18 and 24 h for the fermentations with the larger inoculum and added cellobiose. Clearly, cellulose and soluble carbohydrate appear to be used simultaneously. Adding glucose during the period of active cellulose digestion confirmed the previous suggestion that soluble carbohydrate and cellulose digestion occur simultaneously (Figure 8.1b). Similar results were obtained with both *R. flavefaciens* and *R. albus*. The rate of cellulose digestion decreased markedly after 24 h for *F. succinogenes* in those fermentations containing cellobiose, which suggested a possible pH effect. Figure 8.2 illustrates the effects of initial medium pH and of cellobiose concentration upon pH and cellulose digestion for *R. flavefaciens*. Exposing the cellulolytics to a low pH environment had little effect upon their subsequent ability to digest cellulose (Figure 8.3). The inoculum substrate had little effect on rate of cellulose digestion by the ruminococii; however, rate was much slower for *F. succinogenes* cells grown on soluble carbohydrate as compared to cellulose. Additional experiments comparing cellobiose grown *F. succinogenes* with attached and unattached cellulose grown cells indicated that the increased lag time for *F. succinogenes* was probably related to attachment mechanisms.

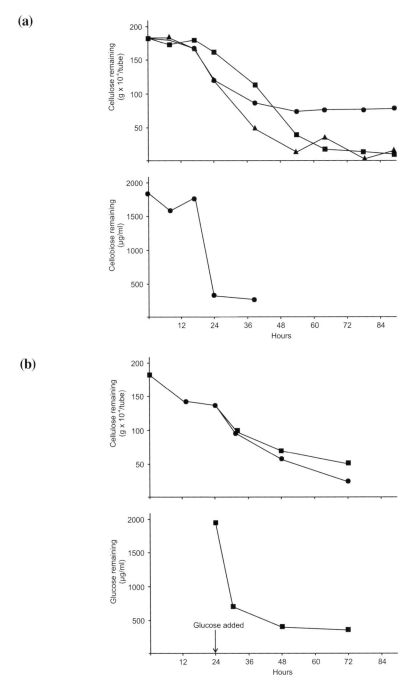

Figure 8.1. (a). Effect of increased inoculum and added cellobiose on purified cellulose digestion by *F. succinogenes*. (■), 0.2 ml inoculum; (▲), 1.0 ml inoculum; (●), 0.2 ml inoculum plus 0.15% cellobiose. (b). Effect of adding glucose after initiation of cellulose digestion by *F. succinogenes*. (●), no glucose (control); (■) 0.15% glucose added. (from Hiltner and Dehority, 1983).

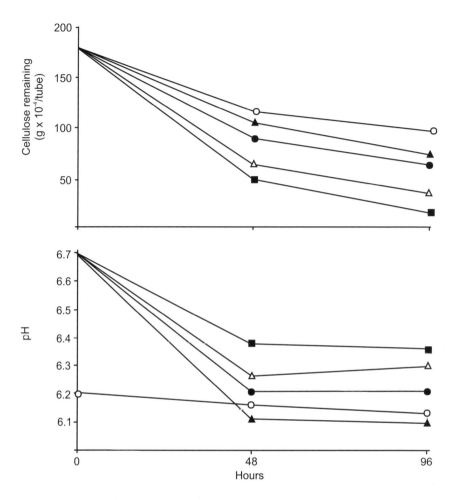

Figure 8.2. Effect of initial medium pH and three levels of cellobiose on cellulose digestion by *R. flavefaciens*. Symbols: (○), low-pH medium, no cellobiose; (■) regular-pH, medium, no cellobiose (control); (△) regular-pH plus 0.05% cellobiose; (●) regular-pH plus 0.1% cellobiose; (▲) regular-pH plus 0.15% cellobiose (from Hiltner and Dehority, 1983).

Factors effecting adhesion and detachment of cellulolytic bacteria to insoluble cellulose substrates

Bhat *et al.* (1990) studied the adhesion of *R. flavefaciens* and *F. succinogenes* to barley straw. They found that maximum adhesion for both organisms occurred at pH 6 during the mid-to late-exponential growth phase. Addition of 0.1% methyl cellulose or carboxymethyl cellulose inhibited adhesion from 24 to 33%. *R. flavefaciens* had no effect on *F. succinogenes* adhesion, while *F. succinogenes* decreased *R. flavefaciens* adhesion by approximately 20%. Two non-cellulolytic species which also adhered to

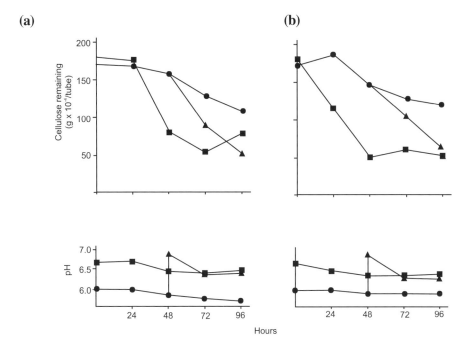

Figure 8.3. Effect of exposing cellulolytic bacteria to a low-pH environment on their subsequent ability to digest cellulose. (a) *Fibrobacter succinogenes*; (b) *Ruminococcus flavefaciens*. (●), low-pH medium; (■) control; (▲) low-pH medium after adjustment to pH 6.9. (from Hiltner and Dehority, 1983).

the straw, *Prevotella ruminicola* and *Selenomonas ruminantium* did not affect adhesion of the two cellulolytic organisms. From these observations, the authors concluded that *R. flavefaciens* and *F. succinogenes* have unique adhesion sites on the barley straw, i.e., specific attachment sites for that organism which are not occupied or blocked by any other organism. It would have been of considerable interest if the authors had included additional strains of the two cellulolytic species, to evaluate whether the attachment sites are strain or species specific.

In a separate study, Roger *et al.* (1990) studied the effects of a number of physiochemical factors on the adhesion of *R. flavefaciens* and *F. succinogenes* to purified cellulose. Adhesion of *R. flavefaciens* to cellulose was almost instantaneous, whereas maximum adhesion of *F. succinogenes* did not occur until about 25 minutes following its addition. In general, adhesion of *F. succinogenes* to purified cellulose appeared to be related to metabolic functions of the cell, i.e., sensitive to low and high temperatures, high concentrations (5%) of glucose or cellobiose, 0.1% hydroxyethyl cellulose, redox potential, pH, lack of monovalent cations, the presence of an inhibitor of membrane ATPases, lasalocid and monensin, or heating to 100°C for 10 minutes. In contrast, *R. flavefaciens* attachment was not affected by any of these parameters, but was sensitive to the removal of divalent cations (Mg^{++} and Ca^{++}), which had no effect on adherence of *F. succinogenes*. The authors suggest that maybe only live cells of *F. succinogenes* are able to attach to cellulose, which could be related to protein and possibly cellulase enzymes on the cell surface. On the other hand, adhesion of *R. flavefaciens* only appears to be influenced by the divalent cations, which could be the link for interaction between the cellulose and large glycocalyx of this species.

Methylcellulose was shown by Rasmussen *et al*. (1988) to inhibit cellulose digestion by *R. flavefaciens*, but not growth on cellobiose or cellulooligosaccharides. Addition of methylcellulose to incubations with bacteria attached to cellulose particles results in their detachment and inhibits growth (Kudo *et al*., 1987). The methylcellulose is not used as a substrate and has no effect when glucose or cellobiose are growth substrates. In a subsequent study, attachment or adherence of *R. flavefaciens* to cellulose was inhibited by formaldehyde, methylcellulose and carboxymethylcellulose (Rasmussen *et al*. (1989).

Mechanisms for adhesion to cellulose

Early studies by Groleau and Forsberg (1981) indicated that the cellulase enzyme of *F. succinogenes* was probably cell-bound, requiring an intimate association between the cell envelope and the substrate for cellulose digestion to occur. In a later study, Forsberg *et al*. (1981) found that *F. succinogenes* appeared to produce subcellular membrane vesicles from blebs, which are formed in pockets between the cells and the cellulose. Shearing forces, including Brownian movement, probably tear the cellulose-bound membrane regions from the cell surface. The membrane fragments then reanneal, forming small vesicles which adhere to the cellulose surface. On the basis of their studies, the authors suggested that *F. succinogenes* releases vesicular packets of hydrolytic enzymes, including cellobiase, xylanase and cellulase, which concentrate and localize enzymatic activity on the insoluble substrate. The enzymatic activity of these subcellular particles undoubtedly provides a source of sugars for those rumen microbes which are unable to degrade the polysaccharides.

Blair and Anderson (1999) also observed ultrastructural protuberances on the cell surface of *Eubacterium cellulosolvens*, but only when grown on cellulose. The authors were able to detect lectin-binding sites and a cellulose-affinity protein fraction which would be consistent with the presence of cellulosome complexes.

Based on studies with fungal cellulases, the model developed for extensive hydrolysis of crystalline cellulose requires the synergistic activity of three different cellulase components. These are an endo - 1,4-ß-glucanase (carboxymethyl cellulase), an exo - 1, 4-ß-glucanase (cellobiohydrolase) and a ß-glucosidase (cellobiase) (Huang and Forsberg, 1987). *F. succinogenes* has been shown to produce multiple endoglucanases, 70% of which occur extracellularly, cellobiase, which is cell associated and an exoglucanase, cellobiosidase, which is located in the periplasmic space (Groleau and Forsberg, 1981, Huang and Forsberg, 1987). This latter enzyme was shown to be a cellodextrinase, with an exo-type function. *F. succinogenes* also produces an extracellular acetylxylan esterase and a ferulic acid esterase (McDermid *et al.*, 1990). These enzyme activities should markedly enhance the ability of *F. succinogenes* to degrade the cross-links which appear to stabilize the cell wall matrix.

An extensive review on what is presently known about the adhesion mechanisms of the major cellulolytic rumen bacteria, i.e., *Fibrobacter succinogenes, Ruminococcus flavefaciens* and *Ruminococcus albus* has been published by Miron *et al.* (2001). They divided the process of adhesion into four phases: (1) transport or movement of the nonmotile bacteria to the substrate surface; (2) initial nonspecific adhesion to unprotected areas on the substrate surface, generally through constitutive elements in the bacterial glycocalyx; (3) specific adhesion to the substrate with adhesins or by ligand formation, which can involve cellulosome complexes, fimbriae connections, glycosylated epitopes of cellulose-binding protein or glycocalyx and the cellulose-binding domain of enzymes; (4) proliferation of the attached bacteria using energy from the potentially digestible fractions of the substrate.

(1)   Movement of the bacteria to the substrate. Since the three predominant species of rumen cellulolytic bacteria are nonmotile, their contact with the insoluble substrate is dependent on the size of the free-suspended population in rumen fluid and the concentration of available substrate sites.

(2)   Initial nonspecific adhesion to the substrate. The initial nonspecific adhesion of the bacteria takes place when the cell comes within range (2 to 50 nm) of van der Waals forces, i.e., hydrophobic, ionic and electrostatic interactions between the cell surface and solid substrate. Pell and Schofield (1993) have defined this process as a combination of reversible and irreversible processes which do not involve either ligands or specific adhesins between the substrate and bacterial cell wall. This initial binding process also appears to involve the constitutive bacterial glycocalyx. Costerton *et al.* (1981) have defined the bacterial cell glycocalyx as those polysaccharide-, glycoprotein-, protein-containing structures of bacterial origin which lie outside the outer membrane of gram-negative cells and the peptidoglycan of gram-positive cells. The rate at which nonspecific adhesion occurs is relatively fast, ranging from 1 to 5 minutes for the ruminococci and between 15 to 30 minutes for *F. succinogenes*. This nonspecific adhesion is a prerequisite for the next step of specific adhesion.

(3)   Specific adhesion to the substrate. This step is defined as the process by which ligands or adhesins on the surface of the bacterial cell recognize and combine with receptors on the substrate. Based on a number of studies as referenced in Miron *et al.* (2001), adhesins have been observed to include polycellulosome complexes, fimbriae or pili, glycocalyx capsule, cellulosic fibrils, cellulose binding proteins and enzyme binding domains. This close adhesion to the substrate provides a distinct advantage for the bacteria, in that the cellulolytic enzymes are concentrated on the substrate and other microorganisms are excluded from the site. This in turn allows the cellulolytic species ready acess to the products of cellulose

hydrolysis. Additional advantages are that the attached bacteria are fairly resistant to possible engulfment by the rumen protozoa and their cellulolytic enzymes are shielded from free rumen proteases.

(4) Growth and colonization on the plant tissue. In this final stage, the bacteria multiply and form colonies along the digestible areas of the plant substrate.

Factors related to the bacteria (age, envelope and microbial competition), substrate (rupture or breaks in the plant surface) and environmental conditions (temperature, pH, presence of cations and presence of soluble carbohydrates) all can effect bacterial adhesion to plant tissue. In addition, each of the three predominant cellulolytic rumen bacteria appear to have different mechanisms of adhesion to cellulose. *F. succinogenes* binds to plant tissues with adhesins, both the cellulose-binding domain (CBD) of enzymes type and the glycosylated epitopes of cellulose-binding protein (CBP) or glycocalyx type. Based solely on electron microscopy, a cellulosome-complex and fimbriae or pili may also be involved. Two mechanisms play a role in the specific adhesion of *R. flavefaviens*, cellulosome-like complexes and carbohydrate epitopes of the glycocalyx layer. In *R. albus*, a cellusomal-like mechanism and the production of fimbrial-like structures appear to be the principal mechanisms involved in adhesion. Both the glycocalyx, CBP and enzyme CBD may also have a part in the nonspecific phase of adhesion.

Additional insight into the mechanisms involved in bacterial adhesion and digestion of cellulose has been reported by Moon and Anderson (2001). They found that when grown on cellulose, *Eubacterium cellulosolvens* alters its cytoplasmic membrane protein, lipoprotein and fatty acid composition. Membrane protein fractions from cells grown on cellulose differed from those grown on soluble sugars. Also, two lipoproteins were present in the cellulose-grown cells. A higher ratio of oleic acid (unsaturated) to palmitic acid (saturated) was observed in the cells grown on cellulose. This change in fatty acid composition would suggest a possible increase in membrane fluidity which may be necessary for the assembly and function of the proteins in the cellulosome complex.

For those readers interested in more detailed information on the cellulosome complex and its role in the extracellular degradation of insoluble cellulose and other plant polysaccharides, an excellent review has been published by Shoham *et al*. (1999). The authors also suggest that limited evidence indicates that the cellulosome is a paradigm for the degradation of other structural polysaccharides in the plant, i.e., hemicelluloses, pectin, chitin, etc.

Digestion of purified and forage celluloses

In 1963, Halliwell and Bryant studied the digestibility of ground cellulose powder and dewaxed cotton fibers by *F. succinogenes*, *R. albus* and *R. flavefaciens*. Their data is shown in Table 8.4. Activity of all cultures is fairly similar on cellulose powder;

however, *F. succinogenes* was able to extensively solubilize the more resistant cotton fiber cellulose. Van Glyswyk and Labuschagne (1971) studied the rate of digestion of ball-milled filter paper and found the ruminococci were much more active than *B. fibrisolvens*. *R. albus* digested cellulose at a more rapid rate than *R. flavefaciens*.

Using a continuous culture fermentative system, Pavlostathis *et al*. (1988) were able to show that *R. albus* can convert almost all of the carbon from insoluble cellulose to fermentation products and biomass (92-97%). The rate limiting step was shown to be the conversion of the insoluble cellulose to soluble substrates which were then fermented to end products as fast as they were produced.

Table 8.4. SOLUBILIZATION OF PURIFIED CELLULOSE BY PURE CULTURES OF CELLULOLYTIC RUMEN BACTERIA[a]

Organism	Cellulose solubilized, %	
	Ground cellulose powder	Cotton fibers
F. succinogenes S85	88	97
R. albus 7	88	10
R. albus D-89	88	40
R. flavefaciens C-94	72	0
R. flavefaciens FD-1	90	55

[a] Data from Halliwell and Bryant (1963).

Dehority and Scott (1967) investigated the extent of cellulose digestion from intact forages by pure cultures of cellulolytic rumen bacteria. A limiting substrate level was used so that the extent of digestion was controlled either by availability of the cellulose in the forage or the ability of the organism to digest that form of cellulose. Their data is shown in Table 8.5. As you will note, *F. succinogenes* strains were able to digest significantly greater amounts of cellulose from forages than were the other species. Two of the four strains of *R. flavefaciens* had a remarkably reduced ability to digest cellulose from alfalfa. *B. fibrisolvens* digested very little of the forage cellulose, the highest value was only 17.7% with immature or boot stage orchardgrass. Across all organisms and forages the extent of cellulose digestion decreased with forage maturity.

Kock and Kistner (1969) investigated the solubilization of cellulose from lipid extracted teff hay. Of 10 *Butyrivibrio* species, solubilization ranged from 10-37%. Two *Clostridium* species solubilized 10.1 and 10.7% while two strains of *R. albus* solubilized 43 and 56% and two *R. flavefaciens* strains 39 and 66%. These data would appear to be in line with the values obtained previously by Dehority and Scott (1967).

Degradation of intact bermuda grass and orchardgrass by several species of cellulolytic rumen bacteria was investigated by Akin and Rigsby (1985). They found that *L. multiparus* could not degrade plant cell wall components and degradation of these two grasses by *B. fibrisolvens* and *R. albus* ranged only from 0 to 14.9% loss of dry matter.

Table 8.5. EXTENT OF DIGESTIBILITY OF CELLULOSE FROM VARIOUS FORAGES BY PURE CULTURES OF CELLULOLYTIC RUMEN BACTERIA[a]

	Cellulose digested (%)							
	F. succinogenes		*R. flavefaciens*				*R. albus*	*B. fib*[c]
Forage[b]	A3c	S-85	B1a	B34b	C1a	C-94	7	H10b
Orchard-1	70.7	73.1	57.4	57.4	49.4	64.3	54.9	17.7
Orchard-2	54.0	54.3	31.8	31.6	28.1	39.9	33.2	3.5
Brome-1	79.4	81.0	58.1	56.3	48.8	65.3	57.3	14.9
Brome-2	58.2	56.0	31.5	31.4	29.9	37.1	32.8	7.1
Reed Canary-1	74.7	77.3	52.3	51.9	45.2	60.4	54.4	13.2
Reed Canary-2	57.1	56.3	29.6	29.4	26.3	39.0	33.3	6.4
Timothy-1	80.3	81.1	57.9	56.7	48.6	67.6	57.9	14.4
Timothy-2	59.7	57.0	32.7	34.5	30.2	41.4	37.3	9.5
Alfalfa-1	61.6	64.2	25.2	54.1	47.8	28.7	53.4	5.9
Alfalfa-2	51.4	52.1	19.8	48.0	41.5	21.2	43.4	6.0
Alfalfa-3	43.5	46.7	16.0	40.6	36.0	12.3	35.1	3.1
Alfalfa	52.6	52.8	23.6	37.1	29.8	24.9	39.4	2.6

[a] Data from Dehority and Scott (1967).
[b] Agronomic description: Grass - 1 (boot stage) and - 2 (bloom stage); Alfalfa - 1 (prebloom), - 2 (early bloom), and - 3 (late bloom).
[c] B. fib = *Butyrivibrio fibrisolvens*

R. flavefaciens degraded 8.2 and 55.3% of bermuda and orchardgrass, respectively. Based on electron microscopy the authors concluded that only *R. flavefaciens* had a capsule, and this was required for attachment and subsequent digestion. They further suggested that their culture of *R. albus* had lost its ability to produce a capsule, which would appear to be an area they should have investigated further, since earlier studies have clearly demonstrated the ability of this strain (*R. albus* 7) to degrade intact forages.

In 1989 Varel isolated two strains of *Clostridium longisporum*, one from a buffalo and the other from a steer. They occurred in numbers of 5×10^6/ml and 17×10^6/ml, respectively. Degradation of alfalfa cell walls dry matter, cellulose and hemicellulose were measured with the strain isolated from the buffalo and compared to values obtained with mixed rumen fluid, *B. fibrisolvens, R. flavefaciens, F. succinogenes* and *R. albus*. Surprisingly, *C. longisporum* degraded all measured fractions of alfalfa cell walls more extensively than any of the other ruminal cellulolytic isolates tested, and almost equivalent to the mixed culture of rumen fluid. However, in subsequent studies this same strain of *C. longisporum* was found to be very limited in its ability to degrade dry matter from barley straw and ryegrass cell walls as compared to alfalfa cell walls (Varel *et al.*, 1989). Although *C. longisporum* extensively solubilized the hemicellulose fraction of alfalfa cell walls, it was unable to use the products as a source of energy. This is very similar to the situation observed with a number of the common cellulolytic rumen species (Coen and Dehority, 1970).

Studies on the possible synergistic effect of combining two cultures in a single fermentation were conducted with four cellulolytic strains (A3c, 7, B34b and B1a), one weakly cellulolytic strain (H10b) and one non-cellulolytic strain (H8a). Using limiting levels of substrate, all possible combinations of two were tested and a significant increase in the extent of cellulose digestion was consistently observed when the non-cellulolytic organism H8a was combined with any of the four cellulolytic strains (Table 8.6). In a later study, Fondevila and Dehority (1996) observed the same increase in digestibility when *R. flavefaciens* B34b and *Prevotella ruminicola* H2b were co-cultured. However, when the organisms were added sequentially (the first organism killed before adding the second), the increase in cellulose digestion only occurred if *P. ruminicola* was the first organism added. As presented in the next two chapters, most strains of *P. ruminicola* are capable of digesting both hemicelluloses and pectin from intact forages, suggesting that this activity exposes additional cellulose to the cellulolytic species. Combinations with the weakly cellulolytic strain H10b either resulted in no change or a decrease in the mean cellulose digestion. In some cases, combination of two cellulolytic strains resulted in an overall decrease in digestibility, i.e., A3c plus B34b.

Table 8.6. EXTENT OF FORAGE CELLULOSE DIGESTION OBTAINED WITH PURE CULTURES OF RUMEN BACTERIA SINGLY OR IN ALL COMBINATIONS OF TWO[a]

		Cellulose digestion, %[b]					
Organism 1[c]	Organism 2...	A3c	7	B34b	B1a	H10b	H8a
A3c		61.9	63.1	44.7[d]	62.2	63.5	66.2[d]
7			44.4	41.2	39.9[e]	40.3[e]	48.8[d]
B34b				44.1	43.5	46.1	47.0[e]
B1a					36.3	32.1[e]	42.2[d]
H10b						8.7	6.1
H8a							1.6

[a] Data from Dehority and Scott (1967) and Dehority (1973).
[b] Mean value for 12 forages (8 grass and 4 alfalfa samples).
[c] A3c, *Fibrobacter succinogenes*; 7, *Ruminococcus albus*; B34b and B1a, *R. flavefaciens*; H10b, *Butyrivibrio fibrisolvens*; and 8a, *Prevotella ruminicola*.
[d] Within a row, significantly different ($P<0.01$) from the mean cellulose digestion for that culture alone.
[e] Within a row, significantly different ($P<0.05$) from the mean cellulose digestion for that culture alone.

Inhibition between species of cellulolytic bacteria

The reduction or inhibition of cellulose digestion when certain species are co-cultured has subsequently been observed by several other investigators using different strains of the same species as Dehority and Scott (1967). Saluzzi et al. (1993) noted an inhibition between *F. succinogenes* (strains S85 and BL2) and *R. flavefaciens* (strains 17 and FD1) while inhibition between *R. flavefaciens* FD1 and *R. albus* 8 has been reported by Odenyo et al. (1994). One possible explanation for this inhibition would be the production of bacterocin-like compounds by one of the organisms which are inhibitory to the other organism. Odenyo et al. (1994) found that *R. albus* 8 produced a peptide-like substance which had inhibitory activity against *R. flavefaciens* but not against *F. succinogenes*. The inhibitory activity could be destroyed by treatment with proteolytic enzymes but not by boiling for 10 minutes. Based on these observations, the authors suggested that the substance may be a bacterocin. In a later study, Chan and Dehority found that *R. albus* 7 plus two additional strains of *R. albus* (MO2a and MO3g) all produced substances with varying degrees of inhibitory activity against four strains of *R. flavefaciens* (B1a, B34b, C1a and R13e2). However, no inhibition was observed against *F. succinogenes*, *Butyrivibrio fibrisolvens* or *Prevotella ruminicola*. The inhibitory substance(s) was present in cell-free culture filtrates and destroyed by autoclaving (20 min) or treating with a protease. Production of bacterocins by rumen bacteria may be fairly widespread, Kalmokoff and Teather (1997) screened 49 strains of *Butyrivibrio fibrisolvens* for production of bacterocins and found that 25 of them produced substances inhibitory in varying degrees to the other strains.

Fondevila and Dehority (1996) investigated the inhibition in cellulose digestion observed when *Fibrobacter succinogenes* A3c and *Ruminococcus flavefaciens* B34b were combined in the same fermentation. The antagonism or inhibition between these two species appeared to be somewhat different than that which occurs between the species of *Ruminococcus*, particularly since the inhibitory activity was not destroyed by autoclaving at 121 C for 20 minutes. They developed sequential addition procedures which allowed fermentation by one organism, killing that organism (either by aeration or autoclaving) and inoculating with a second organism. Essentially they found that co-culturing *F. succinogenes* and *R. flavefaciens* always reduced cellulose digestion compared to *F. succinogenes* alone; however, when added sequentially in either order, no reduction occurred. A trial was set up to investigate this apparant discrepancy and the results are shown in Table 8.7. These data clearly indicate that *R. flavefaciens* only inhibits cellulose digestion by *F. succinogenes* when the two organisms are cultured together. It would appear that production of the inhibitory substance(s) does not occur when *R. flavefaciens* is cultured by itself.

Cross-feeding of the intermediate products of cellulose digestion

High numbers of noncellulolytic bacteria can occur in ruminants being fed high fiber diets. Russell (1985) found that water-soluble cellodextrins, primarily cellotetraose and cellopentaose, were rapidly utilized by both cellulolytic species and some noncellulolytic species. *Butyrivibrio fibrisolvens, Selenemonas ruminantium* and *Prevotella*

Table 8.7. DIGESTION OF CELLULOSE FROM MATURE ORCHARDGRASS BY *F. SUCCINOGENES* AND *R. FLAVEFACIENS*, CULTURED EITHER SIMULTANEOUSLY OR SEQUENTIALLY

Organisms[a]		Cellulose digestion, %
First	Second	
F. succ.	-	48.9^x
R. flav.	-	29.8^y
F. succ. + R. flav.	-	29.7^y
R. flav.	F. succ.	43.3^x
R. flav.	F. succ. + R. flav.	29.6^y
F. succ. + R. flav.	F. succ.	29.7^y
F. succ. + R. flav	F. succ. + R. flav	29.9^y

[a] *F. succ.* = *Fibrobacter succinogenes* A3c; *R. flav.* = *Ruminococcus flavefaciens* B34b.
[x,y] Within the column, values with different superscripts differ at $P<0.05$.

ruminicola all grew rapidly with the cellodextrins as their sole energy source. *Streptococcus bovis* and *Eubacterium ruminantium* grew well on cellobiose, but little if any growth was observed with cellodextrins as substrates. Since the longer chain cellodextrins were hydrolyzed extracellularly to cellotriose and cellobiose before utilization as a source of energy, crossfeeding by *S. bovis* and *E. ruminantium* could readily occur.

Newer methodologies for characterizing rumen bacteria

Until recently, identification and classification of rumen bacteria, including the cellulolytics, has been based on cultivation and measurement of numerous physiological characteristics. However, guanine plus cytosine (G+C) base contents and sugar composition of extracellular polysaccharides (EPS) along with the newer techniques in molecular biology, i.e., 16S rRNA sequences and DNA hybridization, has allowed for a much more definitive classification of rumen bacteria (Sharpe and Dellaglio, 1977; Stackebrandt and Hippe, 1986; Mannarelli, 1988; Montgomery *et al.*, 1988; Mannarelli *et al.*, 1990, 1991; Avgustin *et al.*, 1994). This has led to renaming several ruminal species, for example, *Bacterioides succinogenes* is now *Fibrobacter succinogenes; Bacteroides ruminicola* is *Prevotella ruminicola* and *Bacteroides amylophilis* is *Ruminobacter amylophilis*. Based on data obtained with these newer methods, it is now possible to identify rumen bacteria which occur in relatively low numbers or those which to date we have been unable to cultivate in the laboratory.

References

Akin, D. E. and L. L. Rigsby. (1985). Degradation of bermuda and orchardgrass by species of ruminal bacteria. *Applied and Environmental Microbiology*, **50**, 825-830.

Allison, M. J. and M. P. Bryant. (1963). Biosynthesis of branched-chain amino acids from branched-chain fatty acids by rumen bacteria. *Archives of Biochemistry and Biophysics*, **101**, 269-277.

Allison, M. J., M. P. Bryant and R. N. Doetsch. (1958). Volatile fatty acid growth factor for cellulolytic cocci of bovine rumen. *Science*, **128**, 474-475.

Avgustin, G., F. Wright and H. J. Flint. (1994). Genetic diversity and phylogenetic relationships among strains of *Prevotella* (*Bacteroides*) *ruminicola* from the rumen. *International Journal of Systematic Bacteriology*, **44**, 246-255.

Bhat, S., R. J. Wallace and E. R. Ørskov. (1990). Adhesion of cellulolytic ruminal bacteria to barley straw. *Applied and Environmental Microbiology*, **56**, 2698-2703.

Blair, B. G. and K. L. Anderson. (1999). Cellulose-inducible ultrastructural protuberences and cellulose-affinity proteins of *Eubacterium cellulosolvens*. *Anaerobe*, **5**, 547-554.

Bryant, M. P. (1959). Bacterial species of the rumen. *Bacteriological Reviews*, **23**, 125-153.

Bryant, M. P. and L. A. Burkey. (1953). Cultural methods and some characteristics of some of the more numerous groups of bacteria in the bovine rumen. *Journal of Dairy Science*, **36**, 205-217.

Bryant, M. P. and R. N. Doetsch. (1954). A study of actively cellulolytic rod-shaped bacteria of the bovine rumen. *Journal of Dairy Science*, **37**, 1176-1183.

Bryant, M. P. and R. N. Doetsch. (1955). Factors necessary for the growth of *Bacteroides succinogenes* in the volatile acid fraction of rumen fluid. *Journal of Dairy Science*, **38**, 340-350.

Bryant, M. P. and I. M. Robinson. (1961). Some nutritional requirements of the genus *Ruminicoccus*. *Applied Microbiology*, **9**, 91-95.

Bryant, M. P. and N. Small. (1956). The anaerobic monotrichous butyric acid-producing curved rod-shaped bacteria of the rumen. *Journal of Bacteriology*, **72**, 16-21.

Bryant, M. P., I. M. Robinson and H. Chu. (1959). Observations on the nutrition of *Bacteroides succinogenes* - a ruminal cellulolytic bacterium. *Journal of Dairy Science*, **42**, 1831-1847.

Bryant, M. P., N. Small, C. Bouma and I. M. Robinson. (1958). Characteristics of ruminal anaerobic cellulolytic cocci and *Cillobacterium cellulosolvens* n. sp. *Journal of Bacteriology*, **76**, 529-537.

Caldwell, D. R. and R. F. Hudson. (1974). Sodium, an obligate growth requirement for predominant rumen bacteria. *Applied Microbiology*, **27**, 549-552.

Cheng, K.-J. and J. W. Costerton. (1987). Ultrastructure of *Butyrivibrio fibrisolvens*: A gram-positive bacterium. *Journal of Bacteriology*, **129**, 1506-1512.

Coen, J. A. and B. A. Dehority. (1970). Degradation and utilization of hemicellulose from intact forages by pure cultures of rumen bacteria. *Applied Microbiology*, **29**, 362-368.

Costerton, J. W., R. T. Irvin and K-J. Cheng. (1981). The bacterial glycocalyx in nature and disease. *Annual Review of Microbiology*, **35**, 299-324.

Dehority, B. A. (1963). Isolation and characterization of several cellulolytic bacteria from *in vitro* rumen fermentations. *Journal of Dairy Science*, **46**, 217-222.

Dehority, B. A. (1966). Characterization of several bovine rumen bacteria isolated with a xylan medium. *Journal of Bacteriology*, **91**, 1724-1729.

Dehority, B. A. (1971). Carbon dioxide requirement of various species of rumen bacteria. *Journal of Bacteriology*, **105**, 70-76.

Dehority, B. A. (1973). Hemicellulose degradation by rumen bacteria. *Federation Proceedings*, **32**, 1819-1825.

Dehority, B. A. (1977). Cellulolytic cocci isolated from the cecum of guinea pigs (*Cavia porcellus*). *Applied and Environmental Microbiology*, **33**, 1278-1283.

Dehority, B. A. (1986). Microbes in the foregut of arctic ruminants. In: *Control of Digestion and Metabolism in Ruminants*. Edited by L. P. Milligan, W. L. Grovum and A. Dobson. Prentice-Hall, Englewood Cliffs, NJ, pp. 307-325.

Dehority, B. A. and Jean A. Grubb. (1977). Characterization of the predominant bacteria occurring in the rumen of goats (*Capra hircus*). *Applied and Environmental Microbiology*, **33**, 1030-1036.

Dehority, B. A. and H. W. Scott. (1967). Extent of cellulose and hemicellulose digestion in various forages by pure cultures of rumen bacteria. *Journal of Dairy Science*, **50**, 1136-1141.

Dehority, B. A., H. W. Scott and P. Kowaluk. (1967). Volatile fatty acid requirements of cellulolytic rumen bacteria. *Journal of Bacteriology*, **94**, 537-543.

Fondevila, M. and B. A. Dehority. (1996). Intreactions between *Fibrobacter succinogenes*, *Prevotella ruminicola* and *Ruminococcus flavefaciens* in the digestion of cellulose from forages. *Journal of Animal Science*, **74**, 678-684.

Forsberg, C. W., T. J. Beveridge and A. Hellstrom. (1981). Cellulase and xylanase release from *Bacteroides succinogenes* and its importance in the rumen environment. *Applied and Environmental Microbiology*, **42**, 886-896.

Gilchrist, F.M.C. and A. Kistner. (1962). Bacteria of the ovine rumen. I. The composition of the population on a diet of poor teff hay. *Journal of Agricultural Science*, **59**, 77-83.

Gill, J. W. and K. W. King. (1958). Nutritional characteristics of a *Butyrivibrio*. *Journal of Bacteriology*, **75**, 666-673.

Groleau, D. and C. W. Forsberg. (1981). Cellulolytic activity of the rumen bacterium *Bacteroides succinogenes*. *Canadian Journal of Microbiology*, **27**, 517-530.

Halliwell, G. and M. P. Bryant. (1963). The cellulolytic activity of pure strains of bacteria from the rumen of cattle. *Journal of General Microbiology*, **32**, 441-448.

Hiltner, P. and B. A. Dehority. (1983). Effect of soluble carbohydrates on digestion of cellulose by pure cultures of rumen bacteria. *Applied and Environmental Microbiology*, **46**, 642-648.

Holdeman, L. V. and W.E.C. Moore. (1974). New genus *Coprococcus*. Twelve new species, and emended descriptions of four previously described species of bacteria from human feces. *International Journal of Systematic Bacteriology*, **24**, 260-277.

Huang, L. and C. W. Forsberg. (1987). Isolation of a cellodextrinase from *Bacteroides succinogenes*. *Applied and Environmental Microbiology*, **53**, 1034-1041.

Huang, L. and C. W. Forsberg. (1990). Cellulose digestion and cellulase regulation and distribution in *Fibrobacter succinogenes* subsp. *succinogenes* S85. *Applied and Environmental Microbiology*, **56**, 1221-1228.

Hungate, R. E. (1944). Studies on cellulose fermentation. I. The culture and physiology of an anaerobic cellulose digesting bacterium. *Journal of Bacteriology*, **48**, 499-513.

Hungate, R. E. (1946). Studies on cellulose fermentation. II. An anaerobic cellulose-decomposing actinomycete, *Micromonospora propionici* n.sp. *Journal of Bacteriology*, **51**, 51-56.

Hungate, R. E. (1947). Studies on cellulose fermentation. III. The culture and isolation of cellulose decomposing bacteria from the rumen of cattle. *Journal of Bacteriology*, **53**, 631-645.

Hungate, R. E. (1950). The anaerobic mesophilic cellulolytic bacteria. *Bacteriological Reviews*, **14**, 1-49.

Hungate, R. E. (1957). Micro-organisms in the rumen of cattle fed a constant ration. *Canadian Journal of Microbiology*, **3**, 289-311.

Hungate, R. E. (1966). *The Rumen and its Microbes*. Academic Press, New York, USA.

Hungate, R. E. and R. J. Stack. (1982). Phenylpropanoic acid: growth factor for *Ruminococcus albus*. *Applied and Environmental Microbiology*, **44**, 79-83.

Jarvis, B.D.W. and E. F. Annison. (1967). Isolation, classification and nutritional requirements of cellulolytic cocci in the sheep rumen. *Journal of General Microbiology*, **47**, 295-307.

Kalmokoff, M. L. and R. M. Teather. (1997). Isolation and characterization of a bacterocin (Butyrivibriocin AR 10) from the ruminal anaerobe *Butyrivibrio fibrosolvens* AR 10: evidence in support of the widespread occurrence of bacterocin -like activity among rumen isolates of *B. fibrosolvens*. *Applied and Environmental Microbiology*, **63**, 394-402.

Kelly, W. J., R. V. Asmundson and D. H. Hopcroft. (1987). Isolation and characterization of a strictly anaerobic spore former: *Clostridium chartatabidum* sp. nov. *Archives of Microbiology*, **147**, 169-173.

Kistner, A. and L. Gouws. (1964). Cellulolytic cocci occurring in the rumen of sheep conditioned to lucerne hay. *Journal of General Microbiology*, **34**, 447-458.

Kock, S. G. and A. Kistner. (1969). Extent of solubilization of α-cellulose and hemicellulose of low-protein teff hay by pure cultures of cellulolytic rumen bacteria. *Journal of General Microbiology*, **55**, 459-462.

Kudo, H., K.-J. Cheng and J. W. Costerton. (1987). Electron microscopic study of the methylcellulose-mediated detachment of cellulolytic rumen bacteria from cellulose fibers. *Canadian Journal of Microbiology*, **33**, 267-272.

Leatherwood, J. M. and M. P. Sharma. (1972). Novel anaerobic cellulolytic bacterium. *Journal of Bacteriology*, **110**, 751-753.

Macy, J. M., J. R. Farrand and L. Montgomery. (1982). Cellulolytic and non-cellulolytic bacteria in rat gastrointestinal tracts. *Applied and Environmental Microbiology*, **44**, 1428-1434.

Maluszynska, G. M. and L. Janota-Bassalik. (1974). A cellulolytic rumen bacterium, *Micromonospora ruminantium* sp. nov. *Journal of General Microbiology*, **82**, 57-65.

Mannarelli, B. M. (1988). Deoxyribonucleic acid relatedness among strains of the species *Butyrivibrio fibrisolvens*. *International Journal of Systematic Bacteriology*, **38**, 340-347.

Manarelli, B. M., R. J. Stack, D. Lee and L. Ericsson. (1990). Taxonomic relatedness of *Butyrivibrio, Lachnospira, Roseburia* and *Eubacterium* species as determined by DNA hybridization and extracellular polysaccharide analysis. *International Journal of Systematic Bacteriology*, **40**, 370-378.

Manarelli, B. M., L. D. Ericsson, D. Lee and R. J. Stack. (1991). Taxonomic relationships among strains of the anaerobic bacterium *Bacteroides ruminicola* determined by DNA and extracellular polysaccharide analysis. *Applied and Environmental Microbiology,* **57**, 2975-2980.

Margherita, S. S. and R. E. Hungate. (1963). Serological analysis of *Butyrivibrio* from the bovine rumen. *Journal of Bacteriology*, **86**, 855-860.

Margherita, S. S., R. E. Hungate and H. Storz. (1964). Variation in rumen *Butyrivibrio* strains. *Journal of Bacteriology*, **87**, 1304-1308.

McDermid, K. P., C. R. MacKenzie and C. W. Forsberg. (1990). Esterase activities of *Fibrobacter succinogenes* S85. *Applied and Environmental Microbiology*, **56**, 127-132.

Miron, J., D. Ben-Ghedalia and M. Morrison. (2001). Adhesion mechanisms of rumen cellulolytic bacteria. *Journal of Dairy Science,* **84**, 1294-1309.

Montgomery, L., B. Flesher and D. Stahl. (1988). Transfer of *Bacteriodes* (Hungate) to *Fibrobacter* gen. nov. as *Fibrobacter succinogenes* comb. nov. and description of *Fibrobacter intestinalis* sp. nov. *International Journal of Systematic Bacteriology*, **38**, 430-435.

Moon, M. and J. L. Anderson. (2001). *Eubacterium cellulosolvens* alters its membrane protein, lipoprotein, and fatty acid composition in response to growth on cellulose. *Anaerobe*, **7,** 227-236.

Moore, W.E.C., E. P. Cato and L. V. Holdeman. (1972). *Ruminococcus bromii* sp. n.

and emendation of the description of *Ruminococcus* Sijpestein. *International Journal of Systematic Bacteriology*, **22**, 78-80.

Moore, W.E.C., J. L. Johnson and L. V. Holdeman. (1976). Emendation of *Bacteroidaceae* and *Butyrivibrio* and descriptions of *Desulfomonas* gen. nov. and ten new species in the genera *Desulfomonas, Butyrivibrio, Eubacterium, Clostridium* and *Ruminococcus*. *International Journal of Systematic Bacteriology,* **26**, 238-252.

Morrison, M., R. I. Mackie and A. Kistner. (1990). 3-phenylpropanoic acid improves the affinity of *Ruminococcus albus* for cellulose in continuous culture. *Applied and Environmental Microbiology*, **56**, 3220-3222.

Odenyo, A. A., R. I. Mackie, G. C. Fahey, Jr. and B. A. White. (1991). Degradation of wheat straw and alkaline hydrogen peroxide-treated wheat straw by *Ruminococcus albus* 8 and *Ruminococcus flavefaciens* FD-1. *Journal of Animal Science*, **69**, 819-826.

Odenyo, A. A., R. I. Mackie, D. A. Stahl and B. A. White. (1994).The use of 16S rDNA-targeted oligonucleotide probes to study competition between ruminal fibrolytic bacteria: development of probes for *Ruminococcus* species and evidence for bacterocin production. *Applied and Environmental Microbiology*, **60**, 3688-3696.

Pavlosthathis, S. G., T. L. Miller and M. J. Wolin. (1988). Fermentation of insoluble cellulose by continuous cultures of *Ruminococcus albus*. *Applied and Environmental Microbiology*, **54**, 2655-2569.

Pell, A. N. and P. Schofield. (1993). Microbial adhesion and degradation of plant cell walls. In: *Forage Cell Wall Structure and Digestibility.* Edited by R. D. Hatfield, H. G. Jung, J. Ralph, D. R. Buxton, D. R. Mertens and P. J. Weimer. ASA-CSSA-SSSA, Madison, WI. USA. pp. 397-423.

Prins, R. A., F. van Vugt, R. E. Hungate and C.J.A.H.V. van Vorstenbosch. (1972). A comparison of strains of *Eubacterium cellulosolvens* from the rumen. *Antonie van Leeuwenhoek Journal of Microbiology and Serology*, **38**, 153-161.

Rasmussen, M. A., B. A. White and R. B. Hespell. (1989). Improved assay for quantitating adherence of ruminal bacteria to cellulose. *Applied and Environmental Microbiology*, **55**, 2089-2091.

Rasmussen, M. A., R. B. Hespell, B. A. White and R. J. Bothast. (1988). Inhibitory effects of methylcellulose on cellulose degradation by *Ruminococcus flavefaciens*. *Applied and Environmental Microbiology*, **54**, 890-897.

Roger, V., G. Fonty, S. Komisarczuk-bony and P. Gouet. (1990). Effects of physiochemical factors on the adhesion to cellulose Avicel of the ruminal bacteria *Ruminococcus flavefaciens* and *Fibrobacter succinogenes* subsp. *succinogenes*. *Applied and Environmental Microbiology*, **56**, 3081-3087.

Russell, J. B. (1985). Fermentation of cellodextrins by cellulolytic and noncellulolytic rumen bacteria. *Applied and Environmental Microbiology*, **49**, 572-576.

Saluzzi, L., A. Smith and C. S. Stewart. (1993). Analysis of bacterial phospholipid markers and plant monosaccharides during forage degradation by *Ruminococcus flavefaciens* and *Fibrobacter succinogenes* in co-culture. *Journal of General Microbiology*, **139**, 2865-2873.

Scott, H. W. and B. A. Dehority. (1965). Vitamin requirements of several cellulolytic rumen bacteria. *Journal of Bacteriology*, **89**, 1169-1175.

Shane, B. S., L. Gouws and A. Kistner. (1969). Cellulolytic bacteria occurring in the rumen of sheep conditioned to low-protein teff hay. *Journal of General Microbiology*, **55**, 445-457.

Sharpe, M. E. and F. Dellaglio. (1977). Deoxyribonucleic acid homology in anaerobic lactobacilli and in possible related species. *International Journal of Systematic Bacteriology*, **27**, 19-21.

Shoham, Y., R. Lamed and E. A. Bayer. (1999). The cellulosome concept as an efficient microbial strategy for the degradation of insoluble polysaccharides. *Trends in Microbiology*, **7**, 275-281.

Sijpesteijn, A. K. (1948). *Cellulose-decomposing Bacteria from the Rumen of Cattle*. Thesis. Leiden Univ. The Netherlands.

Sijpesteijn, A. K. (1951). On *Ruminococcus flavefaciens*, a cellulose-decomposing bacterium from the rumen of sheep and cattle. *Journal of General Microbiology*, **5**, 869-879.

Slyter, L. L. and J. M. Weaver. (1969). Growth factor requirements of *Ruminococcus flavefaciens* isolated from the rumen of cattle fed purified diets. *Applied Microbiology*, **17**, 737-741.

Stack, R. J. and M. A. Cotta. (1986). Effect of 3-phenylpropanoic acid on growth of and cellulose utilization by cellulolytic ruminal bacteria. *Applied and Environmental Microbiology*, **52**, 209-210.

Stack, R. J. and R. E. Hungate. (1984). Effect of 3-Phenylpropanoic acid on capsule and cellulases of *Ruminococcus albus* 8. *Applied and Environmental Microbiology*, **48**, 218-223.

Stack, R. J., R. E. Hungate and W. P. Opsahl. (1983). Phenylacetic acid and stimulation of cellulose digestion by *Ruminicoccus albus* 8. *Applied and Environmental Microbiology*, **46**, 539-544.

Stackebrandt, E. and H. Hippe. (1986). Transfer of *Bacteriodes amylophilis* to a new genus *Ruminobacter* gen. nov. *Systematics of Applied Microbiology*, **8**, 204-207.

Stewart, C. S., C. Paniagua, D. Dinsdale, K.-J. Cheng and S. H. Garrow. (1981). Selective isolation and characteristics of *Bacteroides succinogenes* from the rumen of a cow. *Applied and Environmental Microbiology*, **41**, 504-510.

Teather, R. M. (1982). Isolation of plasmid DNA from *Butyrivibrio fibrisolvens*. *Applied and Environmental Microbiology*, **43**, 298-302.

Van Gylswyk, N. O. (1980). *Fusobacterium polysaccharolyticum* sp. nov., a gram-negative rod from the rumen that produces butyrate and ferments cellulose and starch. *Journal of General Microbiology*, **116**, 157-163.

Van Gylswyk, N. O. and J.P.L. Hoffman. (1970). Characteristics of cellulolytic cillobacteria from the rumens of sheep fed teff (*Eragrostis tef*) hay diets. *Journal of General Microbiology*, **60**, 381-386.

Van Gylswyk, N. O. and J.P.L. Labuschagne. (1971). Relative efficiency of pure cultures of different species of cellulolytic rumen bacteria in solubilizing cellulose *in vitro*. *Journal of General Microbiology*, **66**, 109-113.

Van Gylswyk, N. O. and C.E.G. Roche. (1970). Characteristics of *Ruminococcus* and cellulolytic *Butyrivibrio* species from the rumens of sheep fed differently supplemented teff (*Eragrostis tef*) hay diets. *Journal of General Microbiology*, **64**, 11-17.

Van Gylswyk, N. O., E. J. Morris and H. J. Els. (1980). Sporulation and cell wall structure of *Clostridium polysaccharolyticum* comb. nov. (formerly *Fusobacterium polysaccharolyticum*). *Journal of General Microbiology*, **121**, 491-493.

Varel, V. H. (1989). Reisolation and characterization of *Clostridium longisporum*, a ruminal spore forming cellulolytic anaerobe. *Archives of Microbiology*, **152**, 209-214.

Varel, V. H., A. J. Richardson and C. S. Stewart. (1989). Degradation of barley straw, ryegrass and alfalfa cell walls by *Clostridium longisporum* and *Ruminococcus albus*. *Applied and Environmental Microbiology*, **55**, 3080-3084.

Wegner, G. H. and E. M. Foster. (1963). Incorporation of isobutyrate and valerate into cellular plasmalogen by *Bacteroides succinogenes*. *Journal of Bacteriology*, **85**, 53-61.

CHAPTER 9

SPECIES OF RUMEN BACTERIA ACTIVE IN THE FERMENTATION OF HEMICELLULOSE

Those species of rumen bacteria which appear to be the principal organisms responsible for the digestion of cellulose in the rumen have been discussed in the previous chapter. Their importance was judged on the basis of the numbers at which they occurred, wide spread geographic distribution, metabolic reactions and the ability of these species to digest the cellulosic portion of intact forages.

In addition to cellulose, two other forage polysaccharides, hemicellulose and pectin occur in significant amounts (Whistler and Smart, 1953; Hungate, 1966; Dehority, 1973). These three components constitute the major portion of the total carbohydrate present in forages. With most forages, the percent composition for these three principal polysaccharides would fall within the ranges of 20-30% for cellulose, 15-20% for hemicellulose and 5-10% for pectin. The importance of the hemicellulose and pectin fractions becomes obvious when one considers that they constitute about 40 to 50% of the total carbohydrate in the forage. Cellulose is a linear polymer of ß-1-4 linked D-glucose units, while hemicellulose is quite heterogenous and can roughly be defined as a mixture of water-insoluble cell wall polysaccharides, excluding cellulose and pectin. It is closely associated with cellulose in the plant and is considered to be a part of the cell wall components. The relationship between cellulose and hemicellulose is illustrated in Figure 9.1.

Hemicellulose content is empirically determined on the basis of solubility, i.e., that fraction of plant polysaccharides which is unextracted by water or 0.5% ammonium oxalate solution, but which is extracted by aqueous alkali (Whistler and Smart, 1953). Most investigators use sodium hydroxide solutions ranging in concentration from 10 to 17.5%, since α-cellulose has been defined as that polysaccharide fraction which is insoluble in 17.5% NaOH. Alpha-cellulose has an estimated degree of polymerization greater than 200, and thus shorter polymers of cellulose would be included with the hemicellulose fraction if 17.5% NaOH is used for extraction. The exact nature of the hemicelluloses has not been elucidated; however, they are a mixture of unmodified glycans, composed of pentose or hexose sugar units, plus modified glycans (polyuronides) which contain one or more glycuronic acid units combined in the polysaccharide molecule.

Composition studies on hemicelluloses from various sources have shown that the sugar xylose is generally present in very high quantities, presumably either as the polysaccharide xylan (ß-1-4 linked xylose with occasional branches formed by 1-3

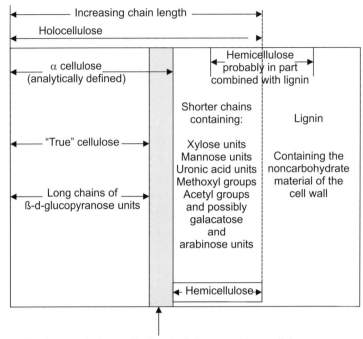

Figure 9.1. Relationship of cellulose, hemicellulose and lignin in the plant cell wall (redrawn from Whistler and Smart, 1953).

linkages) or in mixed polymers with glycuronic acid units. Arabinans, galactans, low molecular weight cellulose, and less often the methyl pentose, L-rhamnose, also occur. Table 9.1 presents the composition of hemicellulose from several different plants, isolated and analyzed by Dr. Fred Smith of the University of Minnesota (Dehority, 1973). Composition data on the hemicellulose extracted from bromegrass by dilute H_2SO_4, as reported by Burdick and Sullivan (1963), is also included.

Hemicellulose fermenting species

In his first work with the cellulose digestors, Hungate (1950) had observed that *B. fibrisolvens* would ferment isolated hemicelluloses, while *F. succinogenes* could not attack these materials. In later studies with the cellulolytic cocci, Hungate (1957) indicated that some strains of these species could also utilize hemicellulose. Butterworth *et al.* (1960), using wheat flour pentosan as a substrate, isolated a xylan-fermenting bacterium from the bovine rumen and tentatively assigned it to the genus *Butyrivibrio*. Cell-free extracts of this species rapidly degraded xylan and pentosan (Howard *et al.*, 1960). A sheep rumen bacterium was isolated by Walker (1961) with the use of a medium containing wheaten hay hemicellulose as the only added carbohydrate. This organism

Table 9.1 COMPOSITION OF HEMICELLULOSES ISOLATED FROM SEVERAL DIFFERENT PLANT SOURCES[a]

Component	Source of hemicellulose					
	Alfalfa, %[b]	Corn hull, %	Flax, %	Fescue, %[c]	Oat hull, %	Bromegrass, %[c]
Arabinose	10.4	35.0	-	20.2	14.0	12.0
Xylose	58.5	48.0	84.7	61.7	66.0	59.3
Glucose	5.9	-	-	9.8	12.0	20.9
Galactose	6.9	7.0	-	8.2	5.0	7.8
Rhamnose	3.9	-	1.5	-	-	
Glucuronic acid[d]	13.5	10.0	13.8		+[e]	

[a] Data on bromegrass taken from Burdick and Sullivan (1963). All other data were obtained by personal communication from F. Smith, University of Minnesota. Blank spaces indicate that the component was not determined; - indicates the component was not present.
[b] Percent of total hemicellulose.
[c] Relative percentages for neutral sugars only.
[d] This fraction consisted of a mixture of several different acidic components.
[e] Present, but only in trace amounts.

was tentatively placed in the genus *Bacteroides*. Hobson and Purdom (1961) isolated two types of xylan-fermenting rumen bacteria from sheep, using the wheat flour pentosan medium previously described by Butterworth *et al.* (1960). One organism was identified as a species of *Butyrivibrio*, and the second organism was not classified. Results of these early studies would suggest that *Butyrivibrio* species are probably quite active in hemicellulose digestion in the rumen; however, other species had also been observed to ferment xylan. In an attempt to gain further information on the important hemicellulose digestors in the rumen, Dehority (1966) isolated 25 cultures from 10^{-8} and 10^{-9} dilutions of bovine rumen contents on a medium containing xylan as the only added energy source. Eight strains were studied in detail. Five were identified as belonging to the species *Butyrivibrio fibrisolvens* and the three remaining strains were identified as *Bacteroides ruminicola*. This latter species, *B. ruminicola* has been reclassified into a new genus *Prevotella* (Shah and Collins, 1990), and will be designated as *P. ruminicola* in the remainder of this text. Six additional cultures were presumptively identified as four strains of *P. ruminicola* and one strain each of *B. fibrisolvens* and *Eubacterium ruminantium*. This study substantiated the probable importance of *B. fibrisolvens* in hemicellulose digestion and indicated the significance of at least one and possibly two additional species.

Clarke *et al.* (1969) subsequently isolated three strains of *B. fibrisolvens* from the rumen of cattle using selective medium, which contained either arabinose or plant hemicellulose fractions other than insoluble xylan as the only added substrate. No other species were isolated in their single series of isolations. In 1985, van Gylswyk and van der Toorn isolated two additional species of *Eubacterium* with a selective xylan medium, *E. uniforme* and *E. xylanophilum*.

Hespell *et al.* (1987) measured the ability of 10 strains of *B. fibrisolvens* plus six other species of rumen bacteria to ferment xylans. Four of the *B. fibrisolvens* strains grew almost as well on the xylans as on a cellobiose-maltose medium, while growth of the remaining six was only moderate. Partial fermentation of the xylans was observed with the other six species (*P. ruminicola, F. succinogenes, R. albus, R. flavefaciens, Succinivibrio dextrinosolvens* and *Selenomonas ruminantium*); however, the xylans appeared to contain small amounts of other carbohydrates which would support growth of non-xylanolytic strains. Xylanase and xylobiase activities were measured for four *B. fibrisolvens* strains. The xylanase activity occurred primarily in the culture fluid while xylobiase activity was associated with the cell. These enzyme activities were found to be both inducible and constitutive, and varied between the different strains.

Thus, from the studies conducted to this time, the species *Butyrivibrio fibrisolvens, Prevotella ruminicola, Ruminococcus flavefaciens,* and *Ruminococcus albus* would appear to be the predominant hemicellulose digesting bacteria in the rumen. *Eubacterium* species would appear to be of somewhat lesser importance. Since the characteristics of *B. fibrisolvens* and the ruminococci were presented in the previous Chapter, only *Prevotella ruminicola* and the three *Eubacterium* species will be described here.

PREVOTELLA RUMINICOLA

The species *Prevotella ruminicola* was established by Bryant *et al.* in 1958. The organism is a gram-negative nonmotile rod, 0.8 to 1.0 µm wide and 0.8 to 8.0 µm long. As with *F. succinogenes*, it is extremely pleomorphic and cells as long as 30 µm have been observed. Many cells appear to be oval. It is a strict anaerobe. Gas is not produced, starch is hydrolyzed, gelatin is liquefied. Cellulose is not fermented. Many of the soluble sugars are fermented. Fermentation products in glucose medium include succinic, formic and acetic acid. Two subspecies were established, subspecies *brevis* for those strains which would grow in a medium in which trypticase and yeast extract replaced rumen fluid, and subspecies *ruminicola* for those strains which would not grow in the absence of rumen fluid. In later work, Bryant and Robinson (1962) found that the rumen fluid requirement of *P. ruminicola* subsp. *ruminicola*, could be satisfied by hemin. Thus, the requirement for hemin is used to classify *P. ruminicola* to the subspecies level.

Several discrepancies with the species description for *P. ruminicola* were noted by Dehority (1966), especially with regard to fermentation products. A detailed study with the three xylan isolated strains and the type strains revealed that propionic acid is a normal fermentation product for *P. ruminicola* when grown in a 40% rumen fluid - 0.5% glucose medium. However, propionate production is negligible when this species is grown in 20% rumen fluid - 0.5% trypticase - 1% glucose medium. Two of the strains isolated by Dehority (1966) were identified as subspecies *brevis* and the third as subspecies *ruminicola*. In addition, one of the subspecies *brevis* strains was found to have an absolute requirement for either isobutyric or 2-methylbutyric acid.

The nitrogen metabolism of *P. ruminicola* is somewhat unusual. In addition to NH_3, it can use enzymatically hydrolyzed casein as a sole source of nitrogen while growth is very limited with acid hydrolyzed casein. Studies by Pittman and Bryant (1964) and Pittman *et al*. (1967) revealed that NH_3 is probably the only low molecular nitrogen source used efficiently by this species for growth. On the other hand, peptides containing four or more amino acid residues can be used quite efficiently. They concluded that *P. ruminicola* possesses a system for the uptake of oligopeptides, but not amino acids, dipeptides or tripeptides. It thus becomes a simple matter of getting the nitrogen into the cell. This differential response to acid and enzymatically hydrolyzed casein is quite useful in characterization of the species.

As with *F. succinogenes*, *P. ruminicola* produces succinic acid as an end-product and thus requires about 0.10% CO_2 in the medium for optimal growth (Dehority, 1971).

Mannarelli *et al*. (1991) used guanine-plus-cytosine (G+C) base contents and DNA hybridization studies to determine the relatedness between 14 strains of *P. ruminicola*. They found a broad range of G+C values, ranging between 37.6 and 50.9 mol %, indicating a number of different species, since previous studies had indicated that strains belonging to the same species had a G+C mol % span of 2.0% or less. Relatedness, based on DNA hybridization, suggested that these 14 strains could be classified as follows: 5 strains in group I, 2 strains in group 2, 1 strain moderately related to group 1 and 6 strains which are unrelated to any of the other strains. The authors concluded that these phenotypically identified strains of *P. ruminicola*, when classified genotypically, probably represent as many as nine separate species.

EUBACTERIUM SPECIES

The species *Eubacterium ruminantium* was established by Bryant in 1959. It is a weakly gram positive, nonmotile, short rod, ranging from 0.4 to 0.7 μm in width by 0.7 to 1.5 μm in length. Strict anaerobe. Catalase negative, indole or H_2S are not produced, nitrate is not reduced, gelatin is not liquefied. Neither starch nor cellulose are fermented. Almost all strains ferment glucose, cellobiose and fructose. The fermentation of xylose, arabinose, lactose, maltose, dextrin, sucrose, and xylan varies between strains. Fermentation products include lactic, formic, acetic and butyric acids. This species has not been studied extensively, and almost all available data have originated from Bryant's lab.

Two new species of *Eubacterium* were isolated with selective xylan medium from rumen contents of sheep fed corn stover by van Gylswyk and van der Toorn (1985). *E. uniforme* constituted from 4 to 6% and *E. xylanophilum* about 1% of the bacteria which produced clearings in xylan agar medium. Total xylanolytic counts were about 6% of the total viable count. *Eubacterium uniforme* (13 strains) fermented a variety of carbohydrates, but not cellulose. End products of xylan fermentation were formic, acetic and lactic acids plus ethanol. *E. xylanophilum* fermented only cellobiose and xylan and produced formic, acetic and butyric acids.

Degradation and utilization of isolated forage hemicellulose by pure cultures of rumen bacteria

In collaboration with Dr. Fred Smith from the University of Minnesota, who was particularly interested in composition and structure of plant hemicelluloses, a study was undertaken by Dehority (1965) on digestibility of isolated forage hemicelluloses by pure cultures of cellulolytic rumen bacteria. It was hoped that partially degraded residues of the hemicellulose might remain after the fermentation which would differ from the oligosaccharides obtained by chemical degradation methods. Such fragments would be of extreme value in studies on hemicellulose structure. Several of the cellulolytic ruminococci (B1a, C-94 and 7), capable of utilizing xylan for growth, plus one strain of *Fibrobacter succinogenes* (B21a) were chosen for the initial studies. Composition of the isolated hemicelluloses was given previously in Table 9.1. On the basis of an increase in optical density, all three strains of ruminococci which digested xylan could utilize the isolated hemicelluloses as energy sources. Growth curves using two of the isolated hemicelluloses as energy sources are shown in Figure 9.2. The extent of digestion for purified xylan and the four isolated hemicelluloses, as determined by pentose loss, is shown in Table 9.2. Considerable variation was noted between both organisms and substrates. No increase in turbidity or loss of total pentose was observed in the fermentations with *F. succinogenes* B21a.

Table 9.2 DIGESTION OF SEVERAL ISOLATED HEMICELLULOSES BY PURE CULTURES OF CELLULOLYTIC RUMEN BACTERIA[a]

Substrate	Hemicellulose digested (%)		
	Ruminococcus flavefaciens		*R. albus*
	B1a	C-94	7
Xylan	64.4	78.9	83.7
Flax hemicellulose	51.6	51.0	81.4
Corn-hull hemicellulose	14.8	39.9	4.8
Oat-hull hemicellulose	45.0	53.9	88.3
Alfalfa hemicellulose[b]	40.2	42.9	63.9

[a] Data from Dehority (1965).
[b] Percent digestion of the soluble portion of alfalfa hemicellulose.

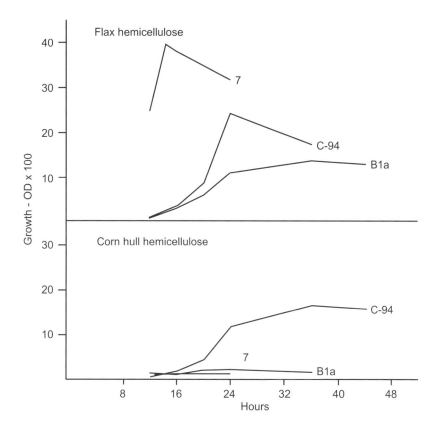

Figure 9.2 Growth of *R. flavefaciens* B1a and C-94 and *R. albus* 7 on isolated flax and corn-hull hemicellulose (from Dehority, 1965).

When these fermentation mixtures were analyzed for hemicellulose residues by Dr. Smith, it was found that only traces of hemicellulose were present in all tubes, including those inoculated with *F. succinogenes* B21a. In addition, all of the fermentation mixtures gave a negative test for reducing sugars. This obvious discrepancy prompted further investigation and subsequent fermentation mixtures were fractionated by precipitation of the residual hemicellulose from an acidified 80% ethanol solution, which were the conditions used in the original hemicellulose isolation procedure. The total pentose concentration was markedly reduced for B1a, C94 and 7, while B21a contained approximately the same amount of total pentose as the control (Table 9.3). Most of the pentose remaining in all four fermentations was found in the ethanol soluble form.

If one considers the loss of total pentose as utilization of the hemicellulose and the conversion of 80% ethanol insoluble pentose to 80% ethanol soluble pentose as degradation, then the data from Table 9.3 can be summarized as shown in Table 9.4.

The three ruminococci, B1a, C94 and 7, all utilized appreciable amounts of the hemicellulose with a concomitant production of organic acid end-products; however,

Table 9.3 PENTOSE CONCENTRATIONS IN THE 80% ETHANOL SOLUBLE AND INSOLUBLE FRACTIONS OF ISOLATED FESCUE GRASS HEMICELLULOSE FERMENTATION MIXTURES[a]

Organism	Total	Pentose concn (mg/ml) Ethyl alcohol-soluble	Ethyl alcohol-insoluble	Recovery from ethyl alcohol precipitation (%)
Blank medium (control)	1.30	0.02	1.14	89.6
Ruminococcus flavefaciens B1a	0.42	0.40	0.03	101.4
Fibrobacter succinogenes B21a	1.22	0.99	0.13	92.3
R. flavefaciens C-94	0.24	0.2	0.02	97.4
R. albus 7	0.25	0.14	0.09	92.1

[a] Data from Dehority (1965).

Table 9.4 EXTENT OF ISOLATED FESCUE GRASS HEMICELLULOSE DEGRADATION (SOLUBILIZATION) AND UTILIZATION BY SEVERAL PURE CULTURES OF RUMEN BACTERIA[a]

Organism	Degradation (%)	Utilization (%)	Total organic acids produced (meq/100 ml)
Ruminococcus flavefaciens B1a	97.5	67.4	1.53
Fibrobacter succinogenes B21a	88.4	5.9	0
R. flavefaciens C-94	98.6	81.8	1.48
R. albus 7	92.3	80.6	0.71

[a] Data from Dehority (1965).

B21a showed little or no utilization and no production of end-products. On the other hand, all organisms extensively degraded the ethanol insoluble hemicellulose into an ethanol soluble form. In addition to organic acids, *R. albus* 7 produces substantial amounts of CO_2, H_2 and ethyl alcohol, which would account for the apparent discrepancy between the level of acids produced by the ruminococci.

Similar experiments were conducted with flax and corn hull hemicellulose and included four additional cellulolytic strains. Results were essentially identical to those obtained with fescue grass hemicellulose. Time curves illustrating the degradation or degradation and utilization of isolated flax and corn hull hemicellulose are shown in Figure 9.3. These data can be compared to the time curves shown in Figure 9.2 which are based on utilization as reflected by growth and an increase in optical density. Thus it would appear that the cellulolytic organisms, regardless of their ability to utilize the substrate, are capable of degrading hemicellulose from an ethanol insoluble to an ethanol soluble form. This ability of the rumen cellulolytic bacteria to degrade hemicellulose was subsequently confirmed in studies by Henning (1979) and Morris and van Gylswyk (1980).

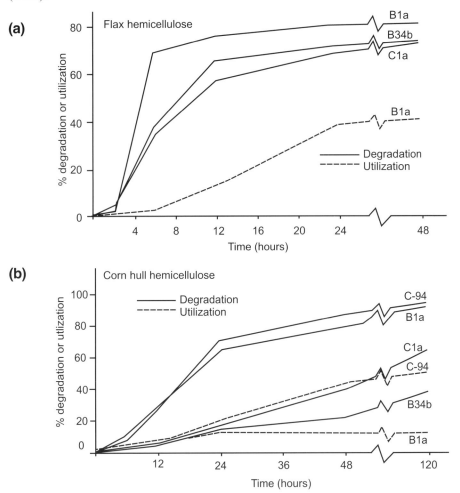

Figure 9.3 Time curves of the degradation or degradation and utilization of isolated (a) flax and (b) corn hull hemicelluloses by *Ruminococcus flavefaciens* strains B1a, B34b, C1a, and C-94. Samples were taken after 0, 6, 12, 24, 48 and 120 hours of incubation (from Dehority, 1967).

The data obtained on degradation of isolated hemicelluloses by the cellulolytic rumen bacteria raised some very interesting questions. First, which organisms are the predominant hemicellulose digestors in the rumen? Secondly, what function, if any, might the cellulolytic species have in hemicellulose fermentation in the rumen itself? In an attempt to determine which species of rumen bacteria might be the predominant hemicellulose digesting organisms, time studies were run comparing the rate and extent of hemicellulose degradation and utilization between the cellulolytic strains and several of the so-called "hemicellulolytic" strains of *B. fibrisolvens* and *P. ruminicola* which had been isolated with a xylan medium. These results are shown in Figure 9.4 (Dehority, 1967).

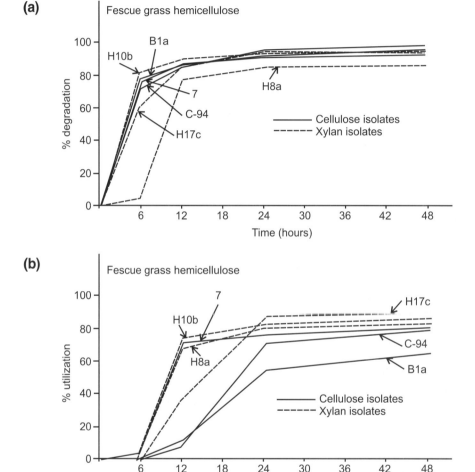

Figure 9.4 Time curves of the (a) degradation and (b) utilization of isolated fescue grass hemicellulose by *Ruminococcus flavefaciens* B1a and C-94, *R. albus* 7, *Butyrivibrio fibrisolvens* H10b and H17c and *Prevotella ruminicola* H8a. Samples were taken after 0, 6, 12, 24 and 48 hours of incubation (from Dehority, 1967).

First, no marked differences were observed in the initial rate of isolated hemicellulose degradation between the hemicellulose utilizing and non-utilizing cellulolytic strains. Secondly, the cellulolytic species could degrade, and where applicable, utilize isolated hemicellulose at a similar rate and extent as observed for the so-called "hemicellulose" digestors. In general, utilization lagged approximately six hours behind degradation.

Results of these experiments suggested that the cellulolytic rumen bacteria, regardless of whether they can utilize the hemicellulose for energy or not, produce a constitutive extracellular enzyme(s) which can degrade or solubilize isolated hemicellulose or xylan. Although the exact nature of this enzyme(s) is unknown, limited observations suggested a similarity to the cellulase enzymes, perhaps a nonspecific cleavage of the ß-1-4 xylosidic linkage of the hemicellulose (Dehority, 1968).

Fermentation of forage hemicellulose

In 1950, Hungate reported that his "less actively cellulolytic" rod, later tentatively classified as *Butyrivibrio fibrisolvens*, produced acid and gas from the fermentation of isolated oat hull, black locust, and white birch hemicellulose. Using alfalfa hay and poor quality grass as substrates, Hungate (1957) later demonstrated a weight loss in the crude "hemicellulose" fraction after fermentation by pure cultures of cellulolytic ruminococci. His "hemicellulose" fraction was that material not soluble in hot water, but soluble in 2% H_2SO_4. He noted that a considerably higher percentage of this "hemicellulose" fraction was digested from alfalfa than from poor quality grass hay.

Dehority and Scott (1967) investigated the extent of hemicellulose digestion by pure cultures in two maturity stages each of intact bromegrass and alfalfa. Substrate concentration was limiting so that the percent digestion should reflect only the capability of the particular species to digest the hemicellulose in a given intact forage. Those strains unable to ferment xylan showed little, if any, digestion of forage hemicellulose (*F. succinogenes* and some ruminococci), while the xylan fermenting strains of ruminococci digested varying but appreciable amounts of hemicellulose from bromegrass. However, the extent of digestion by these cultures was considerably lower with alfalfa as substrate. *Prevotella ruminicola* digested very little hemicellulose from bromegrass, but was able to digest appreciable quantities from alfalfa. *Butyrivibrio fibrisolvens* digested hemicellulose extensively from both bromegrass and alfalfa. Kock and Kistner (1969) from South Africa, estimated the extent of solubilization of cellulose and hemicellulose from lipid extracted low-protein teff hay by pure cultures of bacteria isolated from sheep conditioned to such hay. Their results substantiated the previous findings of Dehority and Scott (1967).

Although some interesting and marked differences were observed in the studies by Dehority and Scott (1967), only those strains capable of utilizing xylan or isolated hemicellulose, utilized the intact forage hemicellulose. Thus, fractionation procedures were developed for estimating degradation or solubilization of intact forage hemicellulose. A limiting substrate level of 0.5% forage was again used, so that the extent of hemicellulose degradation or degradation and utilization would be controlled either by chemical or physical properties of the forage itself or the ability of the particular organism being tested. Ten pure cultures, representing six different species, were used for this study (Coen and Dehority, 1970). Results obtained with two maturity stages of intact bromegrass are presented in the top portion of Table 9.5. All of the cellulolytic strains tested were capable of degrading a considerable amount of the 80% acidified ethanol insoluble pentose to a soluble form. Of the so-called "hemicellulolytic" species, *P. ruminicola* and *B. fibrisolvens*, only the two strains of *B. fibrisolvens*, H10b and H17c, were able to degrade and utilize the intact bromegrass hemicellulose. *L. multiparus* D15d, which cannot utilize either xylan or cellulose could neither degrade or utilize any of the hemicellulose. Degradation, and where applicable utilization, were reduced as the plant matured.

Table 9.5 EXTENT OF DEGRADATION, UTILIZATION OR BOTH OF HEMICELLULOSE FROM TWO MATURITY STAGES OF BROMEGRASS BY PURE CULTURES OF RUMEN BACTERIA[a]

	Forages[b]			
	Bromegrass 1		Bromegrass 2	
Strain[c]	Degradation	Utilization	Degradation	Utilization
		%		
A3c	54.0	2.1	31.8	6.0
S-85	77.3	3.0	62.0	2.4
7	60.9	46.0	40.6	29.4
B1a	56.6	23.0	34.7	17.1
B34b	77.8	0	61.1	0
H10b	51.9	41.3	32.5	27.1
H17c	50.7	44.8	30.2	26.8
H8a	4.7	6.1	5.0	6.1
D31d	4.2	4.1	0.6	0.6
D15d	2.2	4.8	3.1	2.6
B34b+D15d	78.3	3.5	62.9	2.1
B34b+H8a	84.1	80.3	70.3	67.2
B34b+H10b	81.3	69.6	65.8	58.5
B34b+H8a+H10b+D15d	83.5	78.7	70.6	67.3

[a] Data from Coen and Dehority (1970).
[b] Agronomic description: Bromegrass 1 (boot stage); Bromegrass 2 (bloom stage).
[c] Species: A3c and S-85, *Fibrobacter succinogenes*; 7, *Ruminococcus albus*; B1a and B34b, *R. flavefaciens*; H10b and H17c, *Butyrivibrio fibrisolvens*; H8a and D31d, *Prevotella ruminicola*; D15d, *Lachnospira multiparus*.

These results immediately posed the question as to whether the xylan-digesting strains which could not degrade and utilize the intact bromegrass hemicellulose could utilize the material solubilized or degraded by the non-utilizing cellulolytic strains. Fermentations were set up and inoculated with combinations of two or more strains and the results are presented at the bottom of Table 9.5. In all cases, degradation was increased above that obtained with *R. flavefaciens* B34b alone. The most striking effect, however, was noted in the utilization of total pentose by the combination with *P. ruminicola* H8a, in which utilization increased from essentially zero for each organism alone to approximately 80 and 70%, respectively, for maturity stages 1 and 2.

A marked increase in utilization was also observed when B34b and *B. fibrisolvens* H10b were combined. *L. multiparus* D15d was unable to utilize the degraded hemicellulose which would be in agreement with the inability of D15d to use pentoses or xylan as energy sources. When all three organisms, H8a, H10b and D15d were combined with B34b, degradation and utilization were essentially the same as obtained with the highest combination of two strains, i.e., B34b and H8a.

A similar series of experiments were conducted with several maturity stages of intact alfalfa (Table 9.6). Results with the cellulolytic species were essentially similar to those obtained with bromegrass; however, the extent of utilization and/or degradation were generally lower. In contrast to the bromegrass results, strains H8a and D31d of *P.*

Table 9.6 EXTENT OF DEGRADATION, UTILIZATION OR BOTH OF HEMICELLULOSE FROM TWO MATURITY STAGES OF ALFALFA BY PURE CULTURES OF RUMEN BACTERIA[a].

	Forages[b]			
	Alfalfa 1		*Alfalfa 3*	
Strain[c]	*Degradation*	*Utilization*	*Degradation*	*Utilization*
	%			
A3c	60.3	5.1	29.7	0
S-85	62.1	0	28.7	0
7	50.1	26.9	31.6	7.4
B1a	44.6	10.1	26.3	0
B34b	56.3	2.1	26.8	0
H10b	35.4	34.1	27.4	27.0
H17c	28.1	11.4	16.3	12.3
H8a	33.6	33.9	23.6	20.6
D31d	43.4	18.7	35.6	7.0
D15d	49.5	23.2	42.1	14.4
B34b+H8a	59.6	54.8	36.5	33.9
B34b+H10b	61.9	43.2	33.1	19.6
B34b+D15d	61.8	14.9	35.9	0
B34b+D15d+H8a+H10b	61.8	58.4	36.4	34.8

[a] Data from Coen and Dehority (1970).
[b] Agronomic description: Alfalfa 1 (prebloom); Alfalfa 3 (late bloom).
[c] See footnote c, Table 9.5.

ruminicola and strain D15d of *L. multiparus* were able to degrade and utilize the alfalfa pentosans to a limited extent. These data would suggest that there are definite differences in structure (or linkages) of hemicelluloses between intact legumes and grasses. The results with *L. multiparus* were most unusual since, as mentioned earlier, this strain cannot use pentoses, xylan or solubilized bromegrass hemicellulose as energy sources. Additional studies with a second strain of *L. multiparus* confirmed these findings. Synergism studies with the alfalfa substrates gave results quite similar, but of a somewhat lesser magnitude, to those obtained with bromegrass, except for the combination of B34b and D15d, in which case utilization by the combination was decreased. The only explanation for this latter observation would appear to be that B34b may attack different linkages in the hemicellulose than D15d, and at a faster rate. The oligosaccharides or sugars produced by B34b presumably then are not utilized by D15d.

Table 9.7 presents a comparison of hemicellulose degradation, utilization, or both, by several pure cultures of rumen bacteria between fescue grass hemicellulose either in the intact plant or physically isolated from the same forage. In general, the results with intact fescue grass, using single strains or combinations, parallel the pattern observed with bromegrass. On the other hand, except for strain D15d, degradation of the isolated fescue grass hemicellulose was very extensive, as was utilization, where applicable. As might be expected, synergism effects were minimal with the isolated hemicellulose. Thus, either chemical isolation of the hemicellulose or solubilization from the intact forage by a non-utilizing strain allows extensive utilization of the hemicellulose by those xylan-digesting strains which are limited or incapable of attacking the hemicellulose in its native state.

Table 9.7 EXTENT OF DEGRADATION, UTILIZATION OR BOTH OF FESCUE GRASS HEMICCELLULOSE, EITHER ISOLATED OR FROM THE INTACT FORAGE, BY PURE CULTURES OF RUMEN BACTERIA[a]

	Substrate			
	Fescue grass		Isolated fescue hemicellulose	
Strain[b]	Degradation	Utilization	Degradation	Utilization
	%			
B34b	66.6	3.0	88.5	0
H10b	44.8	38.0	87.5	83.8
H8a	2.7	2.0	82.0	80.4
D15d	4.0	1.3	1.7	1.7
B34b+H8a	69.0	67.7	93.9	87.0
B34b+H10b	67.3	64.8	91.3	87.8
B34b+D15d	67.9	3.9	87.0	3.8
B34b+D15d+H8a+H10b	67.6	65.9	87.4	85.7

[a] Data from Coen and Dehority (1970).
[b] See footnote c, Table 9.5.

Osborne and Dehority (1989) carried out a series of experiments using three pure cultures of rumen bacteria, each of which was selective in fermenting only one of the major structural forage polysaccharides. *F. succinogenes* A3c only utilizes cellulose; *Prevotella ruminicola* H2b utilizes only hemicellulose and *Lachnospira multiparus* can only utilize pectin. The data obtained for hemicellulose degradation and utilization from two maturity stages of orchardgrass were very similar to the previous data of Coen and Dehority (1970). Utilization of forage hemicellulose was markedly increased when A3c and H2b were combined. For immature OG, utilization values were 3% and 36% for A3c and H2b, respectively, compared to 74% utilization with the combination. Values with mature OG were 7.0% and 19% alone and 69% combined. In both instances, the increase in utilization is a genuine example of synergism in that the combination of organisms far exceeds the additive effects of each alone. In fact, it is approximately twice the added utilization of the two organisms alone.

In a series of sequential addition experiments, in which one organism was allowed to ferment the forage, then killed and the fermentation tube inoculated with a second organism, Fondevila and Dehority (1994) were able to substantiate previous explanations for the synergism in forage hemicellulose digestion (Coen and Dehority, 1970; Osborne and Dehority, 1989). Utilization of forage hemicellulose as an energy source by *P. ruminicola* is shown in Table 9.8. If *P. ruminicola*, a hemicellulose-utilizing organism, was added at the same time, or sequentially as the second organism, with either *F. succinogenes* or *R. flavefaciens,* hemicellulose-degrading organisms, utilization was higher ($P < 0.05$) than if *P. ruminicola* was the first organism added in sequential addition experiments.

Table 9.8 UTILIZATION OF HEMICELLULOSE FROM INTACT FORAGES BY PURE CULTURES OF RUMEN BACTERIA CULTURED TOGETHER OR SEQUENTIALLY[a]

Organism[b]		Forage		
First	Second	OG 1[a]	OG 2	Alfalfa
		%		
F. succ.+ P. rum.	-	52.8[x]	58.7[x]	30.7[x]
F. succ.	P. rum.	47.7[x]	57.0[x]	28.0[x]
P. rum.	F. succ.	9.7[y]	20.4[y]	14.1[y]
R. Flav.+ P. rum.	-	44.8[x]	36.0[x]	31.5[x]
R. flav.	P. rum.	33.6[y]	34.5[x]	24.8[x]
P. rum.	R. flav.	17.0[y]	26.0[y]	14.6[y]

[a]Data from Fondevila and Dehority (1994).
[b]F. succ.=*Fibrobacter succinogenes* A3c; P. rum.=*Prevotella ruminicola* H2b; R. flav. = *Ruminococcus flavefaciens* B34b.
[c]OG1 = immature orchardgrass; OG2 = mature orchardgrass
[x,y,z]For each pair of organisms, means in the same column followed by different superscripts differ at $P<0.05$.

Thus, as suggested earlier, the synergism observed by combining cultures results from an initial solubilization of hemicellulose from the forage by degrading but essentially non-utilizing organisms and subsequent utilization of the solubilized polysaccharides by the utilizing but non-degrading organism.

Hemicellulose-degrading enzymes of rumen bacteria

Williams and Withers (1981) isolated over 100 bacterial cultures from ovine rumen contents by enrichment techniques in selective xylan, arabinogalactan, pectin and cellulose media. The isolates were screened for their ability to degrade or utilize plant cell wall structural polysaccharides and 35 strains were studied in detail. Based on morphological and biochemical characteristics the authors concluded that most of the strains could be assigned to the genera *Ruminococcus, Butyrivibrio, Prevotella* or *Eubacterium*. Crude enzyme preparations were prepared from both sonicated cells and culture supernatants and used to assay for various activities. Although the isolates varied in their range and level of enzyme activities, the presence of esterase, glycosidase and polysaccharidase enzymes suggested that the organisms would be able to effectively utilize plant cell wall components. This study was the first to present detailed information on glycosidase activity of rumen bacteria.

Williams and Withers (1982a) subsequently determined activity of the principal polysaccharide-degrading enzymes produced by pure cultures of hemicellulolytic rumen bacteria grown on a range of carbohydrate substrates. Enzyme activities (crude enzyme preparations from sonicated cells) were affected by the carbon source used in the growth medium. In general, growth on glucose or cellobiose resulted in reduction or apparent loss of activities, while growth with polysaccharide substrates yielded higher levels of the polysaccharidase. Since enzyme activity was detectable in several isolates after culture on mono- or disaccharides, in the absence of the principal or related polysaccharide substrate, they suggest that certain of the polysaccharidases may be constitutive in nature. Similar results were obtained by these same authors on glycosidase activity of the hemicellulose-degrading rumen bacteria (Williams and Withers, 1982b).

Greve *et al.* (1984b) cultured *R. albus* 8 with isolated alfalfa cell walls as the only carbon source. Assay of the culture broth for muralytic enzymes revealed a wide range of activity. These included ß-glucosidase, ß-xylosidase, α-galactosidase, α-arabinosidase, cellulase, polygalacturonase and ß-1-4 xylanase. Their results suggested that enzyme production was partially regulated by the substrate or products from it. When the monosaccharides contained in alfalfa cell walls were used as substrates in a single fermentation, glucose and xylose were used in preference to the other sugars. Arabinose, galactose, rhamnose and uronic acid were utilized at a much slower rate. Greve *et al.* (1984a) studied the α-L-arabinofuranosidase from *R. albus* 8. This enzyme removes the arabinsyl side chains from hemicellulose and they were able to show a marked increase in the enzymatic degradation of alfalfa cell walls when this purified enzyme was added to incubations with xylanase.

Hespell and O'Bryan-Shah (1988) measured esterase activity in 30 strains of *B. fibrisolvens*. All strains possessed some esterase activity towards acetate, butyrate, caprylate, laurate and palmitate esters. Activity was primarily cell associated. Four strains were also found to possess acetyl xylan esterase activity in the culture fluid. This enzyme activity releases acetate from acetylated xylans and based on several studies, the acetylated xylose residues in grass cell walls are very resistant to digestion. Chemical removal of the acetyl groups markedly increased digestibility, thus suggesting an important role for acetyl xylan esterase type of activity. This esterase had not previously been detected in ruminal bacteria.

Varel *et al.* (1991) incubated several phenolic monomer degrading rumen bacteria in coculture with *F. succinogenes, R. albus* and *C. longisporum*. Although cellulose digestion was not increased by the combinations, increased amounts of hemicellulose were digested. They hypothesized that the lignin and phenolic acids are linked to hemicellulose and not cellulose, therefore, removal of the phenolics should enhance hemicellulose digestion.

Table 9.9 is taken primarily from Hespell and Whitehead (1990) and provides some insight into the enzymatic activities needed to depolymerize and utilize the hemicellulosic fraction of plants. The ability of a given organism to utilize forage hemicellulose thus depends on the number and type of enzymes it produces. The differences observed between the various species probably accounts for the synergism observed in hemicellulose digestion.

Table 9.9 POSSIBLE ENZYMES NEEDED FOR DEGRADATION AND UTILIZATION OF XYLANS (HEMICELLULOSES)[a]

Enzyme activity	Substrates degraded
Celloxylanase[b]	Cellulose; xylan
Xylanase[c]	Xylans; xylooligosaccharides
Arabinosidase	Arabinose sidechains
Acetyl xylan esterase	Acetyl sidechains
Glucuronidase	Methylglucuronate sidechains
Xylodextrinase	Xylooligosaccharides
Xylosidase	Xylooligosaccharides
Xylodextrin phosphorylase	Xylooligosaccharides
Xylobiose phosphorylase	Xylobiose
Xylobiase	Xylobiose

[a] Hespell *et al.* (1987); Hespell and Whitehead (1990).
[b] Readily attacks cellulose or xylans; may function to begin the breakdown of these components in the cell walls to allow better access by the true cellulases and xylanases.
[c] The xylanases appear to attack the xylan molecule at random, producing xylose, xylobiose and long-chain xylooligosaccharides. Sidechains are removed by several enzymes such as acetyl esterase, arabinosidase and glucuronidase.

Conclusions

Our present knowledge concerning the fermentation of hemicelluloses in the rumen might best be summarized as follows: The fermentation of both isolated and intact forage hemicelluloses appears to occur in two stages. The first stage, called degradation, involves a solubilization or depolymerization of the hemicellulose into 80% ethanol soluble oligosaccharides. This is followed by the second stage, utilization of these intermediates for growth. The ability of an organism to utilize the solubilized hemicellulose as an energy source is not necessarily associated with its ability to degrade the hemicellulose. In fact, the most extensive degradation was observed with non-utilizing strains. The situation is further confounded when intact forages are used as substrates, since the species and maturity stage of the forage markedly affect the availability of the hemicellulose for degradation to a given organism. Considerable variation has also been noted between both bacterial species and strains in their ability to degrade and utilize hemicellulose from a particular forage. When the possible synergism between species is included, one can begin to appreciate the complexity of the overall rumen fermentation of hemicellulose.

References

Bryant, M. P. (1959). Bacterial species of the rumen. *Bacteriological Reviews*, **23**, 125-153.

Bryant, M. P. and I. M. Robinson. (1962). Some nutritional characteristics of predominant culturable rumen bacteria. *Journal of Bacteriology*, **84**, 605-614.

Bryant, M. P., N. Small, C. Bouma and H. Chu. (1958). *Bacteriodes ruminicola* n. sp. and *Succinimonas amylolytica* the new genus and species - species of succinic acid-producing anaerobic bacteria of the bovine rumen. *Journal of Bacteriology*, **76**, 15-23.

Burdick, D. and J. T. Sullivan. (1963). Ease of hydrolysis of the hemicelluloses of forage plants in relation to digestibility. *Journal of Animal Science*, **22**, 444-447.

Butterworth, J. P., S. E. Bell and M. G. Garvock. (1960). Isolation and properties of the xylan-fermenting bacterium 11. *Biochemical Journal*, **74**, 180-182.

Clarke, R.T.J., R. W. Bailey and B.D.E. Gaillard. (1969). Growth of rumen bacteria on plant cell wall polysaccharides. *Journal of General Microbiology*, **56**, 79-86.

Coen, J. A. and B. A. Dehority. (1970). Degradation and utilization of hemicellulose from intact forages by pure cultures of rumen bacteria. *Applied Microbiology*, **20**, 362-368.

Dehority, B. A. (1965). Degradation and utilization of isolated hemicellulose by pure cultures of cellulolytic rumen bacteria. *Journal of Bacteriology*, **89**, 1515-1520.

Dehority, B. A. (1966). Characterization of several bovine rumen bacteria isolated with a xylan medium. *Journal of Bacteriology*, **91**, 1724-1729.

Dehority, B. A. (1967). Rate of isolated hemicellulose degradation and utilization by pure cultures of rumen bacteria. *Applied Microbiology*, **15**, 987-993.

Dehority, B. A. (1968). Mechanism of isolated hemicellulose and xylan degradation by cellulolytic rumen bacteria. *Applied Microbiology*, **16**, 781-786.

Dehority, B. A. (1971). Carbon dioxide requirement of various species of rumen bacteria. *Journal of Bacteriology*, **105**, 70-76.

Dehority, B. A. (1973). Hemicellulose degradation by rumen bacteria. *Federation Proceedings*, **32**, 1819-1825.

Dehority, B. A. and H. W. Scott. (1967). Extent of cellulose and hemicellulose digestion in various forages by pure cultures of rumen bacteria. *Journal of Dairy Science*, **50**,1136-1141.

Fondevila, M. and B. A. Dehority. (1994). Degradation and utilization of forage hemicellulose by rumen bacteria, singly in coculture or added sequentially. *Journal of Applied Bacteriology,* **77**, 541-548.

Greve, L. C., J. M. Labavitch and R. E. Hungate. (1984a). α-L-Arabinofuranosidase from *Ruminococcus albus* 8: Purification and possible role in hydrolysis of alfalfa cell wall. *Applied and Environmental Microbiology*, **47**, 1135-1140.

Greve, L. C., J. M. Labavitch, R. J. Stack and R. E. Hungate. (1984b). Muralytic activities of *Ruminococcus albus* 8. *Applied and Environmental Microbiology*, **47**, 1141-1145.

Henning, P. A. (1979). Examination of methods for enumerating hemicellulose - utilizing bacteria in the rumen. *Applied and Environmental Microbiology*, **38**, 13-17.

Hespell, R. B. and P. J. O'Bryan-Shah. (1988). Esterase activities in *Butyrivibrio fibrisolvens* strains. *Applied and Environmental Microbiology*, **54**, 1917-1922.

Hespell, R. B. and T. R. Whitehead. (1990). Physiology and genetics of xylan degradation by gastrointestinal tract bacteria. *Journal of Dairy Science*, **73**, 3013-3022.

Hespell, R. B., R. Wolf and R. J. Bothast. (1987). Fermentation of xylans by *Butyrivibrio fibrisolvens* and other ruminal bacteria. *Applied and Environmental Microbiology*, **53**, 2849-2853.

Hobson, P. N. and M. R. Purdom. (1961). Two types of xylan fermenting bacteria from the sheep rumen. *Journal of Applied Bacteriology*, **24**, 188-193.

Howard, B. H., G. Jones and M. R. Purdom. (1960). The pentosanases of some rumen bacteria. *Biochemical Journal*, **74**, 173-180.

Hungate, R. E. (1950). The anaerobic mesophilic cellulolytic bacteria. *Bacteriological Reviews,* **14**, 1-49.

Hungate, R. E. (1957). Microorganisms in the rumen of cattle fed a constant ration. *Canadian Journal of Microbiology*, **3**, 289-311.

Hungate, R. E. (1966). *The Rumen and Its Microbes*. Academic Press. New York, NY.

Kock, S. G. and A. Kistner. (1969). Extent of solubilization of α-cellulose and hemicellulose of low-protein teff hay by pure cultures of cellulolytic rumen bacteria. *Journal of General Microbiology*, **55**, 459-462.

Mannarelli, B. M., L. D. Ericsson, D. Lee and R. J. Stack. (1991). Taxonomic relationships among strains of the anaerobic bacterium *Bacteroides ruminicola* determined by DNA and extracellular polysaccharide analysis. *Applied and Environmental Microbiology*, **57**, 2975-2980.

Morris, E. J. and N. O. van Gylswyk. (1980). Comparison of the action of rumen bacteria on cell walls from *Eragrostis tef*. *Journal of Agricultural Science*, **95**, 313-323.

Osborne, J. M. and B. A. Dehority. (1989). Synergism in degradation and utilization of intact forage cellulose, hemicellulose, and pectin by three pure cultures of ruminal bacteria. *Applied and Environmental Microbiology*, **55**, 2247-2250.

Pittman, K. A. and M. P. Bryant. (1964). Peptides and other nitrogen sources for growth of *Bacteroides ruminicola*. *Journal of Bacteriology*, **88**, 401-410.

Pittman, K. A., S. Lakshmanan and M. P. Bryant. (1967). Oligopeptide uptake by *Bacteroides ruminicola*. *Journal of Bacteriology*, **93**, 1499-1508.

Shah, H. N. and D. M. Collins. (1990). *Prevotella*, a new genus to include *Bacteroides melaninogenicus* and related species formerly classified in the genus *Bacteroides*. *International Journal of Systematic Bacteriology*, **32**, 271-274.

van Gylswyk, N. O. and J.J.T.K. van der Toorn. (1985). *Eubacterium uniforme* sp. nov. and *Eubacterium xylanophilum* sp. nov., fiber-digesting bacteria from the rumina of sheep fed corn stover. *International Journal of Systematic Bacteriology*, **35**, 323-326.

Walker, D. J. (1961). Isolation and characterization of a hemicellulose fermenting bacterium from the sheep rumen. *Australian Journal of Agricultural and Resource Economics*, **12**, 171-175.

Whistler, R. L. and C. L. Smart. (1953). Polysaccharide Chemistry. Academic Press Inc. New York, NY.

Williams, A. G. and S. E. Withers. (1981). Hemicellulose-degrading enzymes synthesized by rumen bacteria. *Journal of Applied Bacteriology*, **51**, 375-385.

Williams, A. G. and S. E. Withers. (1982a). The production of plant cell wall polysaccharide-degrading enzymes by hemicellulolytic rumen bacterial isolates grown on a range of carbohydrate substrates. *Journal of Applied Bacteriology*, **52**, 377-387.

Williams, A. G. and S. E. Withers. (1982b). The effect of the carbohydrate growth substrate on the glycosidase activity of hemicellulose-degrading rumen bacterial isolates. *Journal of Applied Bacteriology*, **52**, 389-401.

Varel, V. H., H. G. Jung and L. R. Krumholz. (1991). Degradation of cellulose and forage fiber fractions by ruminal cellulolytic bacteria alone and in coculture with phenolic monomer-degrading bacteria. *Journal of Animal Science*, **69**, 4993-5000.

CHAPTER 10

PECTIN-FERMENTING SPECIES OF RUMEN BACTERIA

Of the three principal carbohydrates present in forages, cellulose, hemicellulose and pectin, pectin constitutes the lowest percentage. Values for pectin range from 10 to 20% of the total carbohydrate complex found in grasses and alfalfa, respectively. In general, pectin concentrations are lower and hemicellulose concentrations higher in grasses as compared to legumes. For example, Waite and Gorrod (1959) have reported a complete analysis of several grasses and found young orchardgrass to contain 4.4% pectin, 17.3% hemicellulose and 21.8% cellulose on a dry matter basis. Analysis of two stages of alfalfa by Lagowski *et al.* (1958) revealed 10.4 and 9.4% pectin, 14.2 and 16.5% hemicellulose and 21.2 and 33.2% cellulose. Since appreciable digestion of forage pectin, 75 to 90% has been observed in conventional digestion trials with sheep (Michaux, 1951), it could contribute markedly to the supply of energy available to the rumen microorganisms and in turn the ruminant itself. The ability of mixed cultures of rumen bacteria to ferment isolated pectin has been reported by Howard in 1961 and Dehority *et al.* in 1962.

Pectin, or more correctly termed the pectic substances, which is found in the cell walls and intercellular layers of all plant tissues is primarily galacturonan, a linear polymer of α-1-4 linked galacturonic acid units either fully or partially esterified with methyl alcohol. Lesser amounts of araban and galactan are either linked with the galacturonan through ester groupings or held to one another by the interaction of secondary forces (Whistler and Smart, 1953). As with the hemicelluloses, total pectic substances are empirically determined by solubility methods. Plant materials are extracted with 0.5% ammonium oxalate at 75-80°C and the solubilized pectic substances are precipitated, dried and weighed.

Pectinolytic species

Bryant and coworkers used pectin as a test carbohydrate in their characterization studies on a number of rumen bacteria isolated in non-selective cellobiose-agar medium (Bryant and Doetsch, 1954; Bryant and Small, 1956a,b; Bryant *et al.*, 1958). They found that most strains of *Butyrivibrio fibrisolvens, Prevotella ruminicola, Lachnospira multiparus, Succinivibrio dextrinosolvens* and *Fibrobacter succinogenes* will ferment pectin. To assess the importance of the above named species and determine whether other important pectin fermenting species might be present in the rumen, Dehority (1969) isolated 32 strains of rumen bacteria from the bovine rumen in a medium which contained purified pectin as the only added energy source. Ten strains were selected for characterization, two of which were subsequently identified as *Lachnospira multiparus*, four as *Butyrivibrio fibrisolvens*, three as *Prevotella ruminicola*, and one organism which did not correspond with any previously described species.

The growth response of these ten isolates in a purified pectin medium was compared with a number of previously characterized strains and the results are shown in Table 10.1. Of primary interest was the observation that none of the strains of *F. succinogenes* grew in the medium with pectin as the only added energy source, since strain S85 was one of those strains used in the original study by Bryant and Doetsch (1954) in which they reported that *F. succinogenes* fermented pectin. The ruminococci could not utilize pectin as an energy source. Except for one strain of *P. ruminicola* (H2b), all tested strains of the species *P. ruminicola* and *B. fibrisolvens* grew in a medium with pectin as the only added substrate. However, the growth of two strains of *B. fibrisolvens* not isolated with a pectin medium, H10b and H16a, was minimal.

None of the 22 remaining uncharacterized pectin-fermenting strains, on the basis of morphology and the gram-stain, appeared to resemble either of the other species previously reported as pectin fermentors, i.e., *F. succinogenes* or *Succinivibrio dextrinosolvens*. No particular explanation can be offered for the discrepancy between the study by Dehority (1969) and that of Bryant and Doetsch (1954) on pectin fermentation by *F. succinogenes*. It is of interest that Hungate's type species of *B. succinogenes* did not ferment pectin (1950).

Using a medium with polygalacturonic acid as the only added substrate, Clarke *et al.* 1969) isolated only a single strain of *Lachnospira multiparus*. One of their *B. fibrisolvens* strains, isolated in clover hemicellulose medium, would also grow with polygalacturonic acid as its sole energy source.

Shane *et al.* (1969) reported that several strains of *R. flavefaciens* and *R. albus* isolated in cellulose or cellobiose-xylan-starch agar medium were able to ferment pectin. A subsequent report from this same South African Laboratory by Van Gylswyk and Roché (1970), reported that 24 strains of cellulolytic cocci could all ferment pectin. The report by Dehority (1969) indicated that the ruminococci showed no increase in optical density with pectin as the sole energy source. This observation was confirmed in a later study by Gradel and Dehority (1972); however, it should be noted that although there was no increase in optical density these authors observed a 10-20% decrease in purified pectin concentration, based on galacturonic acid content. In the South African studies pectin fermentation was determined by measuring pH after 6 days incubation in a complex rumen fluid medium. A decrease of more than 0.3 pH units was considered positive. Possibly this may have resulted from release and utilization of small quantities of neutral sugars covalently linked as side chains to the galacturonic backbone.

Nine isolates of *Eubacterium cellulosolvens* from South Africa, studied by Van Gylswyk and Hoffman (1970), plus six strains isolated in the Netherlands by Prins et al. (1972) were pectinolytic. The seventh strain studied by Prins et al. (1972) isolated in California, and the type strain isolated in Maryland (Bryant, 1959), could not ferment pectin.

Table 10.1 GROWTH RESPONSE OF VARIOUS RUMEN BACTERIA IN MEDIUM CONTAINING PURIFIED PECTIN AS THE ONLY ADDED ENERGY SOURCE[a,b]

Organism[c]	Increase in optical density (600 nm)	Organism[c]	Increase in optical density (600 nm)
Prevotella ruminicola		*Butyrivibrio fibrisolvens*	
D28f	0.75 (16)[d]	D16f	0.89 (18)[d]
D31d	1.06 (18)	D23g	0.73 (18)
D42f	0.85 (16)	D29d	0.69 (18)
H2b	0 (112)	D30g	0.24 (16)
H8a	0.78 (16)	H4a	0.70 (16)
H15a	0.82 (16)	H10b	0.13 (16)
23	0.32 (16)	H13b	0.61 (16)
GA33	0.62 (64)	H16a	0.14 (16)
		H17c	0.73 (16)
Fibrobacter succinogenes		*Lachnospira multiparus*	
A3c	0 (168)	D15d	0.25 (16)
B21a	0 (168)	D25e	0.39 (16)
S-85	0 (168)		
Ruminococcus flavefaciens		*Ruminococcus albus*	
B1a	0 (168)	7	0 (168)
B34b	0 (168)		
C1a	0 (168)		
C-94	0 (168)		

[a] Data from Dehority (1969).
[b] A 0.3% pectin medium containing 40% clarified rumen fluid, 0.5% Trypticase, and 0.25% yeast extract.
[c] Strains beginning with the letter D were isolated in a medium containing pectin as the only added energy source; those beginning with H were isolated in a medium containing only xylan; all others were isolated in a nonselective medium containing glucose and cellobiose as energy sources.
[d] The figure in parentheses indicates the hours of incubation required to reach maximum optical density.

It should also be noted that 19 strains of cellulolytic *Butyrivibrio* studied by Shane et al. (1969) and 10 strains studied by Van Gylswyk and Roché (1970), all isolated from sheep fed teff hay in South Africa, were able to ferment pectin.

In studies reported from Poland, Tomerska (1971) used a selective medium containing pectin as the only added source of energy and isolated eight strains of pectin fermenting bacteria. Four strains were identified as *B. fibrisolvens*, two as *S. bovis* and two quite similar to *L. multiparus*. The two *S. bovis* strains were much less active as determined on the basis of cell growth. Subsequent studies from this same lab by Ziolecki *et al.* (1972) revealed that *S. bovis* produces a constitutive pectin lyase which is released into the medium and decomposes pectin to lower oligogalacturonides which it cannot utilize. The streptococci can only utilize the covalently linked sugar side chains of pectin which are released in the course of its degradation.

Isolation of large pectinolytic treponemes from the rumen has been reported several times (Ziolecki, 1979; Paster and Canale-Parola, 1985). Although they have not been considered to be of major importance in the rumen, they appear to satisfy all requirements for consideration as a true rumen organism.

On the basis of the reports cited above, the species *B. fibrisolvens, P. ruminicola* and *Lachnospira multiparus* would appear to be the predominant pectinolytic species occurring in the rumen. Of the three studies in which isolations were made from a selective pectin medium, these were the consistent species isolated. The possible importance of a *Peptostreptococcus* species described by Dehority (1969) cannot be determined at this time, since to date, only a single strain (D43e) has been isolated and characterized. The organism grows quite rapidly with pectin but utilizes few other substrates and then only to a slow and limited degree, thus its isolation would be unlikely on most media. Assessment of the role and activity of the other species in which some strains were found to possess pectin fermenting capabilities, i.e., *F. succinogenes, Succinivibrio dextrinosolvens, R. flavefaciens, R. albus, E. cellulosolvens,* and possibly *S. bovis* awaits a more comprehensive study. The ruminococci and *S. bovis* appear to possess depolymerases but not glycosidases to utilize the oligogalacturonides.

Jensen and Canale-Parola (1985) isolated 42 strains of pectinolytic bacteria from human feces using a selective medium. Three isolates were studied in detail. All three were rods, two were gram-negative and morphologically resembled *Bacteroides* (*Prevotella*?). The third isolate was gram-positive and no identification was attempted. Pectin and polygalacturonic acid were fermented by all strains and two of the three fermented galacturonic and glucuronic acids. No other carbohydrates or amino acids were fermented. They proposed that there is a nutritionally defined group of "pectinophilic bacteria" which to date have only been found in the alimentary tracts of humans and ruminants. They considered these bacteria to be important components of pectin-based food chains and undoubtedly play a significant role in the nutrition of their host.

Description of pectinolytic species

Two of the predominant pectinolytic species, *B. fibrisolvens* and *P. ruminicola* have already been described. Brief descriptions of the third species *L. multiparus* and the *Peptostreptococcus* species isolated by Dehority (1969) will be presented.

LACHNOSPIRA MULTIPARUS

The species was established by Bryant and Small (1956b). The type strain was described as a motile curved rod 0.4 to 0.6 µm wide and 2 to 4 µm long with bluntly pointed ends. Most cells are arranged as singles and pairs. A few very long chains of cells that are only slightly curved and with more rounded ends also occur. Flagellation is monotrichous and polar. Young cultures show many gram positive cells which rapidly become gram-negative. Indole, catalase and H_2S are not produced, nitrate is not reduced, gelatin is not liquefied. Rumen fluid is not required for growth. Glucose, fructose, cellobiose, sucrose and pectin are the common carbohydrates fermented by most strains. Xylan and cellulose are not fermented and starch is not hydrolyzed. Fermentation products include CO_2, ethanol, acetic, formic and lactic acids and small amounts of H_2.

Some interesting data were reported by Rode *et al.* (1981), where they co-cultured *Eubacterium limosum* and *Lachnospira multiparus* in a pectin medium. *L. multiparus* fermented the pectin to acetate, methanol, ethanol, lactate, formate, CO_2 and H_2 in pure culture. *E. limosum* cannot ferment pectin or ethanol, but utilizes methanol, H_2CO_2 and lactate. In co-culture, *E. limosum* utilized the end-products (primarily methanol) of pectin fermentation by *L. multiparus* for growth and end-products produced in the co-culture were acetate, butyrate and CO_2.

TREPONEMES

Ziolecki (1979) reported the isolation of large pectinolytic treponemes from the rumen. The strictly anaerobic spiral organisms were isolated from a 10^{-7} dilution of bovine rumen contents. The organisms are 0.7 µm wide and 12 to 25 µm long, ferment pectin quite rapidly and are also able to ferment arabinose, inulin and sucrose at a much slower rate. None of the other common carbohydrates were fermented. Principal end-products of pectin fermentation were acetic and formic acids.

A new species of pectinolytic rumen spirochete was isolated and described by Paster and Canale-Parola (1985). The antibiotic rifampin was added to the isolation medium as a selective agent and pectin was the sole energy source. The helical cells measured from 0.6 to 0.7 µm in width by 12 to 20 µm in length. In addition to different plant polysaccharides such as pectin, arabinogalactan, starch and inulin, a wide range of carbohydrates were fermented. Pectin fermentation yielded acetate and formate as major end products. The authors proposed the name *Treponema saccharophilum* for this new species of rumen spirochete. Since *T. saccharophilum* not only ferments the plant polysaccharides, but also the building blocks of these polysaccharides, i.e., pentoses, hexoses, uronic acids, etc., this species should be well adapted for growth in the rumen.

PEPTOSTREPTOCOCCUS SPECIES STRAIN D43E

Gram-positive nonmotile coccus, occurring primarily as single cells or diplococci, anaerobic, 1.0 to 1.2 µm in diameter. The organism fermented pectin rapidly, producing acetic acid and hydrogen as the major end products. Small amounts of formic acid were also detected. Aside from very slow and limited growth on glucose, cellobiose, maltose and sucrose, little if any growth occurred on the other energy sources tested.

Enzymatic mechanisms

There are two general types of enzymes which are involved in the breakdown of pectic substances; i.e., the pectinesterases which hydrolyze the methyl ester groups from pectin yielding methanol and pectic acid and the depolymerases which are involved in cleavage of the α-1-4 glycosidic linkages (Deuel and Stutz, 1958). Two types of pectin depolymerizing enzymes have been characterized, hydrolases, which hydrolyze the α-1-4 glycosidic linkage directly, and lyases which function through a trans-elimination mechanism. In general, direct hydrolysis should yield methyl galacturonate and oligogalacturonates, whereas trans-elimination produces unsaturated methyl oligogalacturonates having chain lengths of two or more. In the presence of pectinesterase these would occur as the acid rather than the methyl ester. In addition, both endo- and exoenzyme activity has been observed.

Rumen bacterial species active in the breakdown of pectin have been studied extensively by a group in Poland. Their studies have also included the type of pectic enzymes produced by these bacteria. They have isolated and studied the species *Prevotella ruminicola, Lachnospira multiparus, Streptococcus bovis* and several different types of spirochetes. Enzyme activities were as follows:

Prevotella ruminicola - produces unsaturated oligogalacturonides extracellularly by the action of a trans-elimination mechanism. The degradation products are further metabolized. Galacturonic acid is utilized. Also has some pectinesterase activity (Tomerska, 1971; Wojciechowicz, 1971; Wojciechowicz and Tomerska, 1971).

Streptococcus bovis - Produces an extracellular pectin lyase of the trans-elimination type, which forms unsaturated lower oligogalacturonides that are not further utilized. Galacturonic acid is not utilized. Apparently the streptococci can only utilize the sugars occurring in the pectin molecule which are released during the course of its degradation (Ziolecki *et al.*, 1972).

Lachnospira multiparus - Produces a polygalacturonate lyase of the trans-elimination type, primarily yielding an unsaturated digalacturonide which is utilized. Some galacturonic

Pectin-fermenting species of rumen bacteria 235

acid is produced, but not utilized (Wojciechowicz *et al.*, 1980). Pectinesterase activity is also present (Wojciechowicz and Tomerska, 1971).

Large treponemes - Pectin is decomposed by both trans-elimination and hydrolysis, yielding a mixture of saturated and unsaturated products. Strong pectinesterase activity (Wojciechowicz and Ziolecki, 1979; Ziolecki, 1979). Differs from other bacteria in having a mixture of both types of enzyme activity; however, lyase activity was highest.

Small spirochetes - Polygalacturonate lyase enzyme of the trans-elimination type and pectinesterase (Ziolecki and Wojciechowicz, 1980).

Based on their studies they concluded that the principal pectinolytic enzyme of the pectin-metabolizing rumen bacteria can be classified as an extracellular endopolygalacturonate lyase. It is also of interest that over a period of ten or more years this group of workers in Poland did not isolate *Butyrivibrio fibrisolvens* with their selective pectin medium.

Fermentation of forage pectin

Gradel and Dehority (1972) studied the digestion of both isolated pectin and pectin from intact forages. Since pectin is normally isolated by extraction from the forage and subsequent precipitation with ethanol, suitable methods were developed to allow measurement of 90% acidified ethanol soluble and insoluble pectin in fermentation mixtures. It was postulated that some of the cellulolytic species might possess enzymatic capabilities similar to those observed toward hemicellulose, i.e., depolymerase activity, but no glycosidases to use the oligogalacturonates produced. They found that two strains of ruminococci, *R. flavefaciens* B43b and *R. albus* 7, were able to solubilize or degrade about 30% of the purified pectin and utilize a limited amount of the soluble material. In contrast, *F. succinogenes* A3c and one strain of *B. fibrisolvens* (H10b) could not degrade or utilize purified pectin.

Six cultures were chosen to investigate pectin degradation and utilization from intact forages: *R. flavefaciens* B34b, a pectin degrader but limited utilizer; *P. ruminicola* 23 and D31d; *B. fibrisolvens* D16f; *L. multiparus* D15d and *Peptostreptococcus* strain D43e, all of which could extensively utilize isolated pectin as an energy source. Table 10.2 lists the data on degradation and utilization of pectin from two maturity stages of alfalfa. All strains could degrade and utilize alfalfa pectin. Of particular interest was the limited ability of the *P. ruminicola* strains. Except for B34b, the strains utilized most of what was degraded. Combination of strain B34b with either D31d or D16f in the same fermentation increased degradation above the extent obtained with either strain alone. The most striking effect, however, was with utilization of plant pectin by both combinations. Utilization increased from about 30 and 25% for either B34b or D31d alone to 82 and 74% for maturity stages 1 and 3, respectively. A marked increase, but of lesser magnitude also occurred with the B34b and D16f combination. With bromegrass as a substrate, Table 10.3, results with single strains were somewhat similar to those obtained with alfalfa, except for the two *P. ruminicola* strains and the mature bromegrass, where both degradation and utilization were extremely low, less than 6%. With combinations of the strains (B34b plus D31d or D16f), degradation was not improved on bromegrass 1, and utilization increased only with D31d. Both degradation and utilization were markedly improved on bromegrass 2 with B34b and D31d. Degradation was not improved with the combination of B34b and D16f and utilization was reduced.

Table 10.2 EXTENT OF DEGRADATION, UTILIZATION OR BOTH, OF PECTIN FROM TWO MATURITY STAGES OF ALFALFA BY PURE CULTURES OF RUMEN BACTERIA[a]

	Forages[b]			
	Alfalfa 1		Alfalfa 3	
Organism	Degradation	Utilization	Degradation	Utilization
		%		
Ruminococcus flavefaciens B34b	70.5	30.4	54.3	26.6
Prevotella ruminicola				
23	36.7	36.6	29.5	27.3
D31d	31.3	29.1	29.3	24.1
Butyrivibrio fibrisolvens D16f	67.5	57.3	54.4	53.1
Lachnospira multiparus D15d	62.9	50.4	56.6	45.8
Peptostreptococcus sp. D43e	61.5	49.7	57.0	47.6
R. flavefaciens B34b +				
P. ruminicola D31d	83.2	82.3	74.0	74.3
R. flavefaciens B34b +				
B. fibrisolvens D16f	78.4	74.2	67.4	64.5

[a] From Gradel and Dehority (1972).
[b] Agronomic description: 1 = prebloom; 3 = late bloom.

The different pectinolytic species vary markedly in the amount of pectin they can degrade or solubilize from a specific intact forage; however, if the pectin can be freed from the forage either chemically or by another organism, it is then available for utilization by these organisms. These data also indicate that some of the cellulolytic species, through synergism, could contribute to the overall rumen fermentation of pectin. A similar role was established for the cellulolytics in the rumen fermentation of hemicelluloses (Coen and Dehority, 1970; Fondevila and Dehority, 1994).

Cheng *et al*. (1979) incubated surface-disinfected clover leaflets and ryegrass leaves overnight (17 h) in nutrient medium inoculated with *L. multiparus* D25e. In control flasks without inoculation, clover leaflets showed no sign of breakdown, even with shaking. However, in the inoculated flasks extensive disintegration of the clover leaflets was observed. Transmission electron microscopy (TEM) suggested that *L. multiparus* entered the intercellular spaces of the

Table 10.3 EXTENT OF DEGRADATION, UTILIZATION OR BOTH, OF PECTIN FROM TWO MATURITY STAGES OF BROMEGRASS BY PURE CULTURES OF RUMEN BACTERIA[a]

Organism	Forages[b]			
	Bromegrass 1		Bromegrass 2	
	Degradation	*Utilization*	*Degradation*	*Utilization*
		%		
Ruminococcus flavefaciens B34b	71.3	29.8	35.5	8.1
Prevotella ruminicola				
23	55.0	52.6	5.7	4.9
D31d	43.3	49.7	1.0	2.6
Butyrivibrio fibrisolvens D16f	55.3	49.7	46.7	45.3
Lachnospira multiparus D15d	45.6	43.2	28.3	23.9
Peptostreptococcus sp. D43e	65.5	51.9	29.0	21.2
R. flavefaciens B34b +				
P. ruminicola D31d	72.6	70.1	52.5	53.0
R. flavefaciens B34b +				
B. fibrisolvens D16f	68.8	54.3	43.7	34.8

[a] From Gradel and Dehority (1972).
[b] Agronomic description: 1 = prebloom; 2 = late bloom.

mesophyll tissue and caused a separation of the individual cells. However, there did not appear to be active invasion of plant cells. The main route of colonization of clover appeared to be through cut edges. Similar data were obtained with ryegrass leaves; however, disintegration was much less marked. Pectin content of the ryegrass leaves was also much less than for clover leaflets.

Three cultures of rumen bacteria, each specific in their ability to utilize only one of the structural carbohydrates in forage (cellulose, hemicellulose or pectin), were inoculated singly and in all possible combinations into media containing intact orchardgrass as the only energy source (Osborne and Dehority, 1989). A slight increase in the utilization of cellulose from mature orchardgrass was observed when the cellulolytic culture, *Fibrobacter succinogenes* A3c, was cocultured with either the hemicellulose digester, *Prevotella ruminicola* H2b or the pectin-fermenting culture, *Lachnospira multiparus* D15d, or all three combined. For both maturity stages of orchardgrass, all combinations of A3c with H2b resulted in a synergistic increase in hemicellulose utilization ($P < 0.05$). This data was very similar to the results previously obtained by Coen and Dehority (1970).

However, pectin degradation and utilization from intact orchardgrass was quite different than expected. These results are shown in Table 10.4. Surprisingly, H2b which supposedly cannot utilize pectin was able to degrade and utilize appreciable amounts of pectin from both maturity stages of orchardgrass. On the other hand, the pectinolytic strain, D15d, was quite limited in the amount of pectin it degraded and utilized. Strain A3c, extensively degraded, but could not utilize the forage pectin. Coculture of A3c and H2b increased both degradation and utilization of forage pectin, whereas cocultures of either strain with D15d had little, if any, effect. The authors reinvestigated the ability of these organisms to ferment purified pectin, the criteria on which they had originally been chosen for this study. These data, also shown in Table 10.4, clearly show that only D15d can degrade and utilize this substrate to any extent. These results would suggest that the structure and bonds present in the pectin fractions of intact forages are different than those which occur in purified citrus pectin. More importantly, these limited data might also suggest that the bacterial species we isolate with a purified substrate in selective medium may or may not be the functionally active species in the rumen.

Table 10.4. PERCENT DEGRADATION AND UTILIZATION OF PURIFIED AND FORAGE PECTIN BY PURE CULTURES OF RUMEN BACTERIA, SINGLY AND IN COMBINATION[a]

Organism[b]	Substrate					
	Immature Orchardgrass		Mature Orchardgrass		Purified pectin	
	Deg.[c]	Utl.[d]	Deg.	Utl.	Deg.	Utl.
	%					
A3c	68.5	0	61.2	4.3	17.0	9.5
H2b	54.9	46.1	40.9	29.5	12.1	5.1
D15d	18.0	6.8	28.3	13.1	87.1	73.2
A3c + H2b	83.9	75.3	76.2	61.9	17.9	8.1
A3c + D15d	78.3	0	66.7	4.8	87.8	73.2
H2b + D15d	56.6	49.4	47.2	33.6	87.9	73.4
A3c + H2b + D15d	85.4	76.8	73.1	58.6	88.7	73.5

[a] Data from Osborne and Dehority (1989).
[b] A3c, *Fibrobacter succinogenes*; H2b, *Prevotella ruminicola*; D15d, *Lachnospira multiparus*.
[c] Degradation.
[d] Utilization.

Fermentation of forage polysaccharides in the rumen

Although it has generally been assumed that synergism between the various bacterial species was of importance in the rumen, direct experimental evidence has now been obtained to substantiate this point. Considering only the hemicellulose data where neither of two cultures could utilize any of the hemicellulose from an intact forage and yet 80% was digested by combining the two organisms in the same fermentation, we might conclude that we have an excellent model for rumen synergism based on the combination of just two bacterial cultures. However, in view of the synergism data also obtained on cellulose and pectin digestion involving most of the same strains and species, one must be aware of the scope of interactions involved when considering the *in vivo* fermentation of a complex natural substrate. In other words, the models which we now have on synergism between two organisms may be an over-simplification of true conditions. It should also be kept in mind that we are dealing with extent values in the synergism studies, i.e., total digestibility from a limiting substrate. The *in vivo* fermentation on the other hand is quite dynamic and undoubtedly influenced to a large degree by rates of digestion and passage.

With regard to the bacterial species involved in forage polysaccharide utilization, work in various laboratories using nonspecific and specific cellulose media for isolation suggests that we are dealing with the principal cellulolytic species, i.e., *Fibrobacter succinogenes, Ruminococcus flavefaciens* and *Ruminococcus albus*. Under certain conditions *Butyrivibrio fibrisolvens* may also be of significance. The so-called "hemicellulose" digestors would appear to principally consist of *Prevotella ruminicola, Butyrivibrio fibrisolvens* and possibly certain strains of ruminococci. The numbers at which these species occur, their isolation on a selective xylan medium, and the assay of a large number of non-selectively isolated organisms for xylan digestion would support these conclusions. *Prevotella ruminicola, Butyrivibrio fibrisolvens* and *Lachnospira multiparus* appear to be the predominant pectinolytic species. These observations are again based on total numbers, isolation on a selective pectin medium, and assay of non-selective media isolates for pectin digestion. In general, it is suggested that we are probably working in pure culture with the predominant bacteria active in the overall rumen fermentation. However, some species may exist in the rumen which cannot be isolated, except in media containing the polysaccharide form of carbohydrate. This was brought out in the study by Dehority on isolation of bacteria with a selective pectin medium (Dehority, 1969). One strain subsequently identified as a *Peptrostreptococcus* species was isolated from 10^{-8} g of rumen contents. This organism grew rapidly with pectin as an energy source but showed little, if any, growth on all other carbohydrates. Further work would be required to assess the numbers and potential importance of such species; however, the possibility of their existence should be noted. We may also be able to determine the presence of non-culturable rumen bacteria using the newer techniques of molecular biology. However, at this time we cannot evaluate their potential role in the digestion of forage structural polysaccharides.

References

Bryant, M. P. (1959). Bacterial species of the rumen. *Bacteriological Reviews*, **23**, 125-153.
Bryant, M. P. and R. N. Doetsch. (1954). A study of actively cellulolytic rod-shaped

bacteria of the bovine rumen. *Journal of Dairy Sci*ence, **37**, 1176-1183.
Bryant, M. P. and N. Small. (1956a). The anaerobic monotrichous butyric acid-producing curved rod-shaped bacteria of the rumen. *Journal of Bacteriology*, **72**,16-21.
Bryant, M. P. and N. Small. (1956b). Characteristics of two new genera of anaerobic curved rods isolated from the rumen of cattle. *Journal of Bacteriology*, **72**, 22-26.
Bryant, M. P., N. Small, C. Bouma and H. Chu. (1958). *Bacteroides ruminicola* n. sp. and *Succinimonas amylolytica* the new genus and species - species of succinic acid-producing anaerobic bacteria of the bovine rumen. *Journal of Bacteriology*, **76**,15-23.
Cheng, K.-J., D. Dinsdale and C. S. Stewart. (1979). Maceration of clover and grassleaves by *Lachnospira multiparus*. *Applied and Environmental Microbiology*, **38**, 723-729.
Clarke, R.T.J., R. W. Bailey and B.D. E. Gaillard. (1969). Growth of rumen bacteria on plant cell wall polysaccharides. *Journal of General Microbiology*, **56**, 79-86.
Coen, J. A. and B. A. Dehority. (1970). Degradation and utilization of hemicellulose from intact forages by pure cultures of rumen bacteria. *Applied Microbiology*, **20**, 362-368.
Dehority, B. A. (1969). Pectin fermenting bacteria isolated from the bovine rumen. *Journal of Bacteriology*, **99**, 189-196.
Dehority, B. A., R. R Johnson and H. R. Conrad. (1962). Digestibility of forage hemicellulose and pectin by rumen bacteria *in vitro* and the effect of lignification thereon. *Journal of Dairy Science*, **45**, 508-512.
Duel, H. and E. Stutz. (1958). Pectin substances and pectic enzymes. In: *Advances in Enzymology*. Edited by F. F. Nord. Interscience Publishers, Inc, New York, p. 341-383.
Fondevila, M. and B. A. Dehority. (1994). Degradation and utilization of forage hemicellulose by rumen bacteria, singly in coculture or added sequentially. *Journal of Applied Bacteriology*, **77**, 541-548.
Gradel, C. M. and B. A. Dehority. (1972). Fermentation of isolated pectin and pectin from intact forages by pure cultures of rumen bacteria. *Applied Microbiology*, **23**, 332-340.
Howard, B. H. (1961). Fermentation of pectin by rumen bacteria. *Proceedings of the Nutrition Society*, **20**, xxix-xxx.
Hungate, R. E. (1950). The anaerobic mesophilic cellulolytic bacteria. *Bacteriological Reviews*, **14**, 1-49.
Jensen, N. S. and E. Canale-Parola. (1985). Nutritionally limited pectinolytic bacteria from the human intestine. *Applied and Environmental Microbiology*, **50**, 172-173.
Lagowski, J. M., H. M. Sell, C. F. Huffman and C. W. Duncan. (1958). The carbohydrates in alfalfa (*Medicago sativia*). I. General composition, identification of a non-reducing sugar and investigation of the pectic substances. *Archives of*

Biochemistry and Biophysics, **76**, 306-319.

Michaux, A. (1951). Structural materials of vegetable cellular membranes during digestion by the ewe. *Comptes Rendus des Seances de L'academie D'agriculture de France,* **232**, 121-123.

Osborne, J. M. and B. A. Dehority. (1989). Synergism in degradation and utilization of intact forage cellulose, hemicellulose, and pectin by three pure cultures of ruminal bacteria. *Applied and Environmental Microbiology,* **55**, 2247-2250.

Paster, B. J. and E. Canale-Parola. (1985). *Treponema saccharophilum* sp. nov., a large pectinolytic spirochete from the bovine rumen. *Applied and Environmental Microbiology,* **50**, 212-219.

Prins, R. A., F. van Vugt, R. E. Hungate and C.J.A.H.V. van Vorstenbosch. (1972). A comparison of strains of *Eubacterium cellulosolvens* from the rumen. *Antonie van Leeuwenhoek Journal of Microbiology and Serology,* **38**, 153-161.

Rode, L. M., B.R.S. Genthner and M. P. Bryant. (1981). Syntrophic association by co-cultures of the methanol- and CO_2-H_2 - utilizing species *Eubacterium limosum* and pectin-fermenting *Lachnospira multiparus* during growth in a pectin medium. *Applied and Environmental Microbiology,* **42**, 20-22.

Shane, B. S., L. Gouws and A. Kistner. (1969). Cellulolytic bacteria occurring in the rumen of sheep conditioned to low-protein teff hay. *Journal of General Microbiology,* **55**, 445-457.

Tomerska, H. (1971). Decomposition of pectin *in vitro* by pure strains of rumen bacteria. *Acta Microbiologica Polonica,* **3,**107-115.

Waite, R. and A.R.N. Gorrod. (1959). The comprehensive analysis of grasses. *Journal of the Science of Food and Agriculture,* **10**, 317-326.

Whistler, R. L. and C. L. Smart. (1953). Polysaccharide Chemistry. Academic Press Inc. New York, NY.

Van Gylswyk, N. O. and J.P.L. Hoffman. (1970). Characteristics of cellulolytic cillobacteria from the rumens of sheep fed teff (*Eragrostis tef*) hay diets. *Journal of General Microbiology,* **60**, 381-386.

Van Gylswyk, N. O. and C.E.G. Roché. (1970). Characteristics of *Ruminococcus* and cellulolytic *Butyrivibrio* species from the rumens of sheep fed differently supplemented teff (*Eragrostis tef*) hay diets. *Journal of General Microbiology,* **64**, 11-17.

Wojciechowicz, M. (1971). Partial characterization of pectinolytic enzymes of *Bacteroides ruminicola* isolated from the rumen of a sheep. *Acta Microbiologica Polonica Section A,* **3**, 45-50.

Wojciechowicz, M. and H. Tomerska. (1971). Pectic enzymes in some pectinolytic rumen bacteria. *Acta Microbiologica Polonica Section A,* **3**, 57-61.

Wojciechowicz, M. and A. Ziolecki. (1979). Pectinolytic enzymes of large rumen treponemes. *Applied and Environmental Microbiology,* **37**, 136-142.

Wojciechowicz, M., K. Heinrichova and A. Ziolecki. (1980). A polygalacturonate lyase produced by *Lachnospira multiparus* isolated from the bovne rumen. *Journal* of General Microbiology, **117**, 193-199.

Ziolecki, A. (1979). Isolation and characterization of large treponemes from the bovine rumen. *Applied and Environmental Microbiology*, **37**, 131-135.

Ziolecki, A. and M. Wojciechowicz. (1980). Small pectinolytic spirochetes from the rumen. *Applied and Environmental Microbiology*, **39**, 919-922.

Ziolecki, A., H. Tomerska and M. Wojciechowicz. (1972). Pectinolytic activity of rumen streptococci. *Acta Microbiologica Polonica,* **4**, 183-188.

CHAPTER 11

STARCH DIGESTERS, OTHER LESS NUMEROUS SPECIES, AND FACULTATIVE ANAEROBES IN THE RUMEN

Starch digesting rumen bacteria

A number of the species of rumen bacteria which are cellulolytic, hemicellulolytic or both, are also amylolytic. Almost all strains of *Butyrivibrio fibrisolvens* and *Prevotella ruminicola* are capable of fermenting starch, as are some strains of *Fibrobacter succinogenes* and *Clostridium* species. Additional species of amylolytic bacteria which are not active in the fermentation of forage structural polysaccharides, but occur in reasonably large numbers are *Streptococcus bovis, Ruminobacter amylophilus* (formerly *Bacteroides amylophilus*), *Succinimonas amylolytica,* and *Selenomonas ruminantium*.

STREPTOCOCCUS BOVIS

Streptococcus bovis is a Gram-positive facultatively anaerobic homofermentative streptococcus (Hungate, 1966). It is undoubtedly involved in the fermentation of starch and other soluble carbohydrates in the rumen; however, on the basis of numbers of organisms found it seems probable that under most conditions other groups of bacteria are more significant in starch digestion. Since *S. bovis* does not require a low oxidation-reduction potential, it is generally one of the most commonly isolated species from the rumen. This would be especially so if the investigator's technique and medium did not meet the requirements for growth of the obligate anaerobes. Numbers of *S. bovis* will average about 10^7 per ml and do not tend to deviate as much as other species (Hungate, 1957). Under certain specific conditions, such as feeding an excess of grain or glucose to hay-fed sheep, a rapid marked increase in *S. bovis* has been observed (Hungate *et al.*, 1952). This resulted in the production of very high concentrations of lactic acid, a lowering of rumen pH to values between 4.1 and 4.7 and subsequent death of the animals. Although one might expect high numbers of this organism to occur in grain-fed animals, this is only found occasionally. Their numbers in grain adapted animals and hay-fed animals are similar. Neither Higginbottom and Wheater (1954) nor Hungate (1957) were able to demonstrate the presence of *S. bovis* in hay or ruminant feeds, which would strongly support its being classified as a true rumen organism. Hobson and

Mann (1957) conducted studies with fluorescent antibodies prepared against *S. bovis*, and were able to demonstrate the occurrence of this species in rumen contents from a number of animals. The nutrition of *S. bovis* differs quite markedly from the streptococci growing in other habitats and appears to be well suited to the rumen environment (Hungate, 1966).

Colonies of *S. bovis* are either white, yellow, orange or red in color; however, color does not appear to be a stable characteristic and is apparently not related to culture conditions. Cells are spherical to ovoid in shape, ranging from 0.5 to 1.0 μm in diameter (Buchanan and Gibbons, 1974; Dehority, 1975). In addition to starch, a wide variety of other carbohydrates are fermented by various strains. In general, gelatin is not liquefied and catalase is not produced. Most all strains produce capsules. About 80-85% of the carbohydrate fermented by *S. bovis* is converted to DL-lactic acid. Traces of acetate, formate and CO_2 may also be produced (Hungate, 1957, 1966).

Ford et al. (1958) investigated the vitamin requirements of 26 strains of *S. bovis* isolated from the rumen and found that none of the strains required exogenous vitamins. This appeared to be in contrast with the results reported earlier by Niven et al. (1948). The authors then reinvestigated the vitamin requirements incubating the cultures aerobically, similar to the conditions of Niven. Although growth was less vigorous, various vitamin requirements were observed. However, they concluded that the requirements were imposed by conditions of culture rather than an inability to synthesize these essential vitamins.

Russell and Robinson (1984) have studied the characteristics and composition of seven strains of *S. bovis*, one from California, two from South Africa, three from Scotland and one from Kansas. In general, characteristics of six of the strains were fairly similar; however, the Kansas strain showed marked differences in morphology (coccoid rather than ovoid), final pH (5.5 versus 4.4-4.7) and doubling time (155 min versus 24-27 min). Based on these criteria the authors concluded that classification of the Kansas strain as *S. bovis* was doubtful. The short doubling time and minimum pH for *S. bovis* helps explain its rapid proliferation with resulting acidosis in the animal when large quantities of starch are fed to ruminants. *S. bovis* rapidly ferments starch, producing lactic acid which causes reduction in rumen pH and a reduction in growth rate of the other bacteria. A reduced utilization of lactate by the lactate fermenting species allows pH to fall to levels which can impair animal performance.

Dufva et al. (1982) reported that the Kansas strain of *S. bovis* (later studied by Russell and Robinson, 1984) did not contain the amino acid diaminopimelic acid (DAPA), which has been widely used as a marker for bacterial protein. However, Russell and Robinson (1984) found DAPA in all seven of the *S. bovis* strains. Concentrations of DAPA varied but were in the same range for six of the seven strains (0.026% - 0.032%), while the seventh strain contained three times the amount of DAPA (0.110%). The high DAPA containing strain was one of the strains from Scotland. These data would certainly point out the difficulties, even within a single species, of using DAPA as a marker for bacterial protein.

S. *bovis* was able to grow at pH values ranging from 4.5 to 6.7 (Russell, 1991). Studies suggested that the sensitivity of most rumen bacterial strains to volatile fatty acids at low pH may be more closely related to intracellular pH regulation than an "uncoupling" type of reaction. Intracellular pH decreases in *S. bovis* as extracellular pH decreases, and a rather constant pH gradient is maintained across the cell membrane (0.9 units). Species such as *F. succinogenes* attempt to maintain a near neutral intracellular pH as extracellular pH decreases, and is unable to take up cellobiose or grow at pH below 5.8.

Using 16S rRNA probes and DNA homology, Nelms *et al.* (1995) compared ruminal and human strains of *S. bovis*. Their results indicated that the ruminal strains of *S. bovis* are both genetically and phenotypically distinct from human clinical isolates of this species. The human strains were isolated from individuals with several different diseases, i.e., septicemia, endocarditis or meningitis.

RUMINOBACTER (FORMERLY *BACTEROIDES*) *AMYLOPHILUS*

The species *Bacteroides amylophilus* was first isolated and described by Hamlin and Hungate in 1956. It is a Gram-negative, anaerobic, non-sporeforming, non-motile rod, varying in size from 0.9 to 1.6 µm in width to 1.6 x 4.0 µm in length. Many cells appear to be coccoid to oval in shape and cultures tend to exhibit considerable pleomorphism. Many cells show internal granulation when viewed by phase microscopy. The numbers of this species tend to vary, but they may constitute as much as 17-18% of the total strains isolated on high grain or high roughage diets (Caldwell and Bryant, 1966; Slyter and Putnam, 1967). Gelatin liquefaction is variable for this species. Indole and H_2S are not produced, and nitrate is not reduced. CO_2 is required for growth. The only substrates fermented by this species are starch and maltose, from which acetic, formic and succinic acids plus traces of ethanol are produced. Because of the inability of this species to use glucose or cellobiose as an energy source and possibly other species not yet isolated, starch is now routinely added to non-selective medium for counting and isolations (Bryant and Robinson, 1961).

In 1986, *B. amylophilis* was transferred to a new genus *Ruminobacter*, on the basis of 16S ribosomal RNA sequencing (Stackebrandt and Hippe, 1986). *Ruminobacter amylophilis* groups loosely with the so called gamma subdivision of purple bacteria and their non-phototrophic relatives, which includes enterobacteria, vibrios, oceanospirilla, legionellae and others.

Miura *et al.* (1980) have reported a very interesting study demonstrating the nutritional interdependence among rumen bacteria. They inoculated a basal medium containing starch, glucose and cellobiose with *R. amylophilus, M. elsdenii* and *R. albus*, and observed the successive growth of the three species. Based on data obtained from cocultures with just two species they concluded that *R. amylophilus* grew in the basal medium fermenting the starch and after growth ceased autolysis occurs with the production of branched-chain amino acids. This allows growth of the amino acid requiring *M. elsdenii*, which also produces branched-chain fatty acids. When enough branched-chain fatty acids are produced to meet the requirement of *R. albus*, growth of this species occurs. In the rumen, growth of these species probably occurs simultaneously once the chain is started. Other species of bacteria with similar capabilities would, of course, also be involved.

SUCCINIMONAS AMYLOLYTICA

The genus and species *Succinimonas amylolytica* were established by Bryant *et al.* (1958a). The genus is described as anaerobic, non-sporeforming, Gram-negative, straight rods with rounded ends that are motile with polar flagella. They ferment carbohydrate with the production of large amounts of succinic acid. The type species is an anaerobic Gram-negative, short, rounded end rod to coccoid organism, 1.0 to 1.5 µm wide and 1.2 to 3 µm long with most cells oval in shape. Some bipolar staining and internal granulation are evident in many cells. Motility is by polar, monotrichous flagellation. Glucose, maltose and dextrin are fermented, starch is hydrolyzed. Most of the other common test carbohydrates are not fermented. H_2S, catalase and indole are not produced, nitrate is not reduced, gelatin is not liquefied. Rumen fluid can be replaced by trypticase and yeast extract; however, CO_2 is required. End-products of glucose fermentation are primarily succinic acid, with small amounts of acetic and traces of propionic acid. The numbers of this species tend to be quite limited and never seem to account for more than 2 to 6% of the total isolates on a variety of diets. In the study by Dehority on CO_2 requirements, this species required a higher concentration of CO_2 (>0.10%) than any of the other species tested (Dehority, 1971).

SELENOMONAS RUMINANTIUM

The species *Selenomonas ruminantium* was first described by Certes in 1889, based entirely on morphology, arrangement of flagella and habitat (Hungate, 1966). Physiological characteristics of 11 strains of this species are reported by Bryant (1956). Most strains are curved, crescent-shaped rods usually 0.8 to 1.0 µm in width and 2-7 µm long with bluntly tapered ends. They are Gram-negative, anaerobic and motile. The tuft of flagella has a lateral point of attachment. Two important characteristics of this species are its marked production of H_2S and low minimum pH in poorly buffered medium (4.3 to 4.4). Nitrate is not reduced. Catalase and indole are not produced and gelatin is not liquefied. Cellulose is not hydrolyzed and xylan is generally not fermented. Most strains hydrolyze starch and numerous other soluble carbohydrates. A few strains will ferment lactate. The principal end-products of this species are lactic, acetic and propionic acid, although some butyric, formic and succinic acids are also measurable. CO_2 is produced by some strains and not required by any of those tested; however, under more stringent conditions a low requirement was later found for the type species by Dehority (1971). Replacement of rumen fluid by trypticase and yeast extract varied between strains. The strains studied by Bryant showed considerable variation in physiological characteristics; however, the differences did not appear to be valid criteria for establishing separate species. The only consistent difference was the ability of certain strains to ferment glycerol and lactate, and on this basis, a separate variety was established, *Selenomonas ruminantium* var. *lactilyticas*. Characteristics and end-products of two strains of *Selenomonas ruminantium* isolated from reindeer were similar to those of isolates from domestic ruminants (Dehority, 1975). Numbers of *Selenomonas ruminantium* in the rumen tend to be quite low, accounting for only 1-4% of total isolates. However, in some instances on high concentrate diets, percentages of 20 to 50% have been observed.

Kanegasaki and Takahashi (1967) isolated a strain of *S. ruminantium* var. *lactilyticas* using a lactate medium and found that the organisms requirement for rumen fluid was satisfied by volatile fatty acids in glucose media and biotin in lactate media. Straight chain VFA, C_3 to C_{10} were effective, but valeric acid was the most active. In a later study, these authors found that the radioactivity from n-valeric acid was incorporated into phospholipids and bound lipids (Kanegasaki and Takahashi, 1968).

An interesting method for isolation of *Selenomonas* was reported by Tiwari *et al.* in 1969. Using an anaerobic agar medium containing mannitol as the only added energy source, plus trypticase, yeast extract, n-valerate, acetate, cysteine, minerals and CO_2 gas phase, with a final pH of about 6.0, they were consistently able to isolate *Selenomonas ruminantium* from 10^{-6} to 10^{-8} ml of rumen fluid. The selectivity of their medium appeared to be due to the fact that mannitol is utilized by only a few other species of rumen bacteria and the selenomonads can grow better at a lower pH than most of the more numerous species in the rumen.

In 1971, Prins isolated five strains of a large selenomonad from the rumen of sheep and established a new variety, *Selenomonas ruminantium* var. *bryanti*. The organism is a Gram-negative, motile, crescentic rod with rounded ends and is 2 to 3 µm wide by 5 to 10 µm long. In addition to its large size, this variety fermented fewer carbohydrates than *S. ruminantium*, did not hydrolyze starch, produce H_2S from cysteine, produce gas, or ferment glycerol or lactate.

A ureolytic strain of *Selenomonas ruminantium* was isolated from rumen fluid by John *et al.* (1974). The organism occurred in numbers of 2×10^7 per ml and represented one of the first bacterial species isolated which is of probable importance in rumen urease production.

S. ruminantium can accumulate large quantities of intracellular polysaccharide when grown in a simple defined medium in a chemostat at low dilution rates (Wallace, 1980). The polysaccharide can then be used as an energy source during periods of energy starvation. The polysaccharide contained over 98% glucose, was of the branched glycogen type and had an average chain length of 12 glucose residues. Minor sugar constituents were 0.5% rhamnose, 0.6% arabinose and 0.2% xylose.

Two pathways for ammonia assimilation into glutamate have been found in *S. ruminantium* (Smith *et al.*, 1980). One pathway fixes NH_4^+ through the action of an NADPH-linked glutamate dehydrogenase (GDH). The other pathway fixes NH_4^+ into the amide of glutamine by action of an ATP-dependent glutamine synthetase (GS). GDH activity was highest when NH_4^+ concentrations were not limiting, whereas GS activity was highest under nitrogen limitation. In a subsequent study (Smith *et al.*, 1981) these authors found a high positive correlation between GS and urease activity in *S. ruminantium* which responded to the availability of NH_4^+ in the environment. Both enzyme activities were simultaneously repressed in the presence of excess NH_4^+.

Strobel and Russell (1991) investigated the role of sodium in growth of *Selenomonas ruminantium*. Little, if any NH_3 was utilized as a nitrogen source by *S. ruminantium* in medium containing amino acids; however, if sodium was deleted from the medium, the organism utilized NH_3 as a nitrogen source. No growth occurred in sodium deficient medium when amino acids were the only source of nitrogen. Six, sodium dependent amino acid transport systems were subsequently identified, i.e., aspartate, glutamine, lysine, phenylalanine, serine and valine. Sodium did not appear to be required for intracellular pH control.

In a separate study, Cotta (1990) reported that *S. ruminantium* appears to be fairly unique among the predominant species of rumen bacteria in its ability to ferment RNA.

Relative activity of starch digesting species

The ability of several different species of rumen bacteria to utilize starch was studied by Cotta (1988). Ten strains, representing six different species, were grown in starch medium and their amylase activity was measured. Levels of amylase produced (U/mg protein) in descending order were: *Ruminobacter amylophilus*, 19.67; *S. bovis*, 15.63; *B. fibrisolvens*, 9.80 and 2.87; *P. ruminicola*, 1.24 and 0.80; *S. ruminantium* (2 strains), *S. dextrinosolvens* (1 strain) and *B. fibrisolvens* (1 strain), all ≤ 0.25. In general, amylase activity was fairly similar when either starch or maltose were substrates; however, activity was markedly lower when the cells were grown on glucose. Distribution of amylase activity between cells and culture supernatants was found to vary between species and strains, and was even influenced by growth substrate. For example, with two strains of *B. fibrisolvens*, distribution of amylase activity in cells and fluid were 3 and 97 and 83 and 17, respectively, when cultures were grown on maltose. When grown on starch, distributions were 95 and 6 and 92 and 8, respectively. In contrast, amylase distribution of a *P. ruminicola* strain on starch was 49% cells and 51% fluid. Products of amylose digestion by extracellular amylases were mixed maltooligosaccharides (up to maltoheptaose). Thus, the extracellular amylases are of the endo-splitting type, randomly hydrolyzing internal bonds, similar to the activity of α-amylase.

S. bovis, *R. amylophilus* and *B. fibrisolvens* were all able to digest starch from ground barley, corn and wheat (McAllister *et al.*, 1990). Rate of digestion appeared fastest for *S. bovis*, with the extent of digestion reaching between 40 and 50% for all three grains. *R. amylophilus* digested less, between 25 and 35%. Although *B. fibrisolvens* digested the starch at a slower rate, 50% was digested from both barley and corn. However, digestion of wheat by this species was markedly reduced, barely reaching 20%. Electron microscopy indicated that the three species colonized different areas, i.e., *B. fibrisolvens* on the cell wall material; *S. bovis,* randomly on the endosperm and *R. amylophilus*, starch granules.

Other less numerous species of rumen bacteria

Most of the predominant species of rumen bacteria have been discussed; however, additional species which utilize the less plentiful substrates and occur in low numbers are intermittently or sporadically isolated with non-selective media at high dilutions. Species which only utilize specific substrates such as the end-products of other bacteria have been isolated in selective media. The following species would fit into these categories.

SUCCINIVIBRIO DEXTRINOSOLVENS

The genus *Succinivibrio* was established by Bryant and Small in 1956 to include anaerobic, non-sporeforming, Gram-negative, curved rods with monotrichous polar flagellation. They ferment glucose with the production of a large amount of succinic acid. *Succinivibrio dextrinosolvens* was proposed as the type species. The organism is a small, Gram-negative, helicoidal rod 0.3 to 0.5 µm wide and 1 to 5 µm long. Ends of the cells are pointed. Most cells are short with one or less coils and simply appear to be twisted, while longer cells contain two to three coils. Indole, H_2S and catalase are not produced, gelatin is not liquefied. Starch, cellulose and xylan are not fermented. Substrates fermented are arabinose, xylose, glucose, fructose, galactose, maltose, sucrose, dextrin and pectin. Although CO_2 was not an obligate requirement, growth was markedly improved. Trypticase and yeast extract can replace rumen fluid in the medium. Primary end-products from glucose fermentation are succinic and acetic acids, with strain differences occurring in the production of very small amounts of formic and lactic acids and CO_2.

Although it would appear that this species could be important in the fermentation of intermediates in starch hydrolysis, it generally accounts for only a very small percentage of the cultures isolated. Since most strains of this species have been found to contain urease, it may be the most important ureolytic species on high grain diets (Wozny *et al.*, 1977; Gomez-Alarcon *et al.*, 1982).

Growth of *S. dextrinosolvens* in a basal medium containing glucose, minerals, enzymatic casein hydrolysate, B-vitamins, cysteine and CO_2 required a relatively large inoculum, and was markedly stimulated by rumen fluid (Bryant and Robinson, 1962). Three transfers of *S. dextrinosolvens* through the basal medium were enough to deplete any carry over of the unknown required nutrient in rumen fluid. Addition of 1% rumen fluid or certain vitamin K-like compounds would support good growth of these strains (Gomez-Alarcon *et al.*, 1982). Of the vitamin K-like compounds, 1,4-naphthoquinone supported the best growth. To date this is the only species of rumen bacteria known to have a vitamin K-like requirement.

EUBACTERIUM RUMINANTIUM

This species, described by Bryant in 1959, is a non-motile small short rod (0.4 to 0.7 µm by 0.7 to 1.5 µm) with many cells almost coccoid. Young cultures are weakly Gram-positive, becoming Gram-negative as the culture ages. It is a strict anaerobe. Glucose, cellobiose and fructose are fermented by all strains studied, while cellulose and starch are not hydrolyzed. Fermentation of xylan varied between strains. All strains produced lactic, formic, acetic and butyric acids as end-products. Gas and ethanol are not produced. This species represented from 3.3 to 7.3% of the total isolates in animals fed alfalfa hay, alfalfa silage, fresh alfalfa, alfalfa hay and grain or blue-grass pasture and grain. This species has not been isolated from animals fed all-concentrate rations.

SPIROCHETES

In 1952, Bryant reported the isolation and characterization of a spirochete from bovine rumen contents and classified it as belonging to the genus *Borrelia*. It appeared to be the main spirochete occurring in the rumen of cattle and sheep. The organism is an anaerobic, Gram-negative, motile, spirochete, varying in length from 4 to 14 µm with most cells about 7 µm. Cell diameter varied between 0.3 and 0.5 µm. All strains required rumen fluid for growth. Only soluble carbohydrates were fermented. Carbon dioxide, ethanol, formic acid, acetic acid, lactic acid and succinic acid were all produced from glucose fermentation. The inability of this species to ferment any materials except the soluble sugars probably limits its numbers in the rumen. Normally it comprises 2% or less of the total isolates. Rumen spirochetes were originally placed in the genus *Borrelia*; however, they have subsequently been transferred to the genus *Treponema* (Buchanan and Gibbons, 1974). Only those species of spirochetes which cause relapsing fever are now classified in the genus *Borrelia*.

Dehority (1975) isolated a spirochete from reindeer which differed from the strain described by Bryant (1952) in not requiring rumen fluid for growth, having a lower minimum pH, fermentation of mannitol and dextrin and showing only a very weak fermentation of cellobiose. Organic acid end-products were quite similar. Species designations of rumen spirochetes have not been made because of lack of sufficient information; however, they differ considerably from those species isolated from the mouth and urogenital tract.

Stanton and Canale-Parole (1979) developed a selective medium for the enumeration of rumen spirochetes. They found that growth of many species of rumen bacteria was inhibited by the antibiotic rifampin, whereas the spirochetes were resistant. When rifampin was included in their agar roll tube medium (1 µg/ml), total numbers decreased 5- to 10-fold. However, the percentage of spirochetes increased from 5 to 30 plus percent. They were able to count the numbers of spirochetes because of their unique colony morphology. Viable spirochete numbers ranged from 0.14 to 1.2 x 10^8 cells/ml of rumen fluid. Seven morphological diverse types of spirochetes were isolated, differing in cell size, cell coiling pattern and number of periplasmic fibers per cell. Representative strains of all seven morphological types were found to be resistant to rifampin (1 µg/ml). *S. dextrinosolvens* was also resistant to the antibiotic, whereas *R. albus*, *F. succinogenes* and *Streptococcus* sp. were inhibited. The authors suggest that the spirochetes are resistant to rifampin either because it cannot penetrate the outer sheath that envelopes the spirochetal cell, they can detoxify the antibiotic by enzyme action or the ribonucleic acid polymerases of spirochetes (site of inhibitions for rifampin) are less sensitive than those of other bacteria. In a subsequent study from this same lab (Paster and Canale-Parole, 1982), pure cultures of rumen spirochetes were shown to utilize the plant polymers pectin and xylan plus the hydrolysis products of these polymers. Starch was also fermented. Based on numbers and substrates utilized, the authors conclude that the spirochetes could markedly contribute to the breakdown of plant polysaccharides in the rumen. Most of the previously isolated rumen spirochetes only utilized soluble carbohydrates and their importance in the overall rumen fermentation was considered minimal.

Lactate utilizing bacteria

VEILLONELLA ALCALESCENS

Veillonella alcalescens was first isolated form the rumen of sheep by Johns (1951) using a lactate medium. It is an anaerobic Gram-negative coccus, 0.3 to 0.6 µm in diameter. The species does not ferment sugars but does ferment lactic acid with the production of acetic and propionic acids, CO_2 and H_2. Failure to ferment glucose has been explained by the lack of hexokinase (Rogosa *et al.*, 1965). Numbers of this species reported for two studies in sheep were 1.2 to 5.2 x 10^5 and 1 to 7.4 x 10^6 per ml of rumen fluid (Gutierrez, 1953; Gutierrez *et al.*, 1958). In cattle, numbers of 60 to 2000 per ml were reported (Gutierrez, 1953). This suggests that this species is probably of limited importance in the rumen.

MEGASPHAERA ELSDENII (FORMERLY *PEPTOSTREPTOCOCCUS ELSDENII*)

Megasphaera elsdenii is an anaerobic Gram-negative coccus, 1.2 to 2.4 µm in diameter. In addition to glycerol and lactate, *M. elsdenii* can ferment several soluble sugars (glucose, fructose and maltose) and some amino acids. End-products of lactate fermentation are acetic, propionic, butyric, valeric and caproic acid, CO_2 and H_2 (Elsden *et al.*, 1956; Gutieirrez *et al.* 1958).

Wallace (1986) reported that the amino acids in acid hydrolyzed casein were more extensively catabolized by *Megasphaera elsdenii* than those in enzymatically hydrolyzed casein. His data suggested that amino acid catabolism was energetically of little value to *M. elsdenii*. However, this activity is probably of considerable importance to other organisms in the rumen, supplying NH_3 and branched-chain VFA, both of which are essential for growth of the cellulolytic bacteria.

This species generally occurs in relatively low numbers; however, it is a normal inhabitant of the rumen and intestinal tract of humans and pigs (Marounek *et al.*, 1989). It may be an important fermenter of lactate in the rumen during periods of adaptation, such as adjustment to a high-grain ration when numbers of *S. bovis* and *M. elsdenii* increase markedly. Numbers of both species decrease again after adaptation (Hungate, 1966). In 1971, Rogosa established a new genus, *Megasphaera*, with the type species *Megasphaera elsdenii*, formerly *Peptostreptococcus elsdenii*. The primary reason for establishing the new genus was the discrepancy of the Gram reaction with *P. elsdenii*. All other species in the genus *Peptostreptococcus* were Gram-positive.

Methanogenic bacteria

METHANOBREVIBACTER RUMINANTIUM

Smith and Hungate (1958), using a mixture of 80% H_2 and 20% CO_2 as substrates in a 30% rumen fluid medium, isolated and described a methane producing bacterium *Methanobrevibacter* (formerly *Methanobacterium*) *ruminantium*. The oxidation-reduction potential obtained with the normal anaerobic techniques were unsuitable for growth of this species. A lower O-R potential was achieved by the anaerobic growth of *E. coli* on pyruvic acid in the tube, destruction of *E. coli* by heat and inoculating through the rubber stopper with a needle and syringe. Their work indicated that a pH of 7 and redox potential of -359 mv was required for the growth of this species. They obtained counts of methanogenic bacteria as high as 2×10^8 per ml. Present evidence indicates that practically all of the methane formed in the rumen is produced via CO_2 reduction with H_2 serving as the main source of electrons. The only other substrate used by *M. ruminantium* is formate. Additional studies have indicated that formate is probably decomposed to CO_2 and H_2 during conversion to CH_4.

The organism is a non-motile, non-sporeforming, Gram-positive, cocobacilli about 0.7-1.0 µm wide and 0.8-1.8 µm in length. The organism will not grow in the absence of rumen fluid, and this cannot be replaced by a large number of unknown growth factor sources. Bryant (1965) has studied the nutritional requirements of this species. The regular technique was modified to include both cysteine and Na_2S as reducing agents in the media, inoculation through the stopper and using a 50-50 CO_2-H_2 gas mixture. Additional gas was added twice daily to replenish the energy source. Tubes were incubated on a shaker. They found that the organism required H_2 and CO_2 or formate as an energy source, NH_4^+ as the major nitrogen source, and acetate and 2-methylbutyrate as carbon sources for growth. However, an additional unknown rumen fluid factor was still required. This factor was subsequently identified by Taylor et al. (1974) as coenzyme M (2-mercaptoethane sulfonic acid).

METHANOMICROBIUM MOBILE

In 1968, Paynter and Hungate were attempting to isolate M. ruminantium and obtained cultures of a new species of methane producing bacteria. The organism is a strictly anaerobic, weakly motile, non-sporeforming, Gram-negative rod (0.7 µm x 1.5 to 2.0 µm). Only formate and H_2 plus CO_2 supported growth, and an unknown factor in rumen fluid is required for growth. The new isolate was named *Methanomicrobium mobile* and occurred in concentrations of approximately 2×10^8 cells per ml.

OTHER METHANOGENS

Two other species of rumen methanogens have been isolated and described, *Methanosarcina barkeri* and *Methanobacterium formicicum* (Stewart and Bryant, 1988). These species appear to be of lesser importance in ruminal methanogenisis; however, with improvements in techniques for anaerobiosis, additional methanogens may be found.

Anaerobic lactobacilli

Bryant et al. (1958b) isolated nine strains of Gram-positive rods from young calves. They were non-sporeforming, non-motile cylindrical rods, 0.5 - 0.7 µm wide by 1.8 - 60 µm long, with rounded ends. The presence of many long filaments and chains containing both Gram-positive and Gram-negative elements was characteristic of these isolates. The organisms had a very low minimum pH, produced only lactic acid as a fermentation product, were unable to hydrolyze starch and grew at 22°C. On the basis of these characteristics and sugars fermented, they considered the strains to be similar to organism

123, isolated and described previously by Mann and Oxford (1954) and classified as an anaerobic variety of *Lactobacillus lactis*. Sharpe *et al*. (1973) isolated six *Lactobacillus* cultures which they compared to strains previously isolated by Bryant *et al*. (1958b). On the basis of motility, percentage D(-) and L(+)-lactic acid, and % base composition of their DNA, they established two new species, *L. vitulinus* and *L. ruminis*. Dehority (1975) isolated and characterized a strain of anaerobic *Lactobacillus* from an Alaskan reindeer, which more closely resembled *L. vitulinus*. Surprisingly, the animal had been fed on native pastures and then dried lichens for the two weeks prior to isolating the lactobacillus, which differed markedly from the concentrate diets fed to the previous hosts.

Proteolytic bacteria

Most of the bacteria in the rumen are saccharoclastic, relying on carbohydrates as a source of energy. Many of these species produce smaller quantities of proteinase enzymes, which when added together apparently accounts for the large amount of proteolytic activity measured in rumen contents (Blackburn and Hobson, 1960). Abou Akkada and Blackburn (1963) isolated a number of species of bacteria on a low carbohydrate-high protein medium, and assayed their ability to hydrolyze casein. After four days of incubation, casein digestion ranged from 30-94% for *Ruminobacter (Bacteroides) amylophilus*, 28-97% for *Prevotella ruminicola*, 26-87% for *Butyrivibrio* and 12-96% for *Selenomonas ruminantium*. The products produced were primarily amino acids and peptides and the organisms did not exhibit marked deaminase activity. However, most strains appeared to preferentially use NH_3 as a main source of nitrogen even in the presence of pre-formed amino acids. Studies by Bladen *et al*. (1961) indicated that *P. ruminicola* is one of the most active producers of NH_3 from casein hydrolysate and on the basis of numbers, etc. probably the most important NH_3 producing bacterium in the rumen.

Wallace and Brammal (1985) designed a study to evaluate the probable importance of different proteolytic bacteria in the rumen. Bacteria were isolated from 3 different media: (1) non-selective rumen fluid-medium; (2) same as 1, minus rumen fluid with cysteine and casein as the only nitrogen sources; and (3) same as 2, with maltose as the only carbohydrate source. One point of particular interest was that the selective medium was no more successful for the selection of proteolytic bacteria than the general medium. The following proteolytic isolates were identified: *Ruminobacter amylophilus, Prevotella ruminicola, Butyrivibrio fibrisolvens, Butyrivibrio alactacidigens, Selenomonas ruminantium*, plus strains in the genera *Eubacterium, Fusobacterium* and *Clostridium*. Of these, *R. amylophilus, B. fibrisolvens, B. alactacidigens* and *Fusobacterium* were the most active proteolytic isolates. In a separate study Wallace (1985) found that *B. alactacidigens, B. fibrisolvens, S. ruminantium* and *Streptococcus bovis* grew much better in pairs when casein was the only added nitrogen source. In essence it appears that bacteria with low activity can cooperate to increase activity.

Attempts to select for proteolytic bacteria capable of utilizing resistant soluble proteins were not successful (Wallace et al.,1987). Although feeding different proteins does appear to enrich for different bacterial species, there was no indication that the organisms can alter their proteolytic activity to enhance utilization of the more resistant soluble proteins.

Proteolytic activity and characterization of proteases in *B. fibrisolvens* were investigated by Cotta and Hespell (1986). They found that relative proteolytic activity varied greatly between strains and in most cases, 90% of the proteolytic activity was associated with the culture fluid and not the cells (Table 11.1). Single strains of two additional proteolytic species (*R. amylophilus* and *P. ruminicola*) were included for comparison purposes. Activity of these two species was in the same overall range as *B. fibrisolvens*; however, almost all of the activity was cell associated.

Table 11.1 LEVEL AND DISTRIBUTION OF PROTEOLYTIC ACTIVITY BETWEEN CELLS AND CULTURE FLUID IN RUMEN BACTERIA[a]

Species and strain	Total activity (U/ml of culture)	Relative activity (U/mg of cell protein)	% Distribution in:	
			Fluid	Cells
Ruminobacter amylophilus H18	47	400	8	92
Prevotella ruminicola B$_1$4	21	100	28	72
Butyrivibrio fibrisolvens				
CF4c	54	336	92	7
CF3	33	231	91	9
CF1B	42	186	95	5
49	26	125	87	13
49[b]	72	570	95	5
12	40	250	88	12
H17c	64	590	91	9
AcTF2	12	90	85	15
R28	28	172	59	41
LM8/1B	15	95	77	23
IL631	7	29	79	21
NOR37	7	32	84	16
S2	11	47	91	8
C14	9	54	75	25
X10C34	8	ND[c]	80	20
X6C61	0	ND	ND	ND
E21C	1	6	ND	ND
D16f	1	5	ND	ND
D1	1	10	100	ND

[a] From Cotta and Hespell (1986). All strains grown in a complete medium without rumen fluid.
[b] ND, Not determined.
[c] Grown in complete medium plus 20% rumen fluid.

For *B. fibrisolvens* 49, the distribution of activity between cells and culture fluid did not change during growth, proteolytic activity was produced constitutively, and the level of activity (units per mg of protein) was affected by growth conditions.

Strydom *et al.* (1986) found ten bands of protease activity in culture supernatants of *B. fibrisolvens*. Molecular weights ranged from 32,000 up to 101,000. All of the protease bands had similar properties, being inhibited by the same serum protease inhibitor and requiring similar conditions for optimal activity. From their studies the authors concluded that the bands of protease activity represented serine exoprotease isoenzymes with different molecular weights.

Using a non-selective medium, Attwood and Reilly (1995) isolated 212 strains of bacteria from rumen contents of three New Zealand cows grazing a mixed pasture of mainly ryegrass and clover. When assayed for protein-hydrolyzing activity, 81 strains (38%) were classified as actively proteolytic, 94 strains (44.5%) as less-actively proteolytic and 37 strains (17.5%) as non proteolytic. Forty-three of the actively proteolytic strains were characterized on the basis of morphology, substrate utilization, biochemical tests and fermentation end-products. These data were then analyzed using hierarchical cluster analysis. Their results were: 26 strains - *Streptococcus bovis*; 10 strains - *Eubacterium budayi* (?); 3 strains - *Butyrivibrio fibrisolvens*; 3 strains - *B. fibrisolvens*-like; and 1 strain *Prevotella ruminicola*. They subsequently measured distribution of the proteolytic activity in eight representative strains of their active isolates (Atwood and Reilly, 1996). Surprisingly, proteinase activity in these strains was predominantly cell-bound or cell-associated which differs from the results for *B. fibrisolvens* reported by Cotta and Hespell (1986).

Based on the data available at the present time, the predominant proteolytic species of ruminal bacteria appear to be *Ruminobacter amylophilus, Prevotella ruminicola, Selenomonas ruminantium, Butyrivibrio fibrisolvens* and *Streptococcus bovis*. Of less significance would be the species *Eubacterium, Clostridium*, Gram-positive cocci and *Lachnospira multiparus*.

Acetogenic bacteria

Acetogenic bacteria have recently been found to occur in fairly high numbers in cattle fed both high and low forage diets (Leedle and Greening, 1988). These bacteria are capable of producing acetic acid from hydrogen and carbon dioxide according to the following equation: $4H_2 + 2CO_2 \rightarrow CH_3COOH + 2 H_2O$. Although the acetogens are present in the rumen, their H_2 threshold is 100 times greater than the methanogens, i.e., the methanogens can scavenge H_2 from very dilute solutions and outcompete the acetogens unless H_2 accumulates.

Greening and Leedle (1989) were able to enrich the obligately anaerobic acetogenic bacteria from the rumen in a medium containing bromoethanesulfonic acid, a strong inhibitor for rumen methanogens. The cultures were incubated under a H_2:CO_2

headspace. They subsequently isolated five strains of bacteria which could reduce CO_2 at the expense of hydrogen. All five strains were classified as a new species and were placed in a new genus, *Acetitomaculum*. The type species is *A. ruminis*. It is a Gram-positive, non-sporeforming curved rod, 2.0-40 µm in length x 0.8 -1.0 µm in width. Cells may be flagellated. Obligate anaerobe. Also ferments formate, glucose, cellobiose, fructose and esculin to acetic acid.

Using a nutritionally non-selective medium containing 10% pre-incubated clarified rumen fluid and bromoethanesulfonic acid, H_2-utilizing acetogenic rumen bacteria can be estimated with a most probable number assay. Duplicate serial dilutions are incubated either under a H_2/CO_2 (4:1) or N_2/CO_2 (4:1) headspace atmosphere. After 20 days incubation, the culture supernatants were analyzed for acetate (Doré *et al.*, 1995). Rumen and hindgut contents of various animals along with human feces were analyzed, with acetogenic bacterial concentrations ranging from below 10^2 to above 10^8 per gram wet weight of gut contents.

Several studies have shown a marked competition between the hydrogenotrophic bacteria in the rumen, specifically the acetogens and methanogens. The hydrogen-utilizing sulfate-reducing bacteria do not appear to be involved in the competition (Morvan *et al.*, 1994). Enumeration of methanogens and acetogens in rumen contents from sheep (4), cattle (10), buffaloes (4), deer (3), stomach contents from llama (6) and cecal contents from horses (10) revealed the presence of methanogens in all samples, whereas the acetogens were absent in several samples from each animal (Morvan *et al.*, 1996). The highest concentrations of acetogens were found in horses and llamas, 1×10^4 and 14×10^4, respectively; however, these concentrations are 10,000 times smaller than that of the methanogens.

LeVan *et al.*(1998) measured acetogen concentrations ranging from 2×10^5 per ml in beef cows fed a high forage diet down to 75 per ml in finishing steers on a high-grain diet. Acetogenic activity was negligible unless methanogenesis was curtailed. The fact that methanogenic and reductive acetogenic bacteria coexist in the rumen, suggests that the acetogens probably utilize other substrates, i.e., glucose, cellobiose, etc.

Several additional species of acetogens have been isolated from rumen contents. Rieu-Lesme *et al.* (1995) isolated an acetogenic spore-forming Gram-negative bacteria from the rumen of a mature deer. It appeared to be able to compete quite sucessfully for H_2 with methanogens. More recently, Rieu-Lesme *et al.* (1996) described another acetogen, isolated from the rumen of suckling lambs. It is a coccobacillus with a Gram-positive type cell wall, and has been classified as *Ruminococcus schinkii*.

Facultative anaerobes

Many different species of facultative anaerobes have been isolated from rumen contents; however, very little, if any, evidence exists to indicate that these organisms are of numerical importance. The main groups of organisms which are generally found belong either to the coliform group, *Bacillus, Propionibacterium, Lactobacillus* or *Streptococcus*. The principal coliform isolated from the rumen is *E. coli*, although *Aerobacter* species also occur. Numbers are generally rather low, in the range of 10^6 per g. Appleby (1955) cultured similar numbers of *Bacillus* species from hay and rumen contents, but found the spore count in the rumen to be much lower; thereby suggesting the numbers were simply a reflection of spore germination. Gutierrez (1953) isolated *Propionibacterium acnes* from rumen contents on a lactate medium, in fairly high numbers; however, he also found relatively high numbers of this species on the hay. Bryant *et al.* (1958b) using similar methods were unable to isolate this species from a number of animals. Facultatively anaerobic *Lactobacillus* species, have been isolated by various investigators (Bryant, 1959).

The range in concentrations reported for facultative anaerobes has been quite large (Jensen *et al.*, 1956). *Streptococci*, primarily *S. bovis*, is the predominant facultatively anaerobic *Streptococcus* isolated from rumen contents. This species has been discussed earlier. The studies reported on facultative anaerobes and their importance might best be summarized as follows: 1) although most of the studies on facultative anaerobes were conducted using conventional anaerobic techniques, very few investigators employed the more rigorous "Hungate" technique. In most studies using the "Hungate" technique, the percent of facultative anaerobes of the total isolates has always been in the range of 1 to 2% (Bryant and Burkey, 1953; Bryant *et al.*, 1958b; Thorley *et al.*, 1968); (2) numbers of the facultative anaerobes appear to be considerably higher in young calves, where a mature type population has not yet been established (Bryant, 1959). This may be a reflection of the redox potential in the rumen of the young animal; (3) most of the facultative anaerobes occur in fairly large numbers in the feed; and (4) studies on attempts to establish these organisms in adult ruminants have been rather unsuccessful.

With regard to this last point, Brownlie and Grau (1967) inoculated the rumens of cattle with *Salmonella* organisms and followed numbers of both salmonella and *E. coli*. If the animals were fed 6.8 kg alfalfa/day or allowed to graze freely, salmonella were rapidly eliminated from the rumen. *E. coli* concentrations were usually under 10/ml. Decrease of food intake to 2.3 kg/day or starvation for 1 or more days resulted in maintenance or increases of the salmonella and *E. coli* numbers. Refeeding resulted in further increases in numbers which then began to decrease regardless of whether the animals were fed or starved. An interesting observation in this work was that following 2-3 days starvation, infection of the intestines with salmonella generally occurred with organisms being shed in the feces for at least a week. The authors suggest that starvation, or conditions encountered during transport, may be important in development of salmonellosis and infections with enteropathogenic *E. coli*.

Hollowell and Wolin (1965) studied the growth of *E. coli* in a continuous culture *in vitro* system. Addition of a readily available energy source; lactose, in addition to the 50% hay-grain feed, had no effect on growth of *E. coli*. Addition of a large inoculum in the absence and presence of lactose did not establish the species. Anaerobiosis, temperature and pH did not appear to be involved, nor did lysis by a bacteriophage.

However, inhibition assays indicated that rumen fluid contained factors inhibitory to *E. coli*. Subsequent studies by Wolin (1969) indicated that the concentrations of VFA normally found in rumen fluid were toxic to *E. coli*, especially when the pH is 6.5 or lower, and appear to be the primary factor responsible for the exclusion of this species from the rumen.

Adams *et al.* (1966) studied the longevity of selected exogenous microorganisms in the rumen. The times required for 90% loss of viability with an inoculum of approximately 10^8 cells per ml in the rumen were: *Chromobacterium violaceum* - 2 h; laboratory strain of *Serratia marcescens* - 5 h; *Serratia* sp. isolated from the rumen -over 8 h; vegetative cells of *Bacillus Stearothermophilus* - 3 h, spores of this same species - 4 h; and yeasts (*Candida krusei* and *Hansenula anomala*), isolated from high moisture corn - 8 h. Survival time of these exogenous organisms was not affected by the diet of the host animal (steers). Numbers of "background" colonies observed during their experiments suggested that other bacteria are affected in a manner similar to the test organisms. The background on the plates increased after the animals were fed and then decreased until the next feeding.

References

Attwood, G. T. and K. Reilly. (1995). Identification of proteolytic rumen bacteria isolated from New Zealand cattle. *Journal of Applied Bacteriology*, **79**, 22-29.

Attwood, G. T. and K. Reilly. (1996). Characterization of proteolytic activities of rumen bacterial isolates from forage-fed cattle. *Journal of Applied Bacteriology*, **81**, 545-552.

Abou Akkada, A. R. and T. H. Blackburn. (1963). Some observations on the nitrogen metabolism of rumen proteolytic bacteria. *Journal of General Microbiology*, **31**, 461-469.

Adams, J. C., P. A. Hartman and N. L. Jacobson. (1966). Longevity of selected exogenous microorganisms in the rumen. *Canadian Journal of Microbiology*, **12**, 363-396.

Appleby, J. C. (1955). The isolation and classification of proteolytic bacteria from the rumen of the sheep. *Journal of General Microbiology*, **12**, 526-533.

Blackburn, T. H. and P. N. Hobson. (1960). Isolation of proteolytic bacteria from the sheep rumen. *Journal of General Microbiology*, **22**, 282-289.

Bladen, H. A., M. P. Bryant and R. N. Doetsch. (1961). A study of bacterial species from the rumen which produce ammonia from protein hydrolysate. Applied Microbiology, **9**, 175-180.

Brownlie, L. E. and F. H. Grau. (1967). Effect of food intake on growth and survival of *Salmonellas* and *Escherichia coli* in the bovine rumen. *Journal of General Microbiology*, **46**, 125-134.

Bryant, M. P. (1952). The isolation and characterization of a spirochete from the bovine rumen. *Journal of Bacteriology*, **64**, 325-335.

Bryant, M. P. (1956). The characteristics of strains of *Selenomonas* isolated from bovine rumen contents. *Journal of Bacteriology*, **72**, 162-167.

Bryant, M. P. (1959). Bacterial species of the rumen. *Bacteriological Reviews*, **23**, 125-153.

Bryant, M. P. (1965). Rumen methanogenic bacteria. In: *Physiology of Digestion in the Ruminant.* Edited by R.W. Dougherty. Butterworths, Washington, DC, pp 411-481.

Bryant, M. P. and L. A. Burkey. (1953). Cultural methods and some characteristics of some of the more numerous groups of bacteria in the bovine rumen. *Journal of Dairy Science*, **36**, 205-217.

Bryant, M. P. and I. M. Robinson. (1961). An improved nonselective culture medium for ruminal bacteria and its use in determining diurnal variation in numbers of bacteria in the rumen. *Journal of Dairy Science*, **44**, 1446-1456.

Bryant, M. P. and I. M. Robinson. (1962). Some nutritional characteristics of predominant culturable ruminal bacteria. *Journal of Bacteriology*, **84**, 605-614.

Bryant, M. P. and N. Small. (1956). Characteristics of two new genera of anaerobic curved rods isolated from the rumen of cattle. *Journal of Bacteriology*, **72**, 22-26.

Bryant, M. P., N. Small, C. Bouma and H. Chu. (1958a). *Bacteroides ruminicola* n. sp. and *Succinimonas amylolytica* the new genus and species. Species of succinic acid-producing anaerobic bacteria of the bovine rumen. *Journal of Bacteriology*, **76**, 15-23.

Bryant, M. P., N. Small, C. Bouma and I. M. Robinson. (1958b). Studies on the composition of the ruminal flora and fauna of young calves. *Journal of Dairy Science*, **41**, 1747-1767.

Buchanan, R. E. and N. E. Gibbons (Ed.). (1974). Bergey's Manual of Determinative Bacteriology, 8th Ed. The Williams and Wilkens Co., Baltimore, Maryland.

Caldwell, D. R. and M. P. Bryant. (1966). Medium without rumen fluid for non-selective enumeration and isolation of rumen bacteria. *Applied Microbiology*, **14**, 794-801.

Cotta, M. (1988). Amylolytic activity of selected species of ruminal bacteria. *Applied and Environmental Microbiology*, **54**, 772-776.

Cotta, M. (1990). Utilization of nucleic acids by *Selenomonas ruminantium* and other ruminal bacteria. *Applied and Environmental Microbiology*, **56**, 3867-3870.

Cotta, M. A. and R. B. Hespell. (1986). Proteolytic activity of the ruminal bacterium *Butyrivibrio fibrisolvens. Applied and Environmental Microbiology*, **52**, 51-58.

Dehority, B. A. (1971). Carbon dioxide requirement of various species of rumen bacteria. *Journal of Bacteriology*, **105**, 70-76.

Dehority, B. A. (1975). Characterization studies on rumen bacteria isolated from Alaskan reindeer (*Rangifer tarandus* L.). *Proceedings of the 1st International Reindeer and Caribou Symposium,* Special Report Number 1, Biological Papers of the University of Alaska, Fairbanks, pp. 228-240.

Doré, J., B. Morvan, F. Rieu-Lesme, I. Goderel, P. Gouet and P. Pochart. (1995). Most probable number enumeration of H_2-utilizing acetogenic bacteria from the digestive tract of animals and man. *FEMS Microbiology Letters,* **130,** 7-12.

Dufva, G. S., E. E. Bartley, M. J. Arambel, T. G. Nagaraja, S. M. Dennis, S. J. Galtzer and A. D. Dayton. (1982). Diaminopimelic acid content of feeds and rumen bacteria and its usefulness as a rumen bacterial marker. *Journal of Dairy Science,* **65,** 1754-1759.

Elsden, S. R., B. E. Volcani, F.M.C. Gilchrist and D. Lewis. (1956). Properties of a fatty acid forming organism isolated from the rumen of sheep. *Journal of Bacteriology,* **72,** 681-689.

Ford, J. E., K. D. Perry and C.A.E. Briggs. (1958). Nutrition of lactic acid bacteria isolated from the rumen. *Journal of General Microbiology,* **18,** 273-284.

Gomez-Alracon, R. A., C. O'dowd, J.A.Z. Leedle and M. P. Bryant. (1982). 1,4-Napthoquinone and other nutrient requirements of *Succinivibrio dextrivosolvens. Applied and Environmental Microbiology,* **44,** 346-350.

Greening, R. C. and J. A. Z. Leedle. (1989). Enrichment and isolation of *Acetitomaculum ruminis,* gen. nov., sp. nov.: acetogenic bacteria from the bovine rumen. *Archives of Microbiology,* **151,** 399-406.

Gutierrez, J. (1953). Numbers and characteristics of lactate utilizing organisms in the rumen of cattle. *Journal of Bacteriology,* **66,** 123-128.

Gutierrez, J., R. E. Davis, I. L. Lendahl and E. J. Warwick. (1958). Bacterial changes in the rumen during the onset of feedlot bloat of cattle. *Applied Microbiology,* **7,** 16-22.

Hamlin, L. J. and R. E. Hungate. (1956). Culture and physiology of a starch-digesting bacterium (*Bacteroides amylophilus* n. sp.) from the bovine rumen. *Journal of Bacteriology,* **72,** 548-554.

Higginbottom, C. and D. W. Wheater. (1954). The incidence of *Streptococcus bovis* in cattle. *Journal of Agricultural Science,* **44,** 434-442.

Hobson, P. N. and S. O. Mann. (1957). Some studies on the identification of rumen bacteria with fluorescent antibodies. *Journal of General Microbiology,* **16,** 463-471.

Hollowell, C. A. and M. J. Wolin. (1965). Basis for the exclusion of *Escherichia coli* from the rumen ecosystem. *Applied Microbiology,* **13,** 918-924.

Hungate, R. E. (1957). Microorganisms in the rumen of cattle fed a constant ration. *Canadian Journal of Microbiology,* **3,** 289-311.

Hungate, R. E. (1966). *The Rumen and Its Microbes.* Academic Press, New York, NY.

Hungate, R. E., R. W. Dougherty, M. P. Bryant and R. M. Cello. (1952). Microbiological and physiological changes associated with acute indigestion in sheep. *Cornell Veterinarian,* **42,** 423-449.

Jensen, R. G., K. L. Smith, J. E. Edmondson and C. P. Merilan. (1956). The characteristics of some rumen lactobacilli. *Journal of Bacteriology*, **72**, 253-258.

John, A., H. R. Isaacson and M. P. Bryant. (1974). Isolation and characteristics of a ureolytic strain of *Selenomonas ruminantium*. *Journal of Dairy Science*, **57**, 1003-1014.

Johns, A. T. (1951). Isolation of a bacterium, producing propionic acid, from the rumen of sheep. *Journal of General Microbiology*, **5**, 317-325.

Kanegasaki, S. and H. Takahashi. (1967). Function of growth factors for rumen microorganisms. I. Nutritional characteristics of *Selenomonas ruminantium*. *Journal of Bacteriology*, **93**, 456-463.

Kanegasaki, S. and H. Takahashi. (1968). Function of growth factors for rumen microorganisms. II. Metabolic fate of incorporated fatty acids in *Selenomonas ruminantium*. *Biochimica et Biophysica Acta*, **152**, 40-49.

Leedle, J.A.Z. and R. C. Greening. (1988). Postprandial changes in methanogenic and acidogenoic bacteria in the rumens of steers fed high- or low-forage diets once daily. *Applied and Environmental Microbiology*, **54**, 502-506.

LeVan, T.D., J.A. Robinson, J. Ralph, R.C. Greening, W.J. Smolenski, J.A.Z. Leedle and D.A. Schaefer. (1998). Assessment of reductive acetogenesis with indigenous ruminal bacterium populations and *Acetitomaculum ruminis*. *Applied and Environmental Microbiology*, **64**, 3429-3436.

McAllister, T. A., K.-J. Cheng, L. M. Rode and C. W. Forsberg. (1990). Digestion of barley, maize, and wheat by selected species of ruminal bacteria. *Applied and Environmental Microbiology*, **56**, 3146-3153.

Mann, S. O. and A. E. Oxford. (1954). Studies of some presumptive lactobacilli isolated from the rumens of young calves. *Journal of General Microbiology*, **11**, 83-90.

Marounek, M., K. Fliegrova and S. Bartos. (1989). Metabolism and some characteristics of ruminal strains of *Megasphaera elsdenii*. *Applied and Environmental Microbiology*, **55**, 1570-1573.

Miura, H., M. Horiguchi and T. Matsumoto. (1980). Nutritional interdependence among rumen bacteria, *Bacteroides amylophilus, Megasphaera elsdenii* and *Ruminococcus albus*. *Applied and Environmental Microbiology*, **40**, 294-300.

Morvan, B., F. Bonnemoy, G. Fonty and P. Gouet. (1996). Quantitative determination of H_2-utilizing acetogenic and sulfate-reducing bacteria and methanogenic archaea from digestive tract of different mammals. *Current Microbiology*, **32**, 129-133.

Morvan, B., J. Doré, F. Rieu-Lesme, L. Foucat, G. Fonty and P. Gouet. (1994). Establishment of hydrogen-utilizing bacteria in the rumen of the newborn lamb. *FEMS Microbiology Letters*, **117**, 249-256.

Nelms, L. F., D. A. Odelson, T. R. Whitehead and R. B. Hespell. (1995). Differentiation of ruminal and human *Streptococcus bovis* strains by DNA homology and 16s rRNA probes. *Current Microbiology*, **31**, 294-300.

Niven, C. F., M. R. Washburn and J. C. White. (1948). Nutrition of *Streptococcus bovis*. *Journal of Bacteriology*, **56**, 601-606.

Paster, B. J. and E. Canale-Parola. (1982). Physiological diversity of rumen spirochetes. *Applied and Environmental Microbiology*, **43**, 686-693.

Paynter, M.J.B. and R. E. Hungate. (1968). Characterization of *Methanobacterium mobilis*, sp. n., isolated from the bovine rumen. *Journal of Bacteriology*, **95**, 1943-1951.

Prins, R. A. (1971). Isolation, culture, and fermentation characteristics of *Selenomonas ruminantium* var. *bryanti* var. n. from the rumen of sheep. *Journal of Bacteriology*, **105**, 820-825.

Rieu-Lesme, F., G. Fonty and J. Doré. (1995). Isolation and characterization of a new hydrogen-utilizing bacterium from the rumen. *FEMS Microbiology Letters*, **125**, 77-82.

Rieu-Lesme, F., B. Morvan, M. D. Collins, G. Fonty and A. Willems. (1996). A new H_2/CO_2-using acetogenic bacterium from the rumen: Description of *Ruminococcus schinkii* sp. nov. *FEMS Microbiology Letters*, **140**, 281-286.

Rogosa, M. (1971). Transfer of *Peptostreptococcus elsdenii* Guiterrez *et al.* to a new genus, *Megasphaera* [*M. elsdenii* (Guiterrez *et al.*) comb. nov.]. *International Journal of Systematic Bacteriology*, **21**, 187-189.

Rogosa, M., M. I. Krichevsky and F. S. Bishop. (1965). Truncated glycolytic system in *Veillonella*. *Journal of Bacteriology*, **90**, 164-171.

Russell, J. B. (1991). Resistance of *Streptococcus bovis* to acetic acid at low pH: relationship between intracellular pH and anion accumulation. *Applied and Environmental Microbiology*, **57**, 255-259.

Russell, J. B. and P. H. Robinson. 1984. Compositions and characteristics of strains of *Streptococcus bovis*. *Journal of Dairy Science*, **67**, 1525-1531.

Sharpe, E. M., M. J. Latham, E. I. Garvie, J. Zirngibl and O. Kandler. (1973). Two new species of *Lactobacillus* isolated from the bovine rumen, *Lactobacillus ruminis* sp. nov. and *Lactobacillus vitulinus* sp. nov. *Journal of General Microbiology*, **77**, 37-49.

Smith, P. H. and R. E. Hungate. (1958). Isolation and characterization of *Methanobacterium ruminantium* n. sp. Journal of Bacteriology, **75**, 713-718.

Smith, C. J., R. B. Hespell and M. P. Bryant. (1980). Ammonia assimilation and glutamate formation in the anaerobe *Selenomonas ruminantium*. *Journal of Bacteriology*, **141**, 593-602.

Smith, C. J., R. B. Hespell and M. P. Bryant. (1981). Regulation of urease and ammonia assimilatory enzymes in *Selenomonas ruminantium*. *Applied and Environmental Microbiology*, **42**, 89-96.

Slyter, L. L. and P. A. Putnam. (1967). *In vivo* vs *in vitro* continuous culture of ruminal microbial populations. *Journal of Animal Science*, **26**, 1421-1427.

Stackebrandt, E. and H. Hippe. (1986). Transfer of *Bacteroides amylophilus* to a new genus *Ruminobacter* gen. nov., nom. rev. as *Ruminobacter amylophilus* comb.

nov. *Systematic Applied Microbiology*, **8**, 204-207.
Stanton, T. B. and E. Canale-Parola. (1979). Enumeration and selective isolation of rumen spirochetes. *Applied and Environmental Microbiology*, **38**, 969-973.
Stewart, C. S. and M. P. Bryant. (1988). The rumen bacteria. In: *The Rumen Microbial Ecosystem*. Edited by P. N. Hobson. Elsevier Science Publishers Ltd. London, England, pp. 21-76.
Strobel, H. J. and J. B. Russell. (1991). Role of sodium in the growth of a ruminal selenomonad. *Applied and Environmental Microbiology*, **57**, 1663-1668.
Strydom, E., R. I. Mackie and D. R. Woods. (1986). Detection and characterization of extracellular proteases in *Butyrivibrio fibrisolvens* H17c. *Applied Microbiology and Biotechnology*, **24**, 214-217.
Taylor, C. D., B. C. McBride, R. S. Wolfe and M. P. Bryant. (1974). Coenzyme M, essential for growth of a rumen strain of *Methanobacterium ruminantium*. *Journal of Bacteriology*, **120**, 974-975.
Thorley, C. M., M. E. Sharpe and M. P. Bryant. (1968). Modification of the rumen bacterial flora by feeding cattle ground and pelleted roughage as determined with culture media with and without rumen fluid. *Journal of Dairy Science*, **51**, 1811-1816.
Tiwari, A. D., M. P. Bryant and R. S. Wolfe. (1969). Simple method for isolation of *Selenomonas ruminantium* and some nutritional characteristics of the species. *Journal of Dairy Science*, **52**, 2054-2056.
Wallace, R. J. (1980). Cytoplasmic reserve polysaccharide of *Selenomonas ruminantium*. *Applied and Environmental Microbiology*, **39**, 630-634.
Wallace, R. J. (1985). Synergism between different species of proteolytic rumen bacteria. *Current Microbiology*, **12**, 59-64.
Wallace, R. J. (1986). Catabolism of amino acids by *Megasphaera elsdenii* LC1. *Applied and Environmental Microbiology*, **51**, 1141-1143.
Wallace, R. J. and M. L. Brammall. (1985). The role of different species of bacteria in the hydrolysis of protein in the rumen. *Journal of General Microbiology*, **131**, 821-832.
Wallace, R. J., G. A. Broderick and M. L. Brammall. (1987). Protein degradation by ruminal microorganisms from sheep fed dietary supplements of urea, casein or albumin. *Applied and Environmental Microbiology*, **53**, 751-753.
Wolin, M. J. (1969). Volatile fatty acids and the inhibition of *Escherichia coli* growth by rumen fluid. *Applied Microbiology*, **17**, 83-87.
Wozny, M. A., M. P. Bryant, L. V. Holdeman and W.E.C. Moore. (1977). Urease assay and urease producing species of anaerobes in the bovine rumen and human feces. *Applied and Environmental Microbiology*, **33**, 1097-1104.

CHAPTER 12

NUMBERS, FACTORS AFFECTING THE POPULATION AND DISTRIBUTION OF RUMEN BACTERIA

Estimates of bacterial numbers in the rumen are very desirable if one wishes to evaluate treatment or ration effects on the overall rumen fermentation. However, considerable difficulty has been encountered in developing adequate methods for this purpose. In general, two main approaches have been used, direct counts and culture counts, both of which have their respective advantages and disadvantages. Direct microscopic counts, made on suitable dilutions of rumen contents, are fast and relatively simple to carry out. However, such factors as both living and dead cells are included in the count, clumping of cells, distinguishing small feed particles from bacteria, and the difficulties in counting bacteria attached or associated with solids in the ingesta must be considered. Culture or viable counts are usually much lower than direct counts and suffer from the obvious disadvantage that the numbers obtained can only reflect the ability of the investigator to simulate conditions of the natural rumen habitat (Hungate, 1966).

Numbers of rumen bacteria

SAMPLING OF RUMEN CONTENTS

Whether one is interested in direct counts or culture counts, considerable thought should be given to the sampling methods. Hungate (1966) has shown that higher metabolic activity is associated with total rumen contents as compared to rumen fluid. Gas production was used as a criteria, and in subsequent studies he and others have shown this to be directly related to bacterial numbers. In preliminary studies (unpublished), viable or culture counts were made on whole rumen contents and compared with counts obtained in the fluid and particulate fractions of a separate subsample of the same rumen contents filtered through cheesecloth. Based on only two experiments, 51% of the total viable count was present in the fluid fraction and 41.4% in the particulate fraction. The overall recovery in the two fractions was thus 92.4% . Several more recent experiments have substantiated these data. Thus, the need to sample whole rumen contents for a reliable estimate of total numbers is quite evident.

Since the rumen contents are a heterogenous mixture with possible varying degrees of stratification, particularly in cattle on long hay, considerable thought should be given to the procedures used in obtaining a sample representative of the whole contents. Three methods are available for obtaining samples of rumen contents: (a) by stomach tube from a normal animal; (b) through a fistula; or (c) from a slaughtered animal (Bryant, 1959; Hungate, 1966). Each procedure has its advantages and disadvantages.

If one wishes to sample a large number of animals on different rations or specific animals which belong to an individual or institution not associated with your research facility, fistulation or slaughter are obviously not viable procedures. Thus, obtaining a sample of rumen contents by stomach tube would be the only method available under these circumstances. Samples obtained by stomach tube probably represent the more fluid portion of rumen contents and little control can be used on the site of sampling within the rumen. The length of a flexible tube swallowed by the animal was found to be unsatisfactory as a means of controlling sampling site (Forbes *et al.*, 1969). X-ray photographs indicated that marked folding occurred as the length of swallowed tubing increased. More rigid tubes are difficult to swallow and can injure the epithelium of the mouth and esophagus. With coarser feeds, the end of the tube often becomes plugged. On the other hand, if consideration is given to the size of the animal, pliability and diameter of the tubing and a satisfactory source of suction, samples can be obtained. For animals fed long hay, obtaining a representative sample may be difficult; however, samples from animals on ground or finely chopped feeds or concentrates are quite satisfactory.

When sampling sheep through a fistula, a rigid plastic tube is used to obtain samples from various locations within the rumen. A larger sample provides better representation of total contents than a small one; however, this is governed by the number of samples to be taken in a given time period. With cattle the contents can be mixed by hand through the fistula and samples taken at different locations with a suitable container (beaker or jar). Results of two studies have indicated a site difference in the rumen of cattle with respect to bacterial numbers (Wilson and Briggs, 1955; Munch-Peterson and Boundy, 1963). No such differences have been observed with sheep (Munch-Peterson and Boundy, 1963). For routine studies, particularly where frequent time samples are desired, fistulated research animals are almost a necessity.

The disadvantage of slaughtering the animal to obtain a sample of rumen contents is quite obvious; however, it is used for obtaining samples from wild ruminants, and samples from domestic ruminants can be obtained from a slaughter house. With this method, contents of the entire rumen can be thoroughly mixed and subsampled. A combination of the last two procedures has also been used (Burroughs *et al.*, 1946), where the entire contents are removed through the fistula, mixed, subsampled and the remaining contents returned to the rumen. However, the effect on the microbial population has not been determined with much certainty.

DIRECT COUNTS

Two procedures are available for making direct microscopic counts of rumen bacteria

(Hungate, 1966). The first involves dilution of the sample, staining the bacteria and counting the bacteria in a chamber of known volume. In the second procedure, a known quantity of the dilution is spread over a measured area of a slide. The slide is then dried, fixed and stained. Two strips at right angles across the smear are generally counted. Numbers are determined by knowing the diameter of the microscope field, area of the smear and the volume of diluted sample spread over that area.

Warner (1962a), conducted a very thorough study on the techniques used in preparing rumen samples for direct counts. He used three methods for obtaining samples and compared the numbers obtained with each procedure by the counting chamber technique. A flow diagram of his procedures are given in Figure 12.1. For the standard count, about 100 ml of rumen contents were removed through the fistula with a glass tube and suction. The ingesta was strained through bolting cloth with kneading and squeezing and the filtrate was diluted 1:5 with formal saline and counted. The entire rumen contents were either removed through the fistula or taken at slaughter and mixed in a bucket for the true total count. A 50 g aliquot of the well-mixed total contents was then diluted with 200 ml formal saline, mixed and strained as described earlier. This filtrate was called the "strained sample". The solids were resuspended in 100 ml of formal saline and strained again to yield the "washed sample". Fifty ml of formal saline were added to the residual solids and the suspension mixed in a homogenizer for 4 minutes and strained as before. This process was repeated a total of seven times, after which most of the plant material appeared to be disintegrated, and if not, showed very few adherent bacteria. The remaining solids were washed with three additional 50 ml aliquots of formal saline, centrifuged at 50 x g for 5 min and the supernatant and residue strained. All fluid portions were combined and labeled "blended sample". The sum of counts in the strained, washed and blended samples was called the true total count.

The true fluid sample count was obtained by taking 200 g of the entire rumen contents, straining and diluting as for the standard sample. The ratio of the numbers of rumen bacteria counted in the true fluid sample to those counted in the standard sample ranged from 0.85 to 1.16, with a mean ratio of 1.00. Although the data is limited, it suggests that the sample obtained through the fistula compares quite closely with a subsample of the entire contents which have been removed from the animal and mixed well.

Warner reported counts for the strained, washed and blended fractions and found that the highest numbers were obtained in the "blended" fraction (1/2 or more of the total), indicating that a large proportion of the rumen bacteria are closely associated or attached to the feed particles. In general, the true total count for bacteria was 2 to 3 times greater than the numbers obtained by the standard count. Differential bacterial counts, determined from gram-stained smears, were reported from one animal. The author states that for this animal, less than 1/3 of the total bacteria were counted by the standard method; however, numbers and proportions in the standard method were similar to those in the strained sample fraction, to which it would be most comparable. Basically similar patterns were obtained with other animals.

268 Rumen microbiology

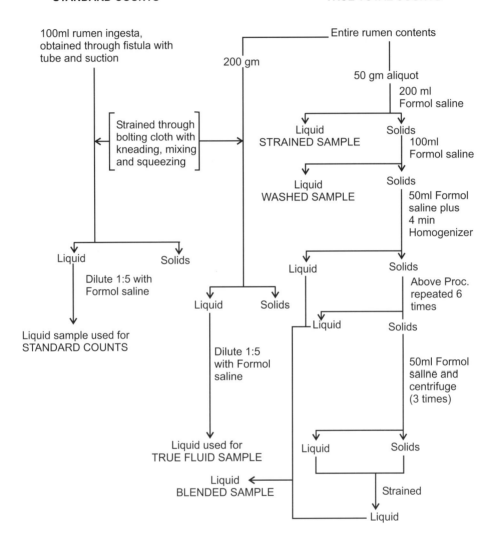

Figure 12.1. Flow diagram of sample preparation procedures used by Warner (1962a) for making direct bacterial counts on rumen contents.

If Warner would have used the "true total count" procedure on a small sample obtained through the fistula prior to removing the entire contents and measuring true total count, some very useful information could have been obtained on how representative the small sample is in relation to the total contents.

CULTURE OR VIABLE COUNTS

In making culture or viable counts, the same problems in sampling rumen contents are encountered as for direct counts. However, there is the added problem of finding a medium which will not be limiting on the basis of environment or nutrition. Most workers have used a habitat-simulating medium containing several different energy sources (Hungate, 1966).

Some of the first comparative work between culture counts and direct counts was reported by Bryant and Burkey (1953a; 1953b). They found higher total counts from the whole contents than from the fluid portion alone. Higher culture counts were also obtained by using a habitat-simulating medium containing rumen fluid, by diluting in an anaerobic versus an aerobic solution or the medium itself, and by mixing the contents in a Waring blender versus shaking 1:10 dilutions vigorously by hand. Comparison of their colony counts and direct microscopic counts revealed that only about 1/10 of the bacteria counted could be cultured. Hungate (1957) reported a comparison of direct counts and culture counts on stomach tube samples from cattle. A 1:10 dilution was shaken vigorously for 30 seconds and then inoculated into a rumen fluid-cellulose-agar medium and a feed extract medium. Direct counts were made on gram-stained smears of the 10X dilution. His results indicated that the total culturable bacteria on the feed extract medium were only 0.1 to 1.0% of the direct count. Even with changes in technique to include rumen fluid in the medium and mixing the samples in a Waring blender, it appeared doubtful that the culture count could be increased to account for more than a few % of the direct count. His counts for cellulolytic bacteria were about 0.01 to 0.025% of the direct count and from 2.5 to 8.0% of the total culturable count.

Maki and Foster (1957) have reported that viable counts of bacteria in the rumen contents of cows fed a high roughage ration represented only 3 - 12% of the number determined by direct count; whereas 57 - 73% of the bacteria from cows fed a ration without roughage (grain plus alfalfa meal) could be cultured. A similar increase in the proportion of viable to direct bacterial count was noted in rumen contents from an all concentrate fed animal by Bryant and Burkey (1953b). These same authors also observed that viable counts were of a similar percentage to direct counts, about 8.4%, whether animals were fed all roughage or a mixture of roughage and concentrate (Bryant and Burkey, 1953a). As mentioned earlier, possible reasons proposed for the discrepancy between direct and viable counts are that the direct count includes dead and clumped cells and that not all organisms can grow in the medium used for the study. The differences between roughage and concentrate fed animals must then be attributed to a higher proportion of dead cells or clumped cells in roughage fed animals, a shift in the population in concentrate fed animals to more organisms which can be grown, or possible sequestration and attachment of the bacterial cells to the fibrous material in hay fed animals, from which they are not readily dislodged by mixing. One additional point to be considered is that in the studies of Bryant and Burkey (1953b) and Maki and Foster (1957) viable colonies were counted after three and four days, respectively. Subsequently,

Bryant and Robinson (1961) have reported that their three-day counts averaged only 67% of seven-day counts. Rumen contents for their study were obtained from a cow fed a 79% alfalfa - 21% grain ration. A similar increase in colony count has been observed in the author's laboratory between five and seven days incubation (unpublished). If those organisms which appear after three to five days incubation are specifically associated with roughage digestion, the differences observed between direct and viable counts on roughage and concentrate type rations may be less than previously reported.

Whitelaw *et al.* (1972) compared total and viable counts in protozoa-free steers fed an 85% barley ration *ad libitum* in period 1 and 70% of *ad libitum* in periods 2 and 3. Two steers were inoculated and had established ciliate populations in period 3. Viable counts, as % of the total count, varied markedly both within and between animals; however, it was of considerable interest that the proportion of bacteria which could be cultured decreased considerably with the establishment of a ciliate population. These results could be confounded by the fact that only starch was used as a substrate for viable counts and counts were made after 3 days incubation.

Media

The media used by Bryant and Burkey (1953a) in their initial studies was a habitat-simulating, non-selective medium which contained 40% rumen fluid, minerals, glucose, cellobiose, agar, cysteine, Na_2CO_3 and a 100% CO_2 gas phase (RGCA). In 1961, Bryant and Robinson investigated the effects of level of rumen fluid, clarification of rumen fluid and incubation time. The three day counts averaged 67% of the 7 day counts (range of 54-75%) and the difference was highly significant ($P < 0.01$). The 7 day counts were 83% of the 14 day counts and apparently not significantly different. The difference in counts between 20% and 40% rumen fluid was significant, but not significant between clarified and whole rumen fluid. They found a mixture of cysteine and Na_2S to be superior as reducing agents. Level of soluble substrates was reduced (0.025% each of glucose and cellobiose) and starch (0.05%) was included in the medium. Their new medium, 98-5, gave significantly higher colony counts than the old RGCA medium, in fact, almost double.

Subsequent studies by Caldwell and Bryant (1966) indicated that counts similar to those in their rumen fluid medium could be obtained if rumen fluid was replaced by hemin, VFA and low levels of trypticase and yeast extract. Species distribution of bacterial strains isolated with this new medium, Medium 10, was very similar to that obtained with rumen fluid medium.

In the author's laboratory both the rumen fluid and non-rumen fluid media developed by Bryant and coworkers were very time consuming to prepare, and particularly laborious was the sterile opening of each tube just prior to use in order to add the reducing agents. The main criticism of the old RGCA medium had been the large amount of particulate matter, which made colony counting difficult. Two possibilities were investigated which might alleviate this problem, i.e., clarification of the rumen fluid, and a reduction of the volume of medium (Grubb and Dehority, 1976). A significant decrease in colony count was found when the rumen fluid was clarified; however, reducing the volume to 4 ml per tube was without effect. With the 4 ml volume, interference from particulate matter was minimal to absent. Colony counts were significantly higher using 0.1% total carbohydrate versus 0.3% and 0% ($P < 0.05$). The ratio of glucose plus cellobiose to starch of 1:1, as compared to 2:1, 4:1 and 9:1, also significantly increased total counts ($P < 0.01$). Thus, the only changes from the old RGCA medium were a reduction in total substrate conc. to 0.1%, addition of soluble starch at a ratio of 1:1 with glucose + cellobiose, and use of 4 ml medium per tube. This medium, designated RGCSA, was then compared to the rumen fluid medium (RFM) and non-rumen fluid medium (Medium 10) previously described by Bryant and coworkers (Bryant and Robinson, 1961; Caldwell and Bryant, 1966), and prepared according to their procedures. The results are shown in Table 12.1. As can be noted, the RGCSA medium colony counts were significantly higher than those with Medium 10 for all rations. They were higher than the RFM medium on all rations, but the difference was significant only with the 60-40 ration. It was thus, concluded, that if rumen fluid is readily available, the RGCSA medium is easier to prepare, faster to inoculate, gives higher colony counts and would be the method of choice.

Table 12.1 COMPARISON OF ROLL TUBE COLONY COUNTS FOR TOTAL VIABLE RUMEN BACTERIA OBTAINED WITH DIFFERENT MEDIA (MEDIUM 10, RFM, AND RGCSA)[a]

	Colony count/10^{-8} g of rumen contents[b]		
Ration	Medium 10[c]	RFM[c]	RGCSA[c]
Alfalfa	19.0	44.1	62.6
Orchardgrass	31.1	54.3	64.2
NU-8[d]	70.4	134.4	150.8
60% corn-40% orchardgrass	90.2	148.6	181.6

[a] From Grubb and Dehority (1976).
[b] All means not underlined by a common line are significantly different ($P < 0.01$). Counts were determined on three replicates at three inoculum levels and four roll tubes per inoculum level, giving a total of 36 roll tubes for each mean value.
[c] Medium 10 (non-rumen fluid medium) and RFM (40% clarified rumen fluid medium) are described by Caldwell and Bryant (1966), 9 ml per tube. RGCSA is described by Grubb and Dehority (1976), 4 ml per tube. For each replicate, RFM and RGCSA media were prepared from the same sample of rumen fluid.
[d] Pelleted diet containing 49% corn cobs, 15% soybean meal, 15% ground corn, 20% dehydrated alfalfa meal plus 1% vitamins, minerals and urea.

Dehority et al. (1989) published a procedure for the simultaneous enumeration of total and cellulolytic bacterial numbers in one single MPN medium. Essentially this involved adding a limited amount of soluble carbohydrates, so that a decrease in medium pH could be measured but the decrease would not be large enough to inhibit digestion of insoluble cellulose included in the same medium. Thus, cellulose digestion is determined by visible loss of cellulose, and growth of total bacteria by decrease in medium pH. A comparison was made of total bacterial concentrations estimated from roll tubes, 3 tube MPN and 5 tube MPN procedures. In summary, the overall mean bacterial concentrations did not differ between the three methods. The procedure for simultaneous MPN estimation of total and cellulolytic bacterial numbers was compared using separate MPN assays for each bacterial group. Samples of rumen contents were obtained from both calves and sheep fed low and high energy diets. Based on 28 samples, concentrations of total and cellulolytic bacteria were not different whether measured alone or simultaneously in the same tube.

SELECTIVE MEDIA

In addition to measuring total viable numbers, Bryant and Burkey (1953a; 1953b) were also interested in determining the composition of the bacterial population in the rumen. They isolated about 50 strains per sample of rumen contents, from tubes inoculated with 1×10^{-8} g or less. On the basis of colony type, morphology, Gram-stain and motility, representative strains from each sample were presumptively identified.

Kistner (1960) was also interested in determining the species composition of the bacterial population on a routine basis and studied the possibilities of using selective media instead of isolation procedures. Kistner was aware of the difficulties involved in sampling, such as the "attached" bacteria, but believed the more rigorous treatments might affect viability. He was interested primarily in comparative counts of functional groups and assumed the strained rumen fluid would be representative and similar between animals. He obtained samples by suction tube through a rumen fistula. From an animal fed solely alfalfa, he investigated such factors as variation in replicate counts from a single sample (C.V. = 3.95%), site of sampling within the rumen (C.V. = 22.67%), and day to day fluctuations (C.V. = 75.2%) on the viable numbers of cellulolytic organisms. Using these methods, with a 30% rumen fluid medium, Gilchrist and Kistner (1962) obtained so-called selective medium (single substrate) counts as follows (no. x 10^6 per ml rumen fluid): cellulose, 3.2; starch, 12.2; glucose, 56, xylose, 59; lactate, 135.

Grubb and Dehority (1975), attempted to follow the numbers of xylan, pectin and starch utilizing bacteria when an animal was changed abruptly from an all roughage ration to a 60% concentrate-40% roughage ration. The regular carbohydrates in the medium, glucose, cellobiose and starch were replaced by either xylan, pectin or starch. Results were expressed as % of the total count obtained with non-selective medium, and values of over 100% occurred on one or more selective media on the same day.

This strongly suggested that they were not using a truly selective medium. Although some species should utilize more than one substrate, values would not be expected to exceed the total count. Gilchrist and Kistner (1962) did not report a total count, so similar calculations cannot be made with their data. Later studies by Grubb and Dehority (1976) indicated that the basal rumen fluid medium without any added substrate would support about 75% of the number of colonies growing in the regular medium. This observation would, at least in part, explain the high counts on this type of selective medium.

Subsequently, Dehority and Grubb (1976) developed a selective medium in which less than 10% of the total bacterial count would grow without added substrate. The basal medium was prepared by anaerobic incubation of all ingredients in RGCSA medium, except the carbohydrates, Na_2CO_3 and cysteine, for 7 days at 38°C. After incubation, substrate(s), Na_2CO_3 and cysteine are added and the medium was tubed and sterilized as in normal medium preparation. When xylose was included with glucose, cellobiose and starch as added carbohydrates in the incubated medium, colony counts were comparable to those obtained in RGCSA medium. Addition of xylose to regular RGCSA medium was without effect. To evaluate the ability of the selective medium to measure differences in bacterial proportions between animals and rations, studies were conducted in which each of the carbohydrates used in the medium for total colony counts was individually added to the basal incubated medium. Both total colony counts and selective medium counts were found to vary considerably between consecutive sampling days. The only obvious trends between the sheep fed 60% corn- 40% hay and the hay-fed sheep were that the animal fed hay appeared to have a higher percentage of cellobiose-fermenting bacteria along with a lower percentage of starch digestors. These differences agreed with earlier results obtained by other workers in which they assayed non-selective medium isolates on these same substrates.

Factors affecting the population

Several aspects of the rumen fermentation have been investigated by means of culture counts. These include studies on the effect of different feeds, time and frequency of feeding, diurnal variation in total count and estimates of the concentration of predominant or functional groups.

FREQUENCY OF FEEDING

Moir and Somers (1957) found that protozoal concentrations were significantly increased by feeding the same total amount of a ration twice or four times daily over the numbers obtained with a single feeding. However, in the same study they observed that bacterial concentrations did not differ between treatments. Similar results were reported by Warner (1966b). Dehority and Tirabasso (2001) found that feeding the same amount of a given diet either once, 6 or 24 times had only a slight effect on the concentration of rumen bacteria. There were no differences on the first sampling day between feeding frequencies, however, concentrations were higher on day 5 with the 24 feedings per day ($P < 0.05$).

LEVEL OF FEEDING

Gilchrist and Kistner (1962) fed a diet of poor teff hay to three sheep for periods of 60, 109 and 42 days, at levels of 1200, 600 and 300 g/day, respectively. No significant differences were observed either in viable counts or functional groups fermenting cellulose, starch, glucose, xylose and lactate over the experimental periods. Warner (1962b) reached the same conclusion with direct counts and the same range of intakes.

Dearth et al. (1974) estimated total viable anaerobic bacterial numbers in lambs fed the same ration at levels equal to either 1.0 or 1.8 times their daily maintenance energy requirement. The experiment was a 4 x 4 Latin square, extra period design. Numbers significantly increased ($P < 0.01$) from 92.8×10^8 per g of rumen contents when the lambs were fed the maintenance level to 115.0×10^8 per g of rumen contents when fed at 1.8 x maintenance. Experimental conditions were controlled much more closely in this study as compared to the previously cited experiments.

DIET EFFECTS

Numerous data are published on the effects of ration and sampling time on rumen bacterial concentrations; however, the methodology used in many of these studies is somewhat questionable. The diurnal growth curves reported by Bryant and Robinson (1961), based on viable counts with their best medium, and those of Warner (1966a; 1966c) obtained by direct counts appear to be reliable estimates. In general, on both hay and concentrate rations, a decrease in bacterial numbers occurs immediately after feeding, presumably resulting from dilution by feed and water intake. This is followed by a gradual, or in some cases, rapid, increase in numbers in response to nutrient availability. Numbers then level off and may actually decrease slightly prior to the next feeding. Warner (1966c) obtained a similar pattern in rumen bacterial concentrations for sheep on pasture, but did observe that they tended to eat most of their daily intake at one period in the morning. Bacterial numbers were higher in animals fed grain as compared to those fed hay (Bryant and Robinson, 1961). Other studies have indicated that 3 to 10 times more bacteria per g or ml are found in rumen contents of animals on high grain rations (Bryant and Burkey, 1953b; Maki and Foster, 1957). If feed intake is not limited and rumen volume is combined with bacterial numbers, the total number of bacteria in the rumen is rather similar on concentrate, pasture and hay rations (Puch, 1977).

Grubb and Dehority (1975) followed total viable bacterial concentrations in three sheep during an abrupt change in ration from 100% orchardgrass hay (OG) to 60% corn-40% OG (Figure 12.2). Both rations were fed at equal dry matter intake. In two of the three sheep a rapid and marked increase in numbers was observed after changing to the high grain ration.

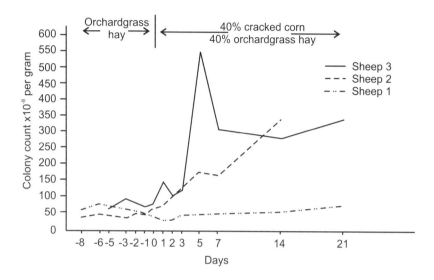

Figure 12.2 Concentration changes in total bacterial numbers associated with an abrupt change in ration in sheep (from Grubb and Dehority, 1975).

Gilchrist and Kistner (1962) and Kistner *et al.* (1962) made some very interesting observations when they compared the rumen bacterial population in sheep fed alfalfa or poor quality teff hay. Species composition of the cellulolytic group, as judged by Gram-stain observation, was quite different. Gram-negative or Gram-variable cocci (*Ruminococcus albus*) were the primary cellulolytic species in the alfalfa hay fed animals, while Gram-negative rods (*Butyrivibrio*) predominated in the sheep fed poor teff hay. Subsequent investigations by Gouws and Kistner (1965) indicated that this was a clearly reversible situation and associated with diet.

Bryant and Robinson (1968) have compared diet effects, sampling time after feeding and position sampled upon viable bacterial numbers. Four rations: chopped alfalfa hay, the same hay ground and pelleted, the same hay plus an equal weight of grain mixture, and hay crop silage were fed. On all rations but the pelleted hay, numbers were lowest at 1 hour after feeding and increased significantly at 2.5 and 5.5 hours. Numbers in the ventral rumen were significantly lower at all times from 1-10 h than in the dorsal rumen. When hay or hay-grain was fed, concentrations in the reticulum were the same as those in the rumen. Concentrations were higher on the pelleted diet ($P < 0.01$) and lower ($P < 0.05$) when silage was fed.

Thorley et al. (1968) investigated the effects of feeding long hay or ground and pelleted hay on total culture counts. Mean viable counts of 15.7 x 10^9 per g were obtained on ground and pelleted grass and 10.5 x 10^9 per g on long grass. Both the clarified rumen fluid and complete medium described earlier (98-5 and Medium 10, respectively) were used for these studies, with higher counts being obtained on the complete medium.

Using the pre-incubated selective medium described earlier, Dehority and Grubb (1976) compared the proportions of the total culturable rumen bacteria capable of fermenting various substrates between sheep fed 100% hay or 60% corn-40% hay. Their results are shown in Table 12.2. The total count and percentage of starch-digesting bacteria were significantly higher in the sheep fed the 60-40 ration. The mean percentages for xylan and pectin-fermenting bacteria were not different; however, the daily variation was quite large with these substrates. Starch utilizers were significantly higher than xylan or pectin-utilizers in the 60-40 fed sheep, while there was no significant difference between the percentages fermenting the different carbohydrates in the hay fed sheep. In a separate set of experiments, lactate, glycerol and mannitol were used as selective substrates. Within each animal, or between rations, no significant differences were found with these three energy sources. However, the percentage of lactate and glycerol utilizing bacteria tended to be higher in the orchardgrass fed sheep. This was rather unexpected since most species of bacteria which are active in the fermentation of starch produce considerable amounts of lactic acid.

Table 12.2 CONCENTRATION AND PERCENTAGE DISTRIBUTION OF RUMEN BACTERIA UTILIZING STARCH, XYLAN AND PECTIN IN SHEEP FED EITHER A 60% CORN - 40% HAY OR AN ALL HAY DIET[a]

Sheep no.	Diet[b]	Concentration[c]	% of total bacteria utilizing:[d]		
			Starch	Xylan	Pectin
1	OG	53.0±4.6^x	60.7±5.4^x	63.5±7.7	59.4±4.4
2	60-40	148.6±13.4^y	95.8±1.8^y	60.5±7.9	60.4±8.3

[a] From Dehority and Grubb (1976). Data for each diet are the mean of four replicates.
[b] OG: orchardgrass hay; 60-40: 60% corn-40% orchardgrass hay
[c] Colony count per 10^{-8} g of rumen contents (Mean ± SE).
[d] Mean ± SE.
[x,y] Means in the same column followed by different superscripts differ at $P < 0.01$.

Mackie and Heath (1979) developed a purified medium for enumeration and isolation of lactate utilizing bacteria from the rumen of sheep. Essentially, their medium contained the usual minerals, agar, $NaHCO_3$, and reducing agents plus 2% lactic acid, 2% Trypticase, 0.2% yeast extract, VFA and hemin. Although they obtained higher counts in medium with lower lactate concentrations, the percentage of their isolates utilizing lactate was higher with the high lactate medium (92% vs 78%). Using this medium, Mackie and Gilchrist (1979) determined the mean numbers of lactate utilizing bacteria during the stepwise adaptation of sheep to a high concentrate diet. In general, the percent lactate-utilizing bacteria increased from 0.2% to 22.3% from the low (10%) to high (71%) - concentrate diet. The percentage of amylolytic bacteria remained below 20% until the animals were fed the 71% concentrate diet for at least three weeks. Lactate-utilizers also increased to about 20% at that time. The authors identified 11 amylolytic and 14 lactate-utilizing strains which they believed to represent the various morphological shapes observed among the cultures isolated. Six genera were identified from the 11 amylolytic strains: *Bacteroides, Selenomonas, Streptococcus, Butyrivibrio, Lactobacillus* and *Eubacterium*. The 14 lactate-utilizing strains were identified as belonging to the genera *Selenomonas, Veillonella, Anaerovibrio, Megasphaera* and *Propionibacterium*. Using morphology, size, Gram reaction and ability to ferment soluble starch with the production of lactate or ability to utilize lactate as criterion (Mackie and Gilchrist, 1979), 350 amylolytic and lactate-utilizing isolates were taken at each sampling date and presumptively identified into one of these genera. For the amylolytic bacteria, *Bacteroides* was predominant during the adaptation phases, but was replaced by *Eubacterium* and *Lactobacillus* on the high-concentrate diet. *Butyrivibrio* was present in a fairly high percentage (20-30%) throughout the whole experiment. For the lactate-utilizers, *Veillonella* and *Selenomonas* were present during low-concentrate feeding but then disappeared. *Anaerovibrio* and *Propionibacterium* were found with all diets and became the predominant genera on the high-concentrate diet.

In the same study, Mackie and Gilchrist (1979) also determined what they termed a "pH6-hour" value, or the time over a 14 h sampling period when rumen pH was below pH 6.0. For one sheep, from day 1 of high-concentrate feeding to day 54, the increase in time below pH 6.0 was 5-6 fold. For all four sheep the mean increase was threefold. Their population shifts appeared to follow this same pattern, i.e., shifting from more acid-sensitive to acid-tolerant genera as percentage concentrate and time below pH 6.0 increased.

A somewhat similar study was conducted by Roxas (1980), in which the numbers of amylolytic and lactate-utilizing bacteria were enumerated during abrupt changes from roughage to high-concentrate rations. The selective medium previously developed by Dehority and Grubb (1976) was used and total concentrations were similar to the data of Mackie and Gilchrist (1979). However, much higher numbers of amylolytic and lactate-utilizing bacteria were obtained. Mackie and Gilchrist (1979) also used a rumen fluid medium for total counts; however, their amylolytic and lactate-utilizing counts were determined on a non-rumen fluid medium. Mackie and Heath (1979) do mention the possibility that their medium might be limiting in growth factors for some species of lactate-utilizers. In the study by Roxas (1980), using a selective starch medium, 72% of the cultures isolated from the all roughage feeding periods were amylolytic, while 92% of the isolates obtained during the corn silage and high-concentrate feeding periods were amylolytic. Using a selective lactate medium, 83% of the cultures isolated from the all roughage periods and 88% of those isolated from the corn silage and high concentrate periods were capable of utilizing lactate. Adjusting the selective medium counts for these percentages, amylolytic and lactate utilizing percentages during roughage feeding were about 50% and 25%, respectively, and during corn silage and high-concentrate periods, 85% and 32%, respectively. These percentages are markedly higher than those reported by Mackie and Gilchrist (1979).

Comparison of the generic distribution of amylolytic isolates from the two studies shows that Roxas (1980) found a larger proportion of *Bacteroides* and *Selenomonas* during high-concentrate feeding. For the lactate-utilizers, *Veillonella* disappeared with high-concentrate feeding in both studies. In contrast to Mackie and Gilchrist (1979), *Selenomonas* was present while the percentage of *Anaerovibrio* was reduced. *Propionibacterium* were present in both studies.

Obviously there are certain dangers in comparing these two studies because of the large methodology differences and the fact that one was a stepwise change and the other an abrupt change from roughage or low-concentrate to a high-concentrate diet. However, the data on adjusted percentages of amylolytic and lactate-utilizing bacteria are probably better estimates of the true values. Roxas (1980) identified a larger number of isolates; however, Mackie and Gilchrist (1979) presumptively classified a much larger number. The questions are whether Roxas identified a representative sample and how accurate were their presumptive identifications. In general, studies of this nature are quite limited because of the time required for identification and classification of bacterial isolates. It is anticipated that studies of this type will be markedly enhanced using the newer techniques of molecular biology.

Leedle and Hespell (1980) developed a basal medium for use in the enumeration of different carbohydrate-utilizing rumen bacteria by plating techniques. Essentially it was a 40% incubated rumen fluid medium using washed agar plus Trypticase, yeast extract, hemin and VFA. Their agar plates were prepared and inoculated in an anaerobic glove box. Suitable aliquots of diluted rumen contents were inoculated onto the surface of the agar plate and dispersed or spread with a sterile bent glass rod. Using various media they compared total colony counts on roll tubes versus plates. On all media, slightly higher colony counts were observed on plates than on roll tubes; however, the authors do not indicate whether this difference is significant. Using pure cultures of 20 different species, agar plates were spot inoculated (10 cultures per plate), allowed to incubate for 48 h and then used as a master plate for replica plating onto the various specific carbohydrate media. Results were well correlated with known substrate specificities of these species, indicating the potential use of this procedure with unknown mixed cultures. Using the plating technique, they determined subgroup profiles of rumen bacteria in a high forage and a high grain fed animal. Some of the diet effects observed were similar to those observed previously by Dehority and Grubb (1976); however, there were also marked differences. A possible explanation other than differences in methods would be sampling procedures. Three to four hours after feeding they manually mixed the rumen contents, removed handfuls and squeezed them through two layers of cheesecloth. The fluid was collected in a flask to one-half the total flask volume after which whole rumen contents were added to completely fill the flask, which was then sealed. The flask contents were subsequently blended for 1 min under CO_2, squeezed through four layers of cheesecloth and the resulting liquid used as an inoculum. To compare results from this procedure to subgroups determined directly on whole rumen contents samples taken just prior to feeding is probably unwise. The authors offer no explanation for their rather unusual method of collecting rumen samples which could markedly influence both numbers and the relative percentages of different subgroups, especially if they differ at all between free and attached populations.

Using the plating and replica plating techniques described above, Leedle *et al.* (1982) studied the diurnal variation in bacterial numbers of specific carbohydrate fermenting subgroups in animals fed low- or high-forage diets. Unexpectedly, diurnal variation in bacterial numbers for these two diets was very similar. The authors concluded that this was probably the result of feeding the diets at equal energy intake, which probably caused only relatively minor changes in the rumen and restricted the amounts of available energy.

Van der Linden *et al.* (1984) compared the numbers of cellulolytic and xylanolytic bacteria in sheep fed varying proportions of corn to roughage. Their results were fairly similar to the results of Leedle *et al.* (1982), in that xylanolytic numbers were more than double the number of cellulolytics and inclusion of corn had little effect on numbers of either group.

Varel and Dehority (1989) measured total and cellulolytic bacterial concentrations in rumen contents from bison, bison hybrids and cattle fed 100% alfalfa, 75% alfalfa - 25% corn, and 50% alfalfa - 50% corn. No differences were found between the three animal types. Percentages of cellulolytic species were determined and % *F. succinogenes* was significantly higher with the 100% and 75% - 25% diets. *Ruminococcus* percentages in bison were higher than in cattle on the 50% - 50% diet. *B. fibrisolvens* percentages were lower in bison than the bison hybrid on the 100% alfalfa diet and lower than in cattle on the 75% - 25% diet.

ANTIBIOTICS

Dawson and Boling (1983) determined total and monensin resistant bacterial numbers in the rumen of steers fed diets with and without monensin. Total counts were not different with monensin added to the diet; however, 63.6% of the population in the monensin supplemented animals were resistant to monensin in the medium compared to 32.8% in the unsupplemented animals. Olumeyan *et al.* (1986) fed salinomycin (a polyether antibiotic) to steers and estimated bacterial numbers and profiles on various diets. They found a two-fold increase in number of ionophore-resistant bacteria and a higher percentage of amylolytic bacteria in the salinomycin fed animals.

Nagaraja and Taylor (1987) measured the susceptibility and resistance of a large number of rumen bacteria to eight antimicrobial feed additives. In general, most of the antimicrobial compounds inhibited the Gram-positive bacteria or those bacteria which

280 *Rumen microbiology*

have a Gram-positive-like cell wall. Gram-negative bacteria were resistant to fairly high concentrations. Those bacteria which produce lactic acid, butyric acid, formic acid or hydrogen appear to be susceptible to the antimicrobial compounds, while those which produce succinate or ferment lactate are resistant. Ionophore type agents seem to be more inhibitory than nonionophore compounds.

Subpopulations of bacteria in the rumen

At least three subpopulations of bacteria appear to be present in the rumen. The first would be those bacteria which are present as single cells or slime enclosed clumps which are not attached to particulate matter. It is assumed that these bacteria would move with the fluid. The second subpopulation are those bacteria or clumps of bacteria which are attached to the particulate matter. These bacteria would pass from the rumen at a much slower rate than the free floating cells. And lastly, the third subpopulation are those bacteria which are attached or adhere to the rumen epithelium. The schematic drawing in Figure 12.3 shows the relationship of these three subpopulations. The experimental data to support the existence of these three subpopulations is certainly adequate; however, there are several additional questions which need to be considered. First, how adequate are our present methods for enumeration and identification of bacteria in the subpopulations and second, what is the role, if any, of each subpopulation in the total rumen ecosystem?

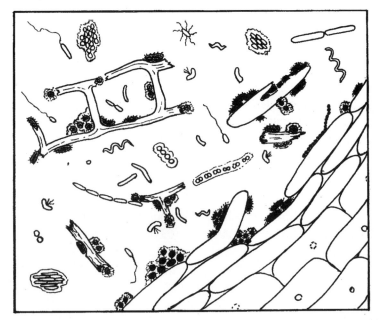

Figure 12.3 Schematic drawing to illustrate the three subpopulations of rumen bacteria: (1) single cells or capsular enclosed clumps; (2) bacteria attached to particulate matter; and (3) bacteria attached to the rumen epithelium.

BACTERIA FLOATING FREE IN RUMEN FLUID

In general, we have used the criteria of numbers or concentration to evaluate the importance of a particular species to the overall rumen fermentation. However, these conclusions may be in error if our procedures are not adequately sampling all subpopulations. As previously discussed, after filtering rumen contents through a double layer of cheesecloth, about 50% of the total bacterial numbers are in the fluid and 50% are associated with the particulate matter. Some of these bacteria can be dislodged and counted if the sample is blended; however, electron microscopy, fluorescent antibody procedures, studies using ^{15}N enrichment and carboxymethylcellulase activity would all indicate that considerable numbers of bacteria are still attached to particulate matter after fairly vigorous physical agitation (Minato *et al.*, 1966; Akin, 1980; Firkins *et al.*, 1991; Bowman and Firkins, 1993).

BACTERIA ASSOCIATED WITH FEED PARTICLES

Since the microscopic studies by Baker and Harriss (1947) we have been aware that rumen bacteria are attached to particulate matter undergoing digestion. Early studies in Ohio showed that greater cellulolytic activity occurred in the bacteria eluted with buffer from pressed rumen ingesta than in strained rumen fluid (Johnson *et al.*, 1958). As discussed previously, Warner (1962a), using direct microscopic counts, found that straining rumen contents through bolting cloth with kneading and mixing and washing the residue by the same procedure left over half of the total bacteria still associated with the particulate matter. Studies using viable counts gave similar results, i.e., after four anaerobic washings of rumen particulate matter about 30-40% of the total countable viable bacteria were still associated with the solid material and could be freed by blending (unpublished).

Dehority and Grubb (1980) conducted some experiments which quantitatively demonstrated that large numbers of bacteria are attached to rumen particulate matter. Anaerobic storage of rumen contents at 0°C for 8 h was unexpectedly found to increase total viable counts. Selective medium counts with glucose, cellobiose, starch and xylose indicated no significant population shifts occurred during cold storage. A number of variables were investigated to explain this increase in viable numbers, i.e., possible growth during storage, variability between subsamples, effect of temperature during blending, bacterial release from inside protozoa, rumen sampling time and blending time, all of which were apparently not involved. The effect of storage time at 0°C was investigated with a graded increase in numbers being observed at 4 and 8 h. Based on these data, storage at 0°C for 6 h was used in future experiments. If rumen contents were filtered through a double layer of cheesecloth, an increase was obtained in numbers after storage of the fluid fraction; however, if the strained rumen fluid was centrifuged at 1000 x g for 10 min, cold storage of the supernatant did not increase the viable count. Storage of diluted rumen contents did not increase viable counts. It was concluded that if there is no multiplication or increase in bacterial numbers during cold storage, and the lowered temperature does not increase percentage viability of the bacteria, the only possible explanation for these data is that there is a strong attachment of the bacteria to particulate matter which is broken down by chilling or that clumps of bacteria held together by capsular material are broken up into smaller clumps or individual cells by chilling. Thus, one would expect a surfactant to have a similar effect to chilling. Addition of Tween 80 to the dilution solution did increase total counts to the same extent as chilling (Table 12.3); however, quite unexpectedly these two treatments were additive. Thus, the data in Table 12.3 clearly indicate that the normal counting procedures are underestimating total bacterial numbers by at least 50%.

Using a pulse dose of ^{15}N as a microbial marker, Craig *et al.* (1987) attempted to quantitate the number of rumen microorganisms associated with particulate matter. As estimated from ^{15}N, only 32 to 52% of particle associated microorganisms could be recovered from particles taken 1, 2, 3, 6, 8 and 10 h after feed was removed. About 70-80% of microbial organic matter in whole rumen contents was associated with the particulate matter. It was also estimated that 50-65% of particle nitrogen and 17-27% of particle dry matter was of microbial origin. These data support the idea that particle-associated microorganisms make up a major portion of the total number of rumen bacteria.

Table 12.3 EFFECT OF ADDING A SURFACTANT UPON TOTAL VIABLE BACTERIAL NUMBERS IN RUMEN CONTENTS STORED FOR 0 OR 6 H AT 0°C[a]

Storage time (h) at 0°C	*Addition to ADS*[b]	*% of zero-time colony count*[c]
0	None	100[x]
0	0.1% Tween 80	144.8 ± 12.8[y]
6	None	146.6 ± 14.1[y]
6	0.1% Tween 80	204.6 ± 24.4[z]

[a] From Dehority and Grubb (1980).
[b] Anaerobic dilution solution.
[c] Mean and standard error of the mean, seven experiments.
[x,y,z] Means followed by different superscripts are significantly different at $P < 0.05$.

Based on the knowledge that a large portion of the rumen bacteria are associated with the particle fraction, several different methods for preparation of *in vitro* inocula have been evaluated. Craig *et al.* (1984) found that enrichment of the inocula with organisms which were washed from the particulate matter increased the rates of neutral detergent fiber digestion and casein degradation. Subsequently, Furchtenicht and Broderick (1987) found it beneficial to chill rumen contents four hours before preparing the inoculum which contained strained rumen fluid enriched with particle-associated microorganisms. The highest microbial dry weight, total bacterial counts and degradation rates for casein and soybean were obtained with the inoculum prepared by this procedure. This information would substantiate the previous results of Dehority and Grubb (1980).

In reality we may be dealing with three subpopulations of particle associated bacteria, i.e., the bacteria associated with particulate matter which can be dislodged by blending, the attached bacteria which can be freed by chilling and the use of surfactants and those bacteria, if any, which are not dislodged by the previous treatments. Further studies are obviously needed to develop methods for the enumeration of the firmly attached subpopulation and to determine if its composition differs from the unattached or readily detached subpopulation.

With the availability of the electron microscope in the 1970's, a number of studies were reported on the rumen bacterial surface layer or cell coat and attachment of the bacteria to particulate matter. Cheng and Costerton (1975) and Cheng et al. (1977) showed that almost all rumen bacteria are surrounded by a fibrous carbohydrate slime that extends away from the cell and probably plays a role in attachment of the bacteria to a surface. Akin and Amos (1975) and Akin (1976, 1980) have observed the attachment of bacteria from whole rumen contents to forage cell walls *in vitro*. The majority of bacteria which were attached and appeared to be degrading the cell walls were encapsulated cocci and irregular shaped bacillus. Morphologically these organisms resembled the major cellulolytic species in the rumen, i.e., *Fibrobacter succinogenes* and the ruminococci. In subsequent studies Latham *et al.* (1978a, 1978b) studied adhesion of pure cultures of these two species to cotton fibers and ryegrass cell walls. *R. flavefaciens* has a thick extracellular glycoprotein coat (65 to 80 nm thick) which firmly binds the cell to insoluble substrates. However, adhesion of *R. flavefaciens* to cotton fibers or plant cell walls appears to be dependent on the availability of cut or otherwise damaged cell walls. In contrast, *F. succinogenes* has an extremely thin cell coat which does not appear to have sufficient mechanical strength to hold the organism against its substrate, particularly during severe physical agitation. Transmission electron microscopy (TEM) of *F. succinogenes* cells attached to plant material indicate that the cell wall is very pliable and allows the cell to conform to the topography of the substrate providing a relatively large area of contact. Using microscopy and fluorescent antibody techniques, Minato *et al.* (1966) have reported that *F. succinogenes* appears to be much more firmly attached to particulate matter than the ruminococcus species. The surface layer or coat of *F. succinogenes* is extremely thin, about 15 nm (Akin, 1976). A schematic drawing of these two species attached to a plant fiber is shown in Figure 12.4. *F. succinogenes* is considered to have a firmly cell-bound cellulase, which in turn might be considerably more effective under these conditions (Forsberg *et al.*, 1981; Groleau and Forsberg, 1981). *F. succinogenes* appears to differ from *R. flavefaciens* by an ability to adhere to undamaged plant surfaces, and this ability may be reflected in the observations that *F. succinogenes* can digest considerably more cellulose from intact forages than ruminococcus species (Dehority and Scott, 1967), 15-20% more in most forages, under limiting substrate conditions.

284 *Rumen microbiology*

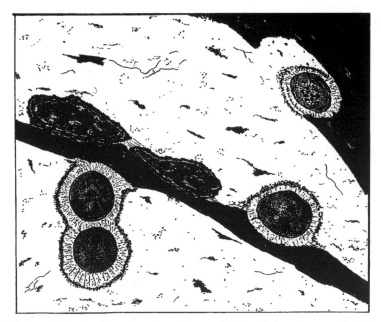

Figure 12.4 Schematic drawing illustrating the attachment of *R. flavefaciens* (coccus with thick capsule) and *F. succinogenes* (bacillus with only a very thin capsular coat) to plant fibers. Note the "pits" or areas of digestion where the cells are attached.

The actual mechanisms by which the cellulolytic species are able to attach to particulate matter, primarily cellulose, has been discussed in Chapter 8. However, several studies have shown that a significant number of non-cellulolytic bacteria are also attached to feed particles (Firkins *et al.*, 1991; Bowman and Firkins, 1993).

BACTERIA ASSOCIATED WITH THE RUMEN EPITHELIUM

In 1975 Bauchop *et al.* studied the epithelium from 14 sites in the sheep rumen by scanning electron microscopy (SEM) and observed a fairly large adherent bacterial population. They also found that both the extent of bacterial cover and morphological types varied between areas; however, bacterial cover was visually estimated to be heaviest on the roof of the dorsal rumen and primarily consisted of rod-shaped cells.

Cheng *et al.* (1979), isolated bacteria from bovine rumen epithelium at various sites within the rumen and found several species of *Micrococcus, Staphyloccus, Streptococcus, Corynebacterium, Lactobacillus, Fusobacterium* and *Propionibacterium*. They concluded that this adherent population was clearly taxonomically distinct from rumen fluid, containing a significant number of Gram-positive organisms. Three main functions were suggested for this adherent population: oxygen scavenging, tissue recycling and digestion of urea. The first two functions were proposed on the basis of their observations that approximately 25% of cattle isolates and 80% of sheep isolates were facultative anaerobes (Cheng et al., 1979; Wallace et al., 1979), and electron microscope studies which showed digestion of dead and keratinized epithelial cells (Cheng et al., 1979). When urease activity of the adherent population was determined, calculations indicated that the adherent population could account for 16 to 50% of the activity of the much larger bacterial population of rumen fluid (Cheng and Wallace, 1978). They suggested that these adherent facultative ureolytic bacteria maintain a localized concentration gradient which serves to increase the rate of diffusion of urea into the rumen.

In contrast to the above studies, Mead and Jones (1981) isolated 161 strains of adherent bacteria from four sites on the rumen epithelial surface of sheep fed hay or a hay-grain ration. Their sites for isolation were roof of the cranial rumen, roof of dorsal rumen, floor of caudodorsal blind sac and floor of caudoventral blind sac. Approximately 95% of their isolates were presumptively identified and assigned to 10 previously described genera of rumen bacteria. Percentages were as follows: *Butyrivibrio* sp., 31.1%; *Bacteroides* sp., 22.4%; *Selenomonas ruminantium*, 9.9%; *Succinivibrio dextrinosolvens*, 8.7%; *Streptococcus bovis*, 8.1%; *Propionibacterium* sp., 4.3%; *Treponema* sp., 3.1%; *Eubacterium* sp., *Lachnospira multiparus* and *Ruminococcus flavefaciens*, 2.5% each. The authors suggested the name "epimural" bacteria for those bacteria adherent or attached to the rumen epithelium.

At about the same time as the studies by Mead and Jones (1981) were being conducted, a somewhat similar study was underway by Dehority and Grubb (1981). Since Bauchop et al. (1975) had found that the roof of the dorsal rumen was the most densely populated area and the bacteria were primarily rod-shaped cells, this appeared to be a promising site for study. Objectives were to quantitate the adherent population in that area and to isolate and identify the bacteria. Table 12.4 presents the data on bacteria attached to the roof of the dorsal rumen in three animals and the effect of repeated washing on their concentration. For comparison, bacterial numbers from the floor of the caudodorsal blind sac were also determined in sheep 1. A total of 95 bacterial strains were isolated from the rumen epithelium on the roof of the dorsal rumen (three animals). These isolates were presumptively identified as follows: *Bacteroides* sp. 38.9%; *Butyrivibrio fibrisolvens*, 36.8%; *Prevotella ruminicola*, 23.2% and *Lactobacillus*, 1.0%. Thus, this area appeared to be primarily colonized by two genera of bacteria, *Butyrivibrio* and *Bacteroides*. This is consistent with the electron microscopy results reported by Bauchop et al. (1975), who observed a dense cover of rod-shaped bacteria in this region of the sheep rumen. Almost 60% of the strains isolated by Mead and Jones (1981) from the roof of the dorsal rumen were presumptively identified in the genera *Butyrivibrio* and *Bacteroides*.

McCowan et al. (1980) examined the same 14 sites in the rumen of cattle as those previously observed by electron microscopy in sheep (Bauchop et al., 1975). Diet variations appeared to influence distribution patterns of tissue-adherent bacteria, but not

Table 12.4 CONCENTRATION OF BACTERIA ATTACHED TO THE RUMEN EPITHELIUM OF SHEEP[a]

Animal[b]	Site	No. of washings	Colony count x $10^7/cm^2$ of rumen wall
1	Roof of dorsal rumen	4	1.91 ±0.13[c]
2	Roof of dorsal rumen	4	0.34 ±0.07
3	Roof of dorsal rumen	4	1.23 ±0.49
3	Roof of dorsal rumen	10	0.084±0.007
1	Floor of caudodorsal blind sac	4	1.34 ±0.08

[a] From Dehority and Grubb (1981).
[b] Rations: animal 1, grazing orchardgrass pasture; animal 2, grass hay; animal 3, mixed hay and corn silage.
[c] Mean and standard deviation.

total numbers. The largest adherent population was observed in the dorsal portion of the rumen, whereas ureolytic activity was predominantly observed in the ventral region. In other studies from this group (McCowan *et al.*, 1978; Dinsdale *et al.*, 1980), based on electron micrographs, they suggest that the adherent bacteria may also play a major part in the digestion of epithelial cells.

The results of Mead and Jones (1981) and Dehority and Grubb (1981) would indicate that the bacterial population adherent to the rumen epithelium is taxonomically and physiologically similar to the population found in rumen contents. In contrast, the results of Cheng and coworkers as cited above suggest that the bacterial population of the rumen wall is taxonomically distinct, containing a high proportion of Gram-positive, facultative, ureolytic, proteolytic bacteria. These organisms usually occur in very low numbers in rumen contents, and their presence suggests that they are carried into the contents attached to sloughed epithelial cells. Although the above results appear to be contradictory with respect to the species of bacteria colonizing the rumen epithelium, these discrepancies may be partially explained on the basis of differences in techniques and sampling. All of the following could be involved: animal species and ration, sampling site in the rumen, procedure and number of washes, methods used to detach the bacteria and whether microscopic or microbiological techniques are used to enumerate the bacteria.

Mueller *et al.* (1984) determined numbers of epimural bacteria from lambs at 1, 2, 4, 6, 8 and 10 weeks of age. Sixty strains were isolated and presumptively identified at each sampling time. In general, they found that the epimural bacteria community of the sheep rumen becomes established shortly after birth and soon reaches population levels similar to adult animals. The epimural bacteria were not markedly different from the bacteria found in rumen contents since most of their isolates could be placed into common rumen genera. These data would support the previous observations of Mead and Jones (1981) and Dehority and Grubb (1981). However, they did note that proportions of certain species differed between the attached and free bacterial populations.

Rieu *et al.* (1990) monitored colonization of the rumen epithelium in newborn lambs by scanning electron microscopy (SEM). A dense epimural population was present in all rumen sacs at two days of age and consisted almost completely of rods. The epimural population was more complex in lambs by 16 to 21 days of age with no particular dominant type present. The authors also observed large numbers of desquamated cells covered by bacteria in the rumen fluid. Regardless of the age of the lamb, lowest numbers of epimural bacteria were found attached to the epithelium of the caudal sac.

Enumeration of the epithelial-attached (epimural) bacterial population poses a somewhat complex problem. After four washings of tissue plugs taken from the rumen wall, Dehority and Grubb (1981) reported numbers of 1.91×10^7, 0.34×10^7 and 1.23×10^7 bacteria per cm^2 of epithelium from the roof of the dorsal rumen of sheep (Table 12.4). Wallace *et al*. (1979), using excised papillae which had been washed and homogenized, reported numbers of bacteria associated with the rumen epithelium ranging from 4.4×10^7 to 2.2×10^8 per g (wet weight) of tissue. However, no details were given concerning site, number of washes or extent of homogenization. Thus, in one case, numbers were based on area and in the other on tissue weight. However, in either case, such factors as size, shape and density of the papillae could markedly affect total numbers. Other parameters such as animal species, site in the rumen, type of feed, number and methods used for washes and extent of homogenization would need to be standardized for direct comparisons. Quantitation of bacterial cover based on actual rumen surface area, including the papillae, would appear to be the solution to this problem.

In the previously mentioned study by Mueller *et al*. (1984), aerobic and anaerobic bacterial numbers were determined on tissue disks taken from four rumen sites in young lambs. The disks were washed three times and then homogenized in a blender, which was very similar to the procedures used by Dehority and Grubb (1981). Their data for total anaerobic counts from the roof of the dorsal rumen ranged from 0.92×10^7 to 1.02×10^7 per cm^2, of rumen wall, which is in a similar range to the values reported by Dehority and Grubb (1981). Also of interest is the observation that after the first two weeks, the aerobic bacteria comprised only 1.5% or less of the total bacterial numbers.

The limited amount of information available on the epithelial attached subpopulation makes it difficult at this time to assess its potential role in the overall rumen fermentation. The epimural bacterial population found by Cheng and coworkers, and their suggested role for this population, have not been substantiated by subsequent studies. With the introduction of newer methodologies, particularly in the area of molecular biology, it should be possible to obtain more definitive information on both numbers and types of bacteria in the different niches. The use of 16S rRNA-targeted oligonucleotide probes and PCR amplification of 16S rDNA sequences should permit estimation of both total bacterial concentrations and the different species present.

Distribution of rumen bacteria

Although not of major importance, the possible distribution of rumen bacterial species in other habitats is of interest. In 1952, Hall isolated seven similar strains of cellulolytic cocci from rabbit cecal contents. Based on carbohydrates fermented and end-products from cellulose fermentation, all strains would appear to belong to the genus *Ruminococcus*. In a study by Dehority (1977), five strains of cellulolytic cocci were isolated from the cecum of the guinea pig. They were classified in the genus *Ruminococcus,* but differed from the two rumen cellulolytic species, *R. flavefaciens* and *R. albus*, and from the strains isolated by Hall from the cecum of the rabbit. Four strains of cellulolytic bacteria were isolated from the large intestine of the horse by Davies (1964), two of which resembled organisms in the genus *Bacteroides*.

Total bacterial numbers in the cecum of sheep were estimated by Lewis and Dehority (1985). Diets ranged from 100% hay to 80% corn-20% hay. Both total bacterial numbers and VFA concentrations were similar to those normally found in rumen contents. Sixteen cultures of cellulolytic bacteria were isolated and characterized from ileal and cecal contents. Seven strains were identified as *B. fibrisolvens* and the remaining nine strains as *Ruminococcus flavefaciens*, all of which were closely related to rumen strains of these particular species.

Bauchop and Martucci (1968) investigated gastric fermentation in the Langur monkey. The stomach of these species is of a diverticular form, which allows a fermentation to occur. Normal pH ranges between 5.0 and 6.7, and high concentrations of short-chain VFA are present. The authors succeeded in isolating two types of cellulolytic bacteria, one a Gram-negative coccus, and the second a Gram-negative rod belonging to the genus *Bacteroides*. In addition, cultures of *Methanobrevibacter ruminantium* were isolated.

Brown and Moore (1960) were able to isolate cultures of *Butyrivibrio fibrisolvens* from human, rabbit and horse fecal samples. This suggested to the authors that adult feces would be a most plausible route for inoculation of young ruminants on pasture.

Nottingham and Hungate (1968) have successfully isolated *Methanobrevibacter ruminantium* from five different human fecal samples. An anaerobic cellulolytic bacterium, identified as a *Bacteroides* sp., was found to be present in 10^{-8} g of feces from one of five human subjects investigated (Betian *et al.*, 1977). The occurrence of these normal rumen bacterial species in human fecal samples is of extreme interest and raises many questions. Of primary concern is how does an obligate anaerobe become established in the intestinal tract of a monogastric? The route of ingestion and viable passage through the digestive system are not immediately obvious.

Anaerobic spirochetes of the genus *Treponema* have been isolated from the human mouth (Socransky *et al.*, 1969) as has *Veillonella alcalescens* (Kafkewitz and Delwiche, 1969). Giesecke *et al.* (1970) have isolated *Megasphaera elsdenii* from the cecum of pigs in numbers corresponding to viable counts of 10^9 per g of cecal contents. Salanitro *et al.* (1974) isolated a number of anaerobes from the chicken cecum which were classified into the genera *Peptostreptococcus, Eubacterium, Bacteroides, Clostridium* and *Propionibacterium*. Strains from these same genera, plus *Fusobacterium* and *Lactobacillus* have also been isolated from the colon of laboratory mice (Harris *et al.*, 1976).

It would thus appear that species of bacteria previously considered to be found only in the rumen may exist in many other habitats. Application of the anaerobic techniques to more thorough investigations of the gastrointestinal tract of other animals as well as molecular techniques may prove most enlightening with regard to the ecology of the rumen population.

References

Akin, D. E. (1976). Ultrastructure of rumen bacterial attachment to forage cell walls. *Applied and Environmental Microbiology*, **31**, 562-568.

Akin, D. E. (1980). Evaluation by electron microscopy and anaerobic culture of types of rumen bacteria associated with digestion of forage cell walls. *Applied and Environmental Microbiology*, **39**, 242-252.

Akin, D. E. and H. E. Amos. (1975.) Rumen bacterial degradation of forage cell walls investigated by electron microscopy. *Applied Microbiology*, **29**, 692-701.

Baker, F. and S. T. Harriss. (1947). The role of the microflora of the alimentary tract of herbivora with special reference to ruminants. 2. Microbial digestion in the rumen (and caecum) with special reference to the decomposition of structural cellulose. *Nutrition Abstracts and Reviews*, **18**, 3-12.

Bauchop, T. and R. W. Martucci. (1968). Ruminant-like digestion of the Langur monkey. *Science*, **161**, 698-699.

Bauchop, T., R.T.J. Clarke and J. C. Newhook. (1975). Scanning electron microscope study of bacteria associated with the rumen epithelium of sheep. *Applied Microbiology*, **30**, 668-675.

Betian, H. G., B. A. Linehan, M. P. Bryant and L. V. Holdeman. (1977). Isolation of a cellulolytic *Bacteroides* sp. from human feces. *Applied and Environmental Microbiology*, **33**, 1009-1010.

Bowman, J.P.G. and J.L. Firkins. (1993). Effects of forage species and particle size on bacterial cellulolytic activity and colonization in situ. *Journal of Animal Science*, **71**, 1623-1633.

Brown, D. W. and W.E.C. Moore. (1960). Distribution of *Butyrivibrio fibrisolvens* in nature. *Journal of Dairy Science*, **43**, 1570-1574.

Bryant, M. P. (1959). Bacterial species of the rumen. *Bacteriological Reviews*, **23**, 125-153.

Bryant, M. P. and L. A. Burkey. (1953a). Cultural methods and some characteristics of some of the more numerous groups of bacteria in the bovine rumen. *Journal of Dairy Science*, **36**, 205-217.

Bryant, M. P. and L. A. Burkey. (1953b). Numbers and some predominant groups of bacteria in the rumen of cows fed different rations. *Journal of Dairy Science*, **36**, 218-224.

Bryant, M. P. and I. M. Robinson. (1961). An improved nonselective culture medium for ruminal bacteria and its use in determining diurnal variation in numbers of bacteria in the rumen. *Journal of Dairy Science*, **44**, 1446-1456.

Bryant, M. P. and I. M. Robinson. (1968). Effects of diet, time after feeding, and position sampled on numbers of viable bacteria in the bovine rumen. *Journal of Dairy Science*, **51**, 1950-1955.

Burroughs, W., P. Gerlaugh, E. A. Silver and A. F. Schalk. (1946). Methods for identifying feeds and measuring their rate of passage through the rumen of cattle. *Journal of Animal Science*, **5**, 272-278.

Caldwell, D. R. and M. P. Bryant. (1966). Medium without rumen fluid for non-selective enumeration and isolation of rumen bacteria. *Applied Microbiology*, **14**, 794-801.

Cheng, K.-J. and J. W. Costerton. (1975). Ultrastructure of cell envelopes of bacteria of the bovine rumen. *Applied Microbiology*, **29**, 841-849.

Cheng, K.-J. and R. J. Wallace. (1978). The mechanism of passage of endogenous urea through the rumen wall and the role of ureolytic epithelial bacteria in the urea flux. *British Journal of Nutrition*, **42**, 553-557.

Cheng, K.-J., D. E. Akin and J. W. Costerton. (1977). Rumen bacteria: interaction with particulate dietary components and response to dietary variation. *Federation Proceedings*, **36**, 193-197.

Cheng, K.-J., R. P. McCowan and J. W. Costerton. (1979). Adherent epithelial bacteria in ruminants and their roles in digestive tract function. *American Journal of Clinical Nutrition*, **32**, 139-148.

Craig, W. M., G. A. Broderick and D. B. Ricker. (1987). Quantitation of microorganisms associated with the particulate phase of ruminal ingesta. *Journal of Nutrition*, **117**, 56-62.

Craig, W. M., B. J. Hong, G. A. Broderick and R. J. Bula. (1984). *In vitro* inoculum enriched with particle-associated microorganisms for determining rates of fiber digestion and protein degradation. *Journal of Dairy Science*, **67**, 2902-2909.

Davies, M. E. (1964). Cellulolytic bacteria isolated from the large intestine of the horse. *Journal of Applied Bacteriology*, **27**, 373-378.

Dawson, K. A. and J. A. Boling. (1983). Monensin-resistant bacteria in the rumens of calves on monensin-containing and unmedicated diets. *Applied and Environmental Microbiology*, **46**, 160-164.

Dearth, R. N., B. A. Dehority and E. L. Potter. (1974). Rumen microbial numbers in lambs as affected by level of feed intake and dietary diethylstilbestrol. *Journal of Animal Science*, **38**, 991-996.

Dehority, B. A. (1977). Cellulolytic cocci isolated from the cecum of guinea pigs (*Cavia porcellus*). *Applied and Environmental Microbiology*, **33**, 1278-1283.

Dehority, B. A. and Jean A. Grubb. (1976). Basal medium for the selective enumeration of rumen bacteria utilizing specific energy sources. *Applied and Environmental Microbiology*, **32**, 703-710.

Dehority, B. A. and J. A. Grubb. (1980). Effect of short term chilling of rumen contents upon viable bacterial numbers. *Applied and Environmental Microbiology*, **39**, 376-381.

Dehority, B. A. and J. A. Grubb. (1981). Bacterial population adherent to the epithelium on the roof of the dorsal rumen of sheep. *Applied and Environmental Microbiology*, **41**, 1424-1427.

Dehority, B. A. and H. W. Scott. (1967). Extent of cellulose and hemicellulose digestion in various forages by pure cultures of rumen bacteria. *Journal of Dairy Science*, **50**, 1136-1141.

Dehority, B.A. and P.A. Tirabasso. (2001). Effect of feeding frequency on bacterial and fungal concentrations, pH, and other parameters in the rumen. *Journal of Animal Science*, **79**, 2908-2912.

Dehority, B. A., P. A. Tirabasso and A. P. Grifo, Jr. (1989). Most-probable-number procedures for enumerating ruminal bacteria, including the simultaneous estimation of total and cellulolytic numbers in one medium. *Applied and Environmental Microbiology*, **55**, 2789-2792.

Dinsdale, D., K.-J. Cheng, R. J. Wallace and R. A. Goodlad. (1980). Digestion of epithelial tissue of the rumen wall by adherent bacteria in infused and conventionally fed sheep. *Applied and Environmental Microbiology*, **39**, 1050-1066.

Firkins, J.L., J.P.G. Bowman, W. P. Weiss and J. Naderer. (1991). Effects of protein, carbohydrate, and fat sources on bacterial colonization and degradation of fiber in vitro. *Journal of Dairy Science,* **74**, 4273-4283.

Forbes, J. M., J. Hodgson and G. R. Lax. (1969). Measurement of rumen volume in pregnant ewes. *Journal of Animal Science*, **29**, 158.

Forsberg, C.W., T.J. Beveridge and A. Hellstrom. (1981). Cellulase and xylanase release from *Bacteroides succinogenes* and its importance in the rumen environment. *Applied and Environmental Microbiology*, **42**, 886-896.

Furchtenicht, J.E. and G.A. Broderick. (1987). Effect of inoculum preparation and dietary energy on microbial numbers and rumen protein degradation activity. *Journal of Dairy Science*, **70**, 1404-1410.

Giesecke, D., S. Wiesmayr and M. Ledinek. (1970). *Peptostreptococcus elsdenii* from the caecum of pigs. *Journal of General Microbiology*, **64**, 123-126.

Gilchrist, F.M.C. and A. Kistner. (1962). Bacteria of the ovine rumen. I. The composition of the population on a diet of poor teff hay. *Journal of Agricultural Science*, **59**, 77-83.

Gouws, L. and A. Kistner. (1965). Bacteria of the ovine rumen. IV. Effect of change of diet on the predominant type of cellulose digesting bacteria. *Journal of Agricultural Science*, **64**, 51-57.

Groleau, D. and C. W. Forsberg. (1981). Cellulolytic activity of the rumen bacterium *Bacteroides succinogenes. Canadian Journal of Microbiology*, **27**, 517-530.

Grubb, J. A. and B. A. Dehority. (1975). Effects of an abrupt change in ration from all roughage to high concentrate upon rumen microbial numbers in sheep. *Applied Microbiology*, **30**, 404-412.

Grubb, J. A. and B. A. Dehority. (1976). Variation in colony counts of total viable anaerobic rumen bacteria as influenced by media and cultural methods. *Applied and Environmental Microbiology*, **31**, 262-267.

Hall, E. R. (1952). Investigations on the microbiology of cellulose utilization in domestic rabbits. *Journal of General Microbiology*, **7**, 350-357.

Harris, M. A., C. A. Reddy and G. R. Carter. (1976). Anaerobic bacteria from the large intestine of mice. *Applied and Environmental Microbiology*, **31**, 907-912.

Hungate, R. E. (1957). Microorganisms in the rumen of cattle fed a constant ration. *Canadian Journal of Microbiology*, **3**, 289-311.

Hungate, R. E. (1966). *The Rumen and Its Microbes*. Academic Press, New York.

Johnson, R. R., B. A. Dehority and O. G. Bentley. (1958). Studies on the *in vitro* rumen procedure: improved inoculum preparation and the effects of volatile fatty acids on cellulose digestion. *Journal of Animal Science*, **17**, 841-850.

Kafkewitz, D. and E. A. Delwiche. (1969). Utilization of D-ribose by *Veillonella*. *Journal of Bacteriology*, **98**, 903-907.

Kistner, A. (1960). An improved method for viable counts of bacteria of the ovine rumen which ferment carbohydrates. *Journal of General Microbiology*, **23**, 565-576.

Kistner, A., L. Gouws and F.M.C. Gilchrist. (1962). Bacteria of the ovine rumen. II. The functional groups fermenting carbohydrates and lactate on a diet of lucerne (*Medicago sativa*) hay. *Journal of Agricultural Science*, **59**, 85-91.

Latham, M. J., B. E. Brooker, G. L. Pettipher and P. J. Harris. (1978a). *Ruminococcus flavefaciens* cell coat and adhesion to cotton cellulose and to cell walls in leaves of perennial ryegrass (*Lolium perenne*). *Applied and Environmental Microbiology*, **35**, 156-165.

Latham, M. J., B. E. Brooker, G. L. Pettipher and P. J. Harris. (1978b). Adhesion of *Bacteroides succinogenes* in pure culture and in the presence of *Ruminococcus flavefaciens* to cell walls in leaves of perennial ryegrass (*Lolium perenne*). *Applied and Environmental Microbiology*, **35**, 1166-1173.

Leedle, J.A.Z. and R. B. Hespell. (1980). Differential carbohydrate media and anaerobic replica plating techniques in delineating carbohydrate-utilizing subgroups in rumen bacterial populations. *Applied and Environmental Microbiology*, **30**, 709-719.

Leedle, J.A.Z., M. P. Bryant and R. B. Hespell. (1982). Diurnal variations in bacterial numbers and fluid parameters in ruminal contents of animals fed low- or high-forage diets. *Applied and Environmental Microbiology*, **44**, 402-412.

Lewis, S. M. and B. A. Dehority. (1985). Microbiology and ration digestibility in the hindgut of the ovine. *Applied and Environmental Microbiology*, **50**, 356-363.

Maki, L. R. and E. M. Foster. (1957). Effect of roughage in the bovine ration on types of bacteria in the rumen. *Journal of Dairy Science*, **40**, 905-913.

Mackie, R. I. and F.M.C. Gilchrist. (1979). Changes in lactate-producing and lactate-utilizing bacteria in relation to pH in the rumen of sheep during stepwise adaptation to a high-concentrate diet. *Applied and Environmental Microbiology*, **38**, 422-430.

Mackie, R. I. and S. Heath. (1979). Enumeration and isolation of lactate-utilizing bacteria from the rumen of sheep. *Applied and Environmental Microbiology*, **38**, 416-421.

McCowan, R. P., K.-J. Cheng and J. W. Costerton. (1980). Adherent bacterial populations on the bovine rumen wall: distribution patterns of adherent bacteria. *Applied and Environmental Microbiology*, **39**, 233-241.

McCowan, R. P., K.-J. Cheng, C.B.M. Bailey and J. W. Costerton. (1978). Adhesion of bacteria to epithelial cell surfaces within the reticulo-rumen of cattle. *Applied and Environmental Microbiology*, **35**, 149-155.

Mead, L. J. and G. A. Jones. (1981). Isolation and presumptive identification of adherent epithelial bacteria ("epimural" bacteria) from the ovine rumen wall. *Applied and Environmental Microbiology*, **41**, 1020-1028.

Minato, H., A. Endo, M. Higuchi, Y. Ootomo and T. Uemura. (1966). Ecological treatise on the rumen fermentation. I. The fractionation of bacteria attached to the rumen digesta solids. *Journal of General Applied Microbiology*, **12**, 39-52.

Moir, R. J. and M. Somers. (1957). Ruminal flora studies. VIII. The influence of rate and method of feeding a ration upon its digestibility, upon ruminal function, and upon the ruminal population. *Australian Journal of Agricultural Research*, **8**, 253-265.

Mueller, R. E., E. L. Iannotti and J. M. Asplund. (1984). Isolation and identification of adherent epimural bacteria during succession in young lambs. *Applied and Environmental Microbiology*, **47**, 724-730.

Munch-Petersen, E. and C.A.P. Boundy. (1963). Bacterial content in samples from different sites in the rumen of sheep and cows as determined in two culture media. *Applied Microbiology*, **11**, 190-195.

Nagaraja, T. G. and M. B. Taylor. (1987). Susceptibility and resistance of ruminal bacteria to antimicrobial feed additives. *Applied and Environmental Microbiology*, **53**, 1620-1625.

Nottingham, P. M. and R. E. Hungate. (1968). Isolation of methanogenic bacteria from feces of man. *Journal of Bacteriology*, **96**, 2178-2179.

Olumeyan, D. B., T. G. Nagaraja, G. W. Miller, R. A. Frey and J. E. Boyer. (1986). Rumen microbial changes in cattle fed diets with or without salinomycin. *Applied and Environmental Microbiology*, **51**, 340-345.

Puch, H. C. (1977). M.S. Thesis. Ohio State University, Columbus, OH.

Rieu, F., G. Fonty, B. Gaillard and P. Gouet. (1990). Electron microscopy study of the bacteria adherent to the rumen wall in young conventional lambs. *Canadian Journal of Microbiology*, **36**, 140-144.

Roxas, D. B. (1980). Effects of abrupt changes in the ration on rumen microflora of sheep. Ph.D. Dissertation, Ohio State University, Columbus.

Salanitro, J. P., I. G. Fairchilds and Y. D. Zgornicki. (1974). Isolation, culture characteristics, and identification of anaerobic bacteria from the chicken cecum. *Applied Microbiology*, **27**, 678-687.

Socransky, S. S., M. Listgarten, C. Hubersak, J. Catmore and A. Clark. (1969). Morphological and biochemical differentiation of three types of small oral spirochetes. *Journal of Bacteriology*, **98**, 878-882.

Thorley, C. M., M. E. Sharpe and M. P. Bryant. (1968). Modification of the rumen bacterial flora by feeding cattle ground and pelleted roughage as determined with culture media with and without rumen fluid. *Journal of Dairy Science*, **51**, 1811-1816.

Van der Linden, Y., N. O. Van Gylswyk and H. M. Schwartz. (1984). Influence of supplementation of corn stover with corn grain on the fibrolytic bacteria in the rumen of sheep and their relation to the intake and digestion of fiber. *Journal of Animal Science*, **59**, 772-783.

Varel, V. H. and B. A. Dehority. (1989). Ruminal cellulolytic bacteria and protozoa from bison, cattle-bison hybrids, and cattle fed three alfalfa-corn diets. *Applied and Environmental Microbiology*, **55**, 148-153.

Wallace, R. J., K.-J. Cheng, D. Dinsdale and E. R. Ørskov. (1979). An independent microbial flora of the epithelium and its role in the ecomicrobiology of the rumen. *Nature*, **279**, 424-426.

Warner, A.C.I. (1962a). Enumeration of rumen microorganisms. *Journal of General Microbiology*, **28**, 119-128.

Warner, A.C.I. (1962b). Some factors influencing the rumen microbial-population. *Journal of General Microbiology*, **28**, 129-146.

Warner, A.C.I. (1966a). Diurnal changes in the concentrations of microorganisms in the rumen of sheep fed limited diets once daily. *Journal of General Microbiology*, **45**, 213-235.

Warner, A.C.I. (1966b). Periodic changes in the concentrations of microorganisms in the rumen of a sheep fed a limited ration every three hours. *Journal of General Microbiology*, **45**, 237-241.

Warner, A.C.I. (1966c). Diurnal changes in the concentrations of microorganisms in the rumen of sheep fed to appetite in pens or at pasture. *Journal of General Microbiology*, **45**, 243-251.

Whitelaw, F. G., J. M. Eadie, S. O. Mann and R. S. Reid. (1972). Some effects of rumen ciliate protozoa in cattle given restricted amounts of a barley diet. *British Journal of Nutrition*, **27**, 425-437.

Wilson, M. K. and C.A.E. Briggs. (1955). The normal flora of the bovine rumen. II. Quantitative bacteriological studies. *Journal of Applied Bacteriology*, **18**, 294-306.

CHAPTER 13

RUMEN FUNGI

In his studies on diurnal changes in the concentrations of rumen microorganisms in sheep fed once daily, Warner (1966) observed that the flagellate protozoa *Neocallimastix frontalis* increased in numbers dramatically after feeding. Population density then decreased rapidly reaching a low point about 10 h after feeding and remained low until the next feeding. To accomplish such marked concentration changes, at least 2-5 divisions of *Neocallimastix* would have to occur within 1 h after feeding, followed by rapid death and lysis. This did not seem likely to Warner who suggested that the flagellates probably sequestered on the rumen wall, returning to the rumen contents by a chemotactic response to feeding and then migrating back to the wall in response to another chemical stimulus. Orpin (1974) investigated this same question and found that the maximum population density of *Neocallimastix frontalis* occurred within 15 to 30 min after feeding. The average increase in population density was 47-fold over 40 experiments. He did not observe any flagellates in washings of the rumen wall or in rumen fluid immediately adjacent to the wall. Population density could be increased *in vivo* by adding an extract of oats to the rumen of sheep which had not been fed for 24 h. He subsequently observed that addition of the oats extract to strained rumen fluid would also increase the concentration of *Neocallimastix* 44-fold within 20 min. Using centrifugation techniques he determined that *Neocallimastix* was associated with the larger feed particles and suggested that the organism sequestered there or that its life cycle involved a multiple reproduction phase which was associated with the large particle fraction of rumen fluid.

In subsequent studies, Orpin (1975) found that the rapid increase in *Neocallimastix* shortly after feeding resulted from stimulation of a reproductive body, on a vegetative phase of the organism, to differentiate and liberate the flagellates. The stimulant was a component of the hosts diet. The flagellates liberated *in vivo* lost motility within an hour and developed into the vegetative phase, thus explaining the rapid decrease in concentration. The author also noted that the vegetative stage was morphologically similar to certain species of aquatic phycomycete fungi. Investigation of the other rumen flagellates revealed that two additional organisms, *Sphaeromonas communis* and *Piromonas communis*, also had similar life cycles and their vegetative stages resembled phycomycete fungi (Orpin, 1976; 1977b). For all organisms, maximum flagellate production occurred at pH 6.5, 39°C, and in the presence of CO_2 and absence of O_2, which are normal rumen conditions.

Since fungi are the only non-photosynthetic microorganisms which contain chitin or cellulose in their vegetative cell walls, Orpin (1977c) analyzed cultures of the three rumen organisms, *N. frontalis, S. communis* and *P. communis*, for these compounds. He found that the vegetative cell walls of all three organisms contained chitin, confirming that they are true fungi despite their ability to grow under low redox potential and in the absence of O_2. The flagellates released from the vegetative stage (sporangia) would thus be correctly called zoospores. The zoospores of these fungi appear to show taxis towards plant tissues surrounding the flowers and seeds (inflorescence tissue), germinating on this tissue with the rhizoids of the developing vegetative stage penetrating into the plant (Orpin, 1977a, 1977b). It is suggested that the zoospores chemotactically respond to materials diffusing from these particular tissues. It was further noted that although the zoospores preferentially invade these tissues, the presence of these tissues is not essential to maintenance of the fungi in the rumen. A diet of grass harvested before flowering maintained 90% of the population density observed with a diet high in inflorescence tissue.

Using scanning electron microscopy, Bauchop (1979) found that large numbers of the phycomycetous fungal zoospores rapidly attached to fibrous plant fragments in the rumen, particularly vascular tissues, and their flagella apparently separate soon after attachment. The small zoospores (6 to 10 μm) then develop with the production of thalli with extensive rhizoids and sporangia up to 175 μm long. Counts of 10^5 sporangial early developmental forms per cm^2 were observed on the surface of the stem vascular cylinder. Based on his observations Bauchop (1979) suggested that the rumen anaerobic fungi may play a significant role in fiber digestion in the rumen.

Classification

Five genera of fungi have been described from rumen contents, they are *Neocallimastix, Caecomyces* (formerly *Sphaeromonas*), *Piromyces* (formerly *Piromonas*), *Orpinomyces* and *Anaeromyces* (synonymous with *Ruminomyces*) (Orpin, 1977c; Heath *et al.*, 1983; Barr, 1988; Gold *et al.*, 1988; Barr *et al.*, 1989; Ho *et al.*, 1990). They are all classified as anaerobic fungi in the class Chytridiomycetes, order Neocallimasticales family Neocallimasticaceae (Heath *et al.*, 1983; Barr, 1988; Li *et al.*, 1993). Four species of fungi have been described and classified in the genus *Neocallimastix*: *N. frontalis* (Heath *et al.*, 1983), *N. patriciarum* (Orpin and Munn, 1986), *N.hurleyensis* (Webb and Theodorou, 1991), and *N. variablis* (Ho *et al.*, 1993a). The genus *Caecomyces* contains two species: *C. communis* and *C. equi* (Orpin, 1976; Gold *et al.*, 1988). A number of *Piromyces* species have been found, seven in all, from a rather diverse group of herbivores, i.e., *P. communis* from sheep rumen (Barr *et al.*, 1989); *P. mae* and *P. citronii* from the horse caecum (Li *et al.*, 1990, Gaillard-Martinie *et al.*, 1995); *P. dumbonica* from the caecum of the elephant (Li *et al.*, 1990); *P. minutus* from deer (Ho *et al.*, 1993b); *P. spiralis* from goat (Ho *et al.*, 1993c); and *P. rhizinflata* from ass (Breton *et al.*, 1991). The remaining two genera are represented by the species *Orpinomyces bovis* (Barr *et al.*, 1989), *O. joyonii* (Breton *et al.*, 1989),

O. intercalaris (Ho, Abdullah and Jalaludin, 1994); *Anaeromyces elegans* (Ho *et al.*, 1990) and *A. mucronatus* (Breton *et al.*, 1990). In 1995, Ho and Barr classified the anaerobic gut fungi based on thallus morphology as observed with the light microscope. Their purpose was to allow functional identification of genera and species. Their classification is shown in Table 13.1. As can be seen, they have proposed that several of the previously described species be classified as synonymous. A more definitive classification should be forthcoming as 18S rRNA sequences are determined for the anaerobic fungi isolated from the gastrointestinal tract of herbivores.

Table 13.1 CLASSIFICATION OF ANAEROBIC FUNGI FROM THE GUT OF HERBIVORES

		Genera/species		
Neocallimastix	Orpinomyces	Anaeromyces	Piromyces[a]	Caecomyces[b]
N. frontalis[c]	*O. joyonii*[d]	*A. mucronatus*	*P. communis*	*C. equi*
N. hurleyensis	*O. intercalaris*	*A. elegans*[e]	*P. mae*	*C. communis*
			P. dumbonicus	
			P. rhizinflatus	
			P. minutus	
			P. spiralis	
			P. citronii	

[a] Formerly *Piromonas*.
[b] Formerly *Sphaeromonas*.
[c] *N. patriciarum* and *N. variabilis* have been classified as synonymous species.
[d] Originally described as *Neocallimastix joyonii*. *O. bovis* is considered synonymous.
[e] Synonomous with *Ruminomyces elegans*.

Characteristics for representative species of these five different genera are listed in Table 13.2. Additional fungal species have been isolated from various hosts, which differ from the those species listed above (Orpin and Joblin, 1998). However, they have not been studied in sufficient detail to allow their description as new species.

Three thallus types occur: endogenous (monocentric), endogenous and exogenous (monocentric) and exogenous (polycentric) (Barr *et al.*, 1989; Gaillard *et al.*, 1989; Ho *et al.*, 1990; Li *et al.*, 1991; Munn *et al.*, 1988). The endogenous species are all monocentric, in that the zoospore cyst retains the nucleus and only a single sporangium develops. The rhizoids are anucleate. Exogenous species may be monocentric or polycentric. The nucleus escapes from the zoospore cyst and the sporangium develops elsewhere in the monocentric type. In the polycentric type, the nucleus escapes but undergoes division and the rhizomycelium is nucleated. Multiple sporangia form on the rhizomycelium.

Table 13.2. CHARACTERISTICS OF THE CHYTRIDOMYCETOUS RUMEN FUNGI

Genus species	Thallus type	Zoospore size (µm)	No. of flagella per zoospore	References[a]
Neocallimastix				
N. frontalis	Monocentric	20.6 x 8.7	7 - 10	1
N. hurleyensis	"	9.6 x 10.7	8 - 16	2
Caecomyces				
C. communis	Monocentric or Polycentric	8 x 10	1	3
C. equi	" "	5 x 7	1	4
Piromyces				
P. communis	Monocentric	7 x 14	1	5
Orpinomyces				
O. joyonii	Polycentric	9 - 15[c]	10 - 25	6, 7, 9
Anaeromyces				
A. elegans[b]	Polycentric	6.5 - 9.0[c]	1	8

[a]References: (1) Orpin, 1975; (2) Webb and Theodorou, 1991; (3) Orpin, 1976; (4) Gold *et al.*, 1988; (5) Orpin 1977b; (6) Barr *et al.*, 1989; (7) Li *et al.*, 1991; (8) Ho *et al.*, 1990; (9) Breton *et al.*, 1989.
[b]May be the same organism as *Anaeromyces mucronatus* (Breton *et al.*, 1990).
[c]Spherical.

Life cycle

The anaerobic fungi have a life cycle which encompasses a motile form (zoospore) and a non-motile vegetative form (thallus). This life cycle is shown diagrammatically in Figure 13.1. The free zoospore is attracted to plant fragments by chemotaxis toward soluble carbohydrates (Orpin and Bountiff, 1978). The zoospore attaches to the plant fragment, which is followed by encystment and then germination. A main rhizoid forms at germination followed by growth of the rhizoid system and development of a single sporangium in the monocentric type or multiple sporangia in the polycentric type. The entire organism (zoospore, rhizoids and sporangium) constitute the thallus. The sporangium enlarges, nuclear division takes place and the zoospores mature. The sporangium ruptures, zoospores are released and the entire cycle begins again. The entire life cycle lasts anywhere from about 8 to 32 h depending upon conditions (Orpin and Joblin, 1988). Zoosporogenesis is induced by a number of labile plant components, with haem-containing compounds being fairly effective *in vitro* (Orpin, 1977d, 1978b).

Rumen fungi 299

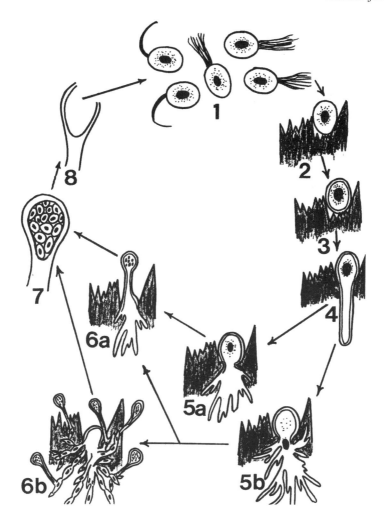

Figure 13.1. Life cycles of anaerobic rumen fungi:

1. Zoospores (both monoflagellate and polyflagellate types are shown).
2. Chemotactic migration to plant particle and attachment.
3. Encystment.
4. Germination.
5. Rhizoid development.
   a. Endogenous, monocentric type.
   b. Exogenous, where nucleus migrates from cyst, monocentric or polycentric type.
6. Sporangium development.
   a. Single sporangium develops in monocentric type.
   b. Polycentric; division and migration of nucleus through rhizomycelium; multiple sporangia develop.
7. Zoospore maturation.
8. Release of zoospores.

Isolation and enumeration

Joblin (1981) published a procedure for the isolation and enumeration of rumen anaerobic fungi. Essentially he used the anaerobic roll tube method of Hungate, including the antibiotics penicillin and streptomycin in his medium. He obtained counts of 2×10^4 viable zoospores per ml of strained rumen fluid which corresponds to the densities of 10^4 to 10^5/ml as determined by direct microscopic count. One point of interest was that when antibiotics were omitted from the medium, fungi were not detected in roll tubes inoculated with rumen fluid.

An endpoint dilution procedure for rumen fungi, based on MPN techniques, was developed by Theodorou et al. (1990). Wheat straw was used as the only substrate. Rumen contents were diluted in basal medium with penicillin and streptomycin but without an energy source. Positive tubes were recorded when zoospores were observed by viewing under an inverted microscope, with eventual appearance of rhizoids and zoosporangia. Thallus forming units (TFU) were reported per gram of sample dry matter. The procedure was not compared to any other enumerative procedures.

Obispo and Dehority (1992) independently developed a MPN procedure for rumen fungi along the lines of the MPN procedure proposed by Dehority et al. (1989) for simultaneous estimation of total and cellulolytic rumen bacterial concentrations. Adding penicillin and streptomycin permitted the growth of fungi, but not bacteria. Tubes were scored on the basis of visible loss of purified, ball-milled cellulose and decrease in pH. Total fungal concentrations ranged from 1.5×10^3 to 1.5×10^6 per g of rumen contents. These concentrations are somewhat higher than reported in previous studies (Orpin, 1974; Joblin, 1981; Ushida et al., 1989; and Theodorou et al., 1990). However, most of these authors used rumen fluid as an inoculum, compared to rumen ingesta in the study by Obispo and Dehority. Cellulolytic fungal concentrations ranged from 4.5 to 8.5×10^3 per gram of rumen contents. The MPN procedure was verified by comparison with the roll tube procedure of Joblin (1981). Similar fungal concentrations were obtained by both methods; however, less than 10% of the total colonies in the roll tubes were fungi. Roll tube counts had to be made with a microscope and were quite time consuming. Adding chloramphenicol or oxytetracycline to the roll tube medium, along with penicillin and streptompycin, completely inhibited bacterial growth; however, fungal numbers were also reduced. The fungi in rumen contents were primarily associated with the particulate fraction, constituting 86.0, 77.2 and 69.0% of the total fungi at 0, 1.5 and 3.0 h after feeding (Figure 13.2). Fungal concentrations were observed to increase after feeding and most of the increase (78%) was associated with the particulate fraction. Concentrations of rumen fungi in sheep decreased as concentrates were included in the diet, which agrees with the more recent data of Kostyukovsky et al. (1991) obtained from zoospore counts in cattle. Frequency of feeding had no consistent effect on diurnal concentration changes with time after feeding (Obispo and Dehority, 1992). In a more recent study, Dehority and Tirabasso (2001) found no differences in fungal concentrations in sheep fed either once, six or twenty four times daily.

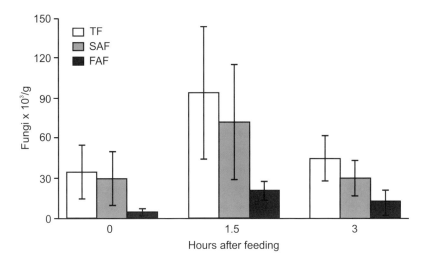

Figure 13. 2 Distribution of rumen fungi between liquid and solid fractions of rumen contents. TF = total fungi; SAF = solids associated fungi; FAF = fluid associated fungi. (from Obispo and Dehority, 1992).

Nutrition

Nutritional and germination requirements of *Neocallimastix patriciarum* were studied by Orpin and Greenwood (1986). In a minimal medium containing minerals, $(NH_4)_2SO_4$, and cellobiose under a CO_2 atmosphere, *N. patriciarum* had an absolute requirement for haemin, thiamin, biotin and a reduced source of sulfur. Growth was markedly improved by the addition of amino acids, acetic acid, isobutyric acid, 2-methylbutyric acid, low concentrations of long-chain fatty acids (C_{14} to C_{18}), nicotinic acid, nicotinamide, cyanocobalamin, riboflavin, inositol, pyridoxine hydrochloride, pyridoxal phosphate and pyridoxamine. Germination of zoospores suspended in an anaerobic salts solution was stimulated by soluble sugars (glucose, galactose, fructose, sucrose, cellobiose and maltose), increasing as the carbohydrate concentration increased from 0.1 to 1 molar. Acetic acid was the only additional nutrient found which stimulated germination in the presence of soluble carbohydrates. Optimum conditions for germination were pH values between 5.5 - 6.4 and temperatures between 38 - 40°C.

Lowe *et al*. (1985) isolated several anaerobic fungi using a plate culture technique. One isolate, studied in some detail, was first grown on a complete medium minus rumen fluid and subsequently on a defined medium from which Trypticase peptone and yeast extract were omitted. Most of the studies on fungal isolates, to determine biochemical activities and growth characteristics, have used the semi-defined medium (medium B) described by Lowe *et al*. (1985). Workers in Australia used medium 10 previously developed by Caldwell and Bryant (1966) for enumeration of rumen bacteria (Phillips and Gordon, 1988, 1989). Essentially these media differ only in that medium B contains trace minerals and coenzyme M. These two media, or slight modifications of them, have been used in most studies where the fungi are cultured without rumen fluid in the medium.

Reviews of the nutrition and biochemistry of anaerobic Chytridiomycetes have been published by Orpin (1988) and Theodorou et al. (1988). Most information is based on studies with *Neocallimastix* sp. grown *in vitro*.

Fermentation

Since the anaerobic fungi can degrade cellulose, as well as starch, xylan and other hemicelluloses (Orpin and Letcher, 1979), their possible role in rumen fiber digestion becomes an important question. Obviously their contribution would be very dependent upon the rate at which they can degrade these structural polysaccharides. The studies by Orpin and Letcher (1979) indicated that *N. frontalis* did not degrade cellulose until the glucose in the culture media had been utilized and concluded that *in vivo* the organism was likely to preferentially utilize soluble carbohydrates. Mountfort and Asher (1983) studied the utilization of soluble sugars by *N. frontalis* and also tested pairs of sugars to determine whether they were used simultaneously or sequentially. Glucose was the preferred substrate when compared with fructose and xylose. Cellobiose and sucrose were preferentially utilized compared with fructose and glucose; however, fructose and maltose appeared to be used simultaneously. When glucose was added in the middle of fructose or xylose fermentations, it was preferentially utilized, suggesting catabolite regulation, i.e., the synthesis of enzyme(s) for the utilization of one substrate is controlled by the presence of another substrate. Morrison et al. (1990) found that cellulolysis by a *Piromyces*-like sp. was catabolite regulated by glucose, cellobiose and soluble starch.

Lowe et al. (1987a) determined growth of a *Neocallimastix* sp. on a variety of carbon sources and found that growth occurred on inulin, pullulan, starch and xylan but not on carboxymethyl cellulose or pectin. The organism also grew on the trisaccharide raffinose and the disaccharides cellobiose, lactose (poorly), maltose and sucrose. Of eight monosaccharides tested, growth occurred on fructose, glucose and xylose but not on arabinose, galactose, mannose, rhamnose or ribose.

In studies from New Zealand (Mountfort and Asher, 1985, 1988, 1989; Pearce and Bauchop, 1985), cellulose, CMC, starch and xylan were hydrolyzed by cell-free culture supernatants of *N. frontalis*. The intracellular fraction (supernatant after homogenization of cellular material) was inactive, while the insoluble or membrane fraction had lesser amounts of the same activities occurring in the extracellular or cell-free culture supernatant. Polygalacturonic acid was not hydrolyzed by any of these fractions. Evidence also indicated that glucose and other soluble sugars were not as effective as cellulose as inducers of CMCase production.

Williams and Orpin (1987a, b) surveyed polysaccharide degrading and glycoside hydrolase enzymes from *Neocallimastix patriciarum, Piromyces communis* and an unidentified fungal isolate. From their studies they were able to conclude that a wide range of polysaccharide-degrading enzymes are produced by the rumen fungi, very similar to the profiles previously observed in rumen bacteria and protozoa. Enzyme activities were found in supernatants of sonicated vegetative material and zoospores as well as cell-free culture supernatants. The fungi were also found to contain a very broad spectrum of glycoside hydrolase activity to further utilize the products of the polysaccharide depolymerases. Enzyme activity was again present in the vegetative stage, cell-free culture supernatant and zoospores. These results were confirmed in a subsequent study by Hébraud and Fèvre (1988). They measured polysaccharidase and glycosidase activities in *N. frontalis, P. communis* and *C. communis* and found a wide range of activities, with most of the activity occurring extracellularly.

Using a *Neocallimastix* sp. isolate, Lowe *et al.* (1987b) found that xylanase activity was constitutive and was mainly associated with the cellular fraction. Borneman *et al.* (1991) have reported a p-coumaroyl esterase in *Neocallimastix*, which apparently acts to free carbohydrates which are ester linked to phenolics in the forage and are otherwise not available.

Wallace and Joblin (1985) observed extracellular proteolytic activity in cultures of *Neocallimastix frontalis*. The level of activity was low compared to aerobic fungi, but comparable to that of the most active proteolytic rumen bacteria. When Michel *et al.* (1993) surveyed seven strains of anaerobic rumen fungi for proteolytic activity (2 strains of *Neocallimastix frontalis* and an undetermined sp.; 2 strains of *Piromyces* sp.; 2 unknown strains; and 1 strain of *Caecomyces* sp.)., only one strain, belonging to the genus *Piromyces*, was able to degrade ^{14}C-labelled casein. The activity for this strain was extracellular, occurring both in the culture supernatant and bound to the mycelium; however, specific activity was 8-fold lower than previously observed by Wallace and Joblin (1985) for *N. frontalis*. All strains exhibited aminopeptidase activity; two had an endopeptidase activity; and none demonstrated any carboxypeptidase activity. The authors concluded that their data was contrary to the commonly accepted idea that the rumen fungi make a large contribution to *in vivo* rumen proteolysis. In reality, the ability to degrade proteins was limited to only a few strains, and was relatively weak when it did occur.

Early studies indicated that the rumen anaerobic fungi were unable to utilize galacturonic acid, polygalacturonic acid or pectin as an energy source, and no pectin depolymerase activity could be detected in cultures (Orpin and Letcher, 1979; Pearce and Bauchop, 1985; Williams and Orpin, 1987a; Phillips and Gordon, 1988). However, Gordon and Phillips (1992) have recently obtained evidence to indicate that *Neocallimastix* sp. LM1, produces an endopectin lyase. No endopolygalacturonate lyase activity could be detected. The authors suggest that the fungi might aid in the penetration of the pectin-containing middle lamella, located between plant cells.

Digestion of forages

Data on digestion of dry matter and several structural polysaccharides from intact forages by rumen fungi are shown in Table 13.3. Digestion of pectin is probably the result of pectin depolymerization and subsequent hydrolysis and utilization of neutral sugar side chains from the pectin backbone (Williams and Orpin, 1987b). Dry matter disappearance from barley straw stems was 37% and 42% for two strains of *N. frontalis* and 43% and 50% for two strains of *P. communis* (Joblin *et al.*, 1989). Thus, strain differences do occur among the fungi as well as rumen bacteria (Dehority and Scott, 1967).

Table 13.3 DIGESTION OF DRY MATTER AND STRUCTURAL POLYSACCHARIDES FROM FORAGES BY PURE CULTURES OF RUMEN FUNGI

Component digested	Fungal species		
	Neocallimastix frontalis	*Piromyces communis*	*Caecomyces communis*
	Wheat straw leaves[a]		
Dry matter, %	45.2	42.3	30.1
Cellulose, %	58.1	50.4	39.4
Hemicellulose, %	52.3	55.0	39.6
Pectin, %	20.5	47.3	16.3
	Perennial rye-grass[b]		
Dry matter, %	42	45	31
	Mixed hay[b]		
Dry matter, %	32	34	29
	Wheat straw[c]		
Cellulose, %	55.2	53.4	38.4

[a] Data from Orpin (1983/1984).
[b] Data from Orpin and Hart (1980).
[c] Data from Gordon and Phillips (1989).

Theodorou *et al.* (1989) found that 30-35% of dry matter from Italian ryegrass was digested in 72 h by *Neocallimastix,* which increased to approximately 53% by 120 h. Dry matter digestion was almost entirely the result of decreases in the concentration of the four major cell wall sugars (arabinose, galactose, glucose and xylose), which are the principal constituents of the structural polysaccharides cellulose and hemicellulose. The sugars appeared to be removed from the cell walls at similar rates; however, the extent of removal or digestion varied, i.e., arabinose (84.1%), galactose (76.2%), glucose (75.0%) and xylose (65.8%).

Digestion of grains

Barley, corn, and wheat kernels, ground to pass through a 2-mm screen but retained on a 0.85-mm screen, were used as the sole substrate for *in vitro* fermentations with three species of anaerobic rumen fungi: *O. joyonii, N. patriciarum* and *P. communis* (McAllister *et al.*, 1993). All three species were able to digest 40-50% of the starch from corn; however, only *O. joyonii* was able to digest more than 20% of the starch from the other two grains (approximately 35% from barley and 45% from wheat). Extent of digestion was reflected in medium pH and gas production. For all grains, maximum digestion generally occurred between 96 and 120 h. The concentration of ammonia decreased in cultures which utilized appreciable starch, suggesting that all three strains assimilate ammonia.

Electron microscopy revealed that digestion of the grains varied both between the three grain types and three fungal strains. Rhizoids from all of the strains penetrated the protein matrix of corn, but not the starch granules. Extracellular amylases appeared to degrade the starch granule as evidenced by pitting. Penetration of the protein matrix in wheat and barley by rhizoids of *N. patriciarum* and *P. communis* was extremely slow and limited as compared to *O. joyonii* and subsequent digestion of starch granules was very low for these two strains. The authors concluded that the ability of rumen fungi to digest cereal grains is a function both of the type of grain and species of fungi. Whether strain differences might also occur in the rumen fungal species also needs to be investigated.

SYNERGISM

Bauchop and Mountfort (1981) studied the fermentation of cellulose by *Neocallimastix frontalis* alone and in combination with rumen methanogens. After 100 h, less than 10% of the cellulose had been degraded in the fungus fermentation versus more than 70% in the coculture. At the end of fermentation these values were 82% cellulose degradation in the coculture (200 h) and 53% in the monoculture (300 h). For both fermentations, pH decreased from an initial value of 6.9 to 6.0. Fermentation products of cellulose degradation by the fungus alone were acetate, lactate, formate, ethanol, CO_2 and H_2. The cocultures produced acetate, CO_2 and CH_4, plus lesser amounts of ethanol and lactate. The authors suggested that the increased cellulose degradation in the cocultures, primarily occurring between 50 and 100 h, might be explained by higher energy yields resulting from a shift in fungal metabolic pathways favoring the production of acetate and methane via H_2 at the expense of the electron-sink products such as lactate and ethanol or simply removal of inhibitory fungal fermentation products by the methanogens. These results were subsequently repeated with a triculture of *Methanobrevibacter* sp., *Methanosarcina barkeri* and *N. frontalis* (Mountfort *et al.*, 1982). As found previously, end-products shifted from H_2, ethanol and lactate to increased methane and acetate. Similar observations on end-product shifts have now been made with isolates of *N. frontalis, P. communis* and *C. communis* in coculture with methanogens (Fonty *et al.*, 1988; Joblin *et al.*, 1989). Cellulose digestion and solubilization of dry matter were also increased by coculture.

Joblin and Williams (1991) cocultured *Methanobrevibacter smithii* with either *P. communis* or *N. frontalis* on alfalfa stems. Both fungi removed pentoses and hexoses simultaneously either in monoculture or coculture with *M. smithii*. Percent dry matter (DM) digestion by *N. frontalis* in monoculture and coculture with *M. smithii*, was 7.8 and 18.2 after 65 h and 31.2 and 30.4 after 233 h, respectively. For *P. communis*, DM digestion was 4.8 and 15% after 65 h and 35.4 and 36.4% after 233 h, respectively. Only rate of digestion appears to have been affected, probably because of a decrease in catabolite repression in the cocultures. In all fermentations, more arabinose was removed from the alfalfa stems (68-80%) than glucose (52-70%) or xylose (25-42%). The specific activity of extracellular hydrolytic enzymes increased 2-10 fold in the cocultures. The increased level of cell wall degrading enzymes in coculture was not reflected by an increase in fungal degradation of alfalfa stems.

The rate and extent of xylan utilization were both increased when *N. frontalis* was cocultured with *Methanobrevibacter smithii* (Joblin *et al.*, 1990). As observed in previous studies, coculture resulted in interspecies hydrogen transfer with an increase in the production of methane and acetic acid and a decrease in formic acid, lactic acid and ethanol. The authors concluded that the stimulation or increased enzyme activities observed when fungi are cocultured with methanogenic bacteria primarily occurs with the polysaccharidases and glycohydrolases. They speculated that the adverse effect of fungal end-products are less in cocultures and the fungi are better able to utilize the sugars produced, which lowers the extent of catabolite repression on enzyme formation.

Marvin-Sikkema *et al.* (1990) cocultured *Neocallimastix* with several methanogens and *S. ruminantium*, a rumen bacterium capable of utilizing H_2. Cellulose hydrolysis increased for all cocultures. It was not determined whether the increase from coculture with *S. ruminantium* resulted from lowered concentrations of H_2 or use of free sugars by *S. ruminantium* which may have inhibited cellulolysis by the fungi in monoculture. Similar increases in the digestion of filter paper had been observed by Richardson *et al.* (1986) when *N. frontalis* was cocultured with *V. alcalescens* and *M. elsdenii*, both of which ferment lactate.

Negative effects between fungi and bacteria

The fungus *Neocallimastix* digested more purified cellulose alone than *F. succinogenes* or *R. flavefaciens* (Bernalier *et al.*, 1988). Cellulose digestion was reduced by combining *R. flavefaciens* with *Neocallimastix* while essentially no difference was found when *F. succinogenes* and the fungus were combined. Addition of *S. ruminantium* to *Neocallimastix* appeared to increase the rate but not extent of purified cellulose digestion.

Richardson *et al.* (1986) obtained similar results in synergism studies on straw digestion. Digestion was increased by coculture of *N. frontalis* PK2 with *F. succinogenes* and decreased with either *R. flavefaciens* or *R. albus*. Digestion was reduced in all cocultures with *N. frontalis* RK21.

Degradation and utilization of purified xylan was measured with *N. frontalis* in monoculture and in coculture with several species of fibrolytic and saccharolytic rumen bacteria (Williams *et al.*, 1991). A synergistic increase in xylan utilization occurred with *N. frontalis* plus *Prevotella ruminicola, Succinivibrio dextrinosolvens,* and *Selenomonas ruminantium. Lachnospira multiparus* and *Streptococcus bovis* cocultures resulted in a marked decrease in utilization. Both the increases and decreases in xylan utilization appeared to be related to the final concentration of reducing sugars in the media, which agreed with the theory of catabolite repression by monosaccharides upon fungal polysaccharidases and glycohydrolysases (Joblin *et al.*, 1990).

Several investigators have observed a decrease in purified cellulose digestion or dry matter digestion from forages when ruminococci are cocultured with fungi. Bernalier *et al.* (1992) observed that cocultures of *N. frontalis* or *P. communis* with *R. flavefaciens* digested less purified cellulose than the fungi alone but more than *R. flavefaciens* in monoculture. Coculture with *F. succinogenes* was similar to the fungus alone, but higher than the bacterium alone. In contrast, cellulose digestion by *C. communis* plus *R. flavefaciens* was greater than either organism alone. The *C. communis - F. succinogenes* coculture was similar to *F. succinogenes* in monoculture and greater than the fungus alone.

Stewart *et al.* (1992) observed an inhibition of cellulolysis by adding the cell-free supernatant from cultures of *R. albus* or *R. flavefaciens* to *N. frontalis* fermentations. However, growth of the fungus on glucose was not affected by addition of the supernatants. The factor was destroyed by autoclaving and after concentration and partial purification, appeared to consist of several polypeptides. In a separate study, Bernalier *et al.* (1993) found that the antagonistic effect of *R. flavefaciens* upon cellulose digestion by *N. frontalis* was an extracellular factor produced and released into the culture supernatant by *R. flavefaciens*. The factor was destroyed by heating above 60°C and found to be protein in nature. The factor appeared to inhibit fungal cellulase, but had no cellulase activity itself. The two studies would certainly appear to substantiate each other.

The effect of normal fermentation end products upon fungal cellulolysis was studied by Joblin and Naylor (1993). Hydrogen, formate, lactate, ethanol, acetate and malate inhibited cellulose digestion; succinate was variable, from slightly stimulatory to inhibitory; and propionate and butyrate were without much effect. Inhibition was minimal at low concentrations, 30%, increasing to 50% at high concentrations. The authors concluded that removal of inhibition by formate, lactate, ethanol and H_2 probably accounts for the increased cellulolysis by coculture with the methanogens. However, they thought it unlikely that the inhibition observed with *R. flavefaciens* was the result of bacterial fermentation products.

The effects of coculturing either *R. flavefaciens* or *F. succinogenes* with *N. frontalis* or *O. joyonii* on wheat straw or maize stem was studied by Roger *et al.* (1993). Both fungi digested similar amounts of dry matter (DM) from the two plants (about 39% from wheat straw and 59% from maize stems). With wheat straw, combining *N. frontalis* with *R. flavefaciens* significantly decreased DM digestion from that of the fungus alone and similar to *R. flavefaciens* alone. The combination of *O. joyonii* and *R. flavefaciens* was the same as *O. joyonii* in monoculture and no inhibition occurred when either fungus was combined with *F. succinogenes*. Results with maize stem as the substrate were slightly different. Combination of *R. flavefaciens* with either fungi resulted in an inhibition of DM digestion which was significantly lower than any of the organisms in monoculture. As before, cocultures with *F. succinogenes* were not inhibited.

Role of the rumen fungi

Using the warm-season forage *Digitaria pentzii* as a substrate for *in vitro* studies, Akin *et al.* (1983) investigated the possible role of rumen fungi in degrading plant tissue. Another variable in their studies was that the *D. pentzii* had been grown with and without sulfur fertilization. The authors observed no differences in the bacterial populations between sheep fed the two forages. Microscopic observation indicated that fungal sporangia were prevalent on the cut ends of leaf blades and also on leaf surfaces of leaves incubated *in vitro* with rumen fluid from the animal fed fertilized forage (antibiotics were added to the fermentation). Rumen fungi were absent or in extremely low numbers in rumen fluid from sheep fed the unfertilized forage; however, fungi were present at 3.5 - 4.5 x 10^3/ml in sheep fed the sulfur fertilized forage. Nylon bag studies indicated that fungi preferentially colonized the lignified cells of blade sclerenchyma. In the presence of antibiotics, marked fungal growth was observed *in vitro* with as much as 63% loss in dry matter in 48 h for the sulfur fertilized forage. Other than possible nutritional deficiency of sulfur for the fungi, no explanation for the differences observed with sulfur fertilized and unfertilized forage was proposed. The authors did conclude that rumen fungi can be significant degraders of fiber in the rumen, specifically attacking and weakening lignocellulose tissues.

In a later study, Windham and Akin (1984) attempted to determine the role of individual rumen microbial groups in degrading fiber and to quantitate fiber degradation by the rumen fungal population. The antibiotics penicillin (P) and streptomycin (S) were used to inhibit bacterial growth and cycloheximide (C) was used to selectively inhibit rumen fungi. Alfalfa (ALF) and Coastal Bermuda grass (CBG) were used as substrates and feed for the inoculum donor animals. *In vitro* digestibility values, or adjusted digestibility coefficients (ADC), using whole rumen fluid (WRF) with the above treatments were determined by a two-stage, 48 h procedure. The bacterial fraction (WRF + cycloheximide) degraded as much dry matter (DM), neutral detergent fiber (NDF), acid-detergent fiber

(ADF) and cellulose as the total population in whole rumen fluid. However, the fungi alone (WRF + antibiotics) degraded less than the total population or bacterial fraction. No loss of lignin was observed with any treatment. A small amount of DM and NDF digestion were noted with S-P-C treatment on the ALF substrate. Since protozoa were visually observed in the S-P-C treatment fermentations, it was suggested that they were responsible for this loss. The authors concluded that rumen bacteria appeared to be the most active fiber degraders and that high numbers of rumen fungal sporangia associated with plant particles does not necessarily indicate increased digestion. This conclusion was substantiated in a later study by Akin and Benner (1988), in which decomposition of forage polysaccharides by the bacteria was similar to that of whole rumen fluid. Degradation by the fungi was significantly less ($P < 0.05$). Thus, there are several unanswered questions regarding the potential role of the fungi in the overall rumen fermentation. Information on the rate and extent of fiber degradation by fungi as well as the quantity of fungal tissue produced in the rumen, in the presence and absence of the other rumen microorganisms, would help to evaluate whether or not they make a significant contribution.

Rumen fungi were observed to physically disrupt the lignified tissues in plant stems, which may in turn facilitate breakdown during rumination and actually increase fiber utilization (Akin *et al.*, 1989). The physical strength of plant stem residues was reduced after fermentation with fungi. These observations clearly support the earlier study by Ho *et al.* (1988), where the rhizoids of anaerobic rumen fungi were able to penetrate the plant cell walls of guinea grass and rice straw. When the fungal rhizoids came into contact with undamaged rigid plant cell walls, they produced appressorium-like structures which in turn produced fine penetration pegs at the point of contact. These pegs actually penetrated through the cell wall, continued to grow inside the cell and developed into normal rhizoids. This should weaken and disrupt the plant tissues, increasing their susceptibility to degradation by both the fungi and bacteria. It has been suggested that this may be the true contribution of fungi to forage digestion in the rumen (Dehority, 1993).

Dehority and Tirabasso (2000) focused studies on establishing the role of the fungi in the overall rumen fermentation. Using either purified cellulose or an intact forage (alfalfa) as a substrate, *in vitro* fermentations were run with and without antibiotics (penicillin and streptomycin). A 1:10 dilution of whole rumen contents was used as an inoculum. In the control fermentations, appreciable cellulose digestion took place in the first 24 h and continued to increase up thru 72 h (Figure 13.3). When antibiotics were added, both the rate and extent of cellulose digestion were markedly decreased. Within 24 h, fungal numbers had essentially dropped to zero in the control fermentations, whereas bacterial numbers increased markedly and then decreased up to 72 h (Table 13.4). In the antibiotic fermentations, the bacteria were almost completely inhibited while fungal numbers increased steadily up to 72 h, paralleling cellulose digestion quite closely. It would appear that the fungi cannot grow and multiply in the presence of the mixed bacterial population.

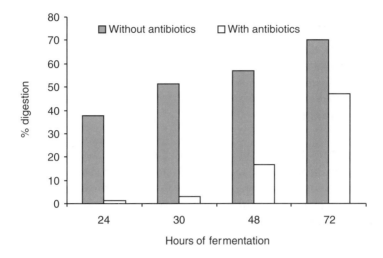

Figure 13.3 *In vitro* cellulose digestion by whole rumen contents, with and without added antibiotics (penicillin and streptomycin). At all sampling times, cellulose digestion in the control was higher than with the added antibiotics ($P < 0.02$). Data from Dehority and Tirabasso (2000).

Table 13.4 CHANGES IN BACTERIAL AND FUNGAL CONCENTRATIONS DURING THE FERMENTATION OF PURIFIED CELLULOSE BY RUMEN CONTENTS IN THE PRESENCE AND ABSENCE (CONTROL) OF ANTIBIOTICS[a]

	No. of bacteria/ml (10^7)		No. of fungi/ml (10^2)	
Time (h)	Control	Antibiotics[b]	Control	Antibiotics[b]
0	9.4±3.1	9.4±3.1	11.9±4.1	11.9±4.1
24	1000±489	0.0004±0.0001	0.01±0.01	15.5±9.7
30	451±231	0.0023±0.0011	0.02±0.01	50.3±33.4
48	290±214	0.0044±0.0010	0	229.8±86.1
72	38.2±4.8	0.0029±0.0014	0	510±80.0

[a] Data from Dehority and Tirabasso (2000).
[b] Penicillin and streptomycin.

In further investigations, the control fermentation of purified cellulose was stopped after 18-20 h, and the microbial population killed either by oxidation or autoclaving. Antibiotics were added to some of the tubes, and all tubes were reinoculated with a 1:10 dilution of rumen contents. Those tubes without antibiotics digested considerably more cellulose, whereas the antibiotic containing tubes digested little or no additional cellulose. The authors concluded that: (1) fermentation of cellulose or forages with mixed rumen contents produces a factor(s) inhibitory to rumen fungi; (2) the factor(s) is probably not the normal bacterial fermentation products, since the extent of fermentation is small after 18 h and even in higher concentrations, end-products did not cause complete inhibition (Joblin and Naylor, 1993); (3) the factor(s) is different than that produced by pure cultures of ruminococci (Stewart *et al.*, 1992; Bernalier *et al.*, 1993), since the inhibitory activity is heat stable.

Distribution of fungi

Numbers of anaerobic fungal zoospores were measured in the rumen, duodenum, cecum and feces of cows by Grenet *et al.* (1989). Concentrations were much higher in the rumen compared to the other sites, varied markedly with diet fed to the animal and were highest with alfalfa hay or corn silage plus monensin. A similar relationship in fungal concentrations between these same sites was observed by Davis *et al.* (1993) in dairy cows, growing steers and mature steers all fed ryegrass silage based diets. They also determined concentrations in the omasum and abomasum, and in the dairy cattle and growing steers, observed concentrations in the omasum higher than those in the rumen (based on thallus forming units per gram of DM).

Anaerobic fungi have now been observed in rumen contents, intestinal contents or feces of numerous ruminant and non-ruminant herbivores. Animal species include sheep, cattle, camel, vicuña, guinea pig, deer, impala, goat, reindeer, muskox, kangaroo, llama, gaur, bongo, greater kudu, blue duiker, antelope, elephant, zebra, rhinoceros (Orpin, 1978a, 1988; Milne *et al.*, 1989; Dehority and Varga, 1991; Teunissen *et al.*, 1991).

Lowe *et al.* (1987c) and Milne *et al.* (1989) have shown that fungi occur in both saliva and feces, which is probably their principal route of transfer between animals. Anaerobic fungi could not be isolated from moist sheep feces stored in plastic bags in air either at 20° or 39°C for longer than a day. Surprisingly, viable fungi could be recovered from sheep feces dried in air at 20°C or 39°C and stored in air at 20°C or 39°C for up to 128 days. Also, viable fungi were found in sun-baked and dried feces of Ethiopian sheep and cattle. Viable fungi could also be isolated from sheep saliva which had been stored in air at 39°C for periods up to 8 h.

Percent recovery of viable fungi after drying intestinal contents or feces from growing steers in air for 7 days at room temperature were as follows: reticulo-rumen, 0.004%; omasum, 2.2%; abomasum, 10.2%; small intestine, 0%; cecum, 7.7%; large intestine, 6.8% and feces, 24.5% (Davies *et al.*, 1993). Survival time for fungi in each site were as follows: reticulo-rumen, 7 days; omasum, 56 days; abomasum, 21 days; cecum, 106 days; large intestine and feces, 252 days. The authors have postulated that when conditions for vegetative fungal growth become unfavorable, a thick-walled resistant type of sporangium is formed. They consider this to be an aero-tolerant survival stage.

Wubah *et al.* (1991) observed structures in axenic culture of a *Neocallimastix* sp. which they termed resistant sporangium (RS). As their cultures aged, the development of the fungi shifted from the production of zoosporangia to the production of RS. The mature RS were dark brown from the presence of the pigment melanin and contained a high concentration of DNA. Unfortunately, the authors were unable to germinate these RS. At this point, it is suggested that the life cycle of the anaerobic rumen fungi includes three stages: the motile zoospore, the vegetative thallus and a resistant sporangium which germinates in the proper environment (Davis *et al.*, 1993).

References

Akin, D. E. and R. Benner. (1988). Degradation of polysaccharides and lignin by ruminal bacteria and fungi. *Applied and Environmental Microbiology*, **54**, 1117-1125.

Akin, D. E., G.L.R. Gordon and J. P. Hogan. (1983). Rumen bacterial and fungal degradation of *Digitaria pentzii* grown with and without sulfur. *Applied and Environmental Microbiology*, **46**, 738-748.

Akin, D. E., C. E. Lyon, W. R. Windham and L. L. Rigsby. (1989). Physical degradation of lignified stem tissues by ruminal fungi. *Applied and Environmental Microbiology*, **55**, 611-616.

Barr, D.J.S. (1988). How modern systematics relate to the rumen fungi. *BioSystems*, **21**, 351-356.

Barr, D.J.S., H. Kudo, K. D. Jakober and K.-J. Cheng. (1989). Morphology and development of rumen fungi: *Neocallimastix* sp., *Piromyces communis*, and *Orpinomyces bovis* gen. nov., sp. nov. *Canadian Journal of Botany*, **67**, 2815-2824.

Bauchop, T. (1979). Rumen anaerobic fungi of cattle and sheep. *Applied and Environmental Microbiology*, **38**, 148-158.

Bauchop, T. and D. O. Mountfort. (1981). Cellulose fermentation by a rumen anaerobic fungus in both the absence and presence of rumen methanogens. *Applied and Environmental Microbiology*, **42**, 1103-1110.

Bernalier, A., G. Fonty and Ph. Gouet. (1988). Dégradation et fermentation de la cellulose par *Neocallimastix* sp. seul ou associé à quelques espèces bactériennes du rumen. *Reproduction Nutrition Development*, **28**, 75-76.

Bernalier, A., G. Fonty, F. Bonnemoy and P. Gouet. (1992). Degradation and fermentation of cellulose by the rumen anaerobic fungi in axenic cultures or in association with cellulolytic bacteria. *Current Microbiology*, **25**, 143-148.

Bernalier, A., G. Fonty, F. Bonnemoy and P. Gouet. (1993). Inhibition of the cellulolytic activity of *Neocallimastix frontalis* by *Ruminococcus flavefaciens*. *Journal of General Microbiology*, **139**, 873-880.

Borneman, W. S., L. G. Ljungdahl, R. D. Hartley and D. E. Akin. (1991). Isolation and characterization of p-coumaroyl esterase from the anaerobic fungus *Neocallimastix* strain MC-2. *Applied and Environmental Microbiology*, **57**, 2337-2344.

Breton, A., A. Bernalier, F. Bonnemoy, G. Fonty, B. Gaillard and P. Gouet. (1989).

Morphological and metabolic characterizations of a new species of strictly anaerobic rumen fungus: *Neocallimastix joyonii. FEMS Microbiology Letters,* **58**, 309-314.

Breton, A., A. Bernalier, M. Dusser, G. Fonty, B. Gaillard-Martinie and J. Guillot. (1990). *Anaeromyces mucronatus* nov. gen., nov. sp. A new strictly anaerobic rumen fungus with polycentric thallus. *FEMS Microbiology Letters,* **70**, 177-182.

Breton, A., M. Dusser, B. Gaillard-Martinie, J. Guillot, L. Millet and G. Prensier. (1991). *Piromyces rhizinflata* nov sp, a strictly anaerobic fungus from faeces of the Saharan ass; a morphological, metabolic and ultrastructural study. *FEMS Microbiology Letters,* **82**, 1-8.

Caldwell, D. R. and M. P. Bryant. (1966). Medium without rumen fluid for nonselective enumeration and isolation of rumen bacteria. *Applied Microbiology,* **14**, 794-801.

Davies, D. R., M. K. Theodorou, M.I.G. Lawrence and A.P.J. Trinci. (1993). Distribution of anaerobic fungi in the digestive tract of cattle and their survival in faeces. *Journal of General Microbiology,* **139**,1395-1400.

Dehority, B. A. (1993). Microbial ecology of cell wall fermentation. IN: *Forage Cell Wall Structure and Digestibility.* Edited by H. G. Jung, D. R. Buxton, R. D. Hatfield and J. Ralph. ASA-CSSA-SSSA, 677 S. Segoe Rd., Madison, WI 53711, USA. pp. 425-453.

Dehority, B. A. and H. W. Scott. (1967). Extent of cellulose and hemicellulose digestion in various forages by pure cultures of rumen bacteria. *Journal of Dairy Science,* **50**, 1136-1141.

Dehority, B. A. and P. A. Tirabasso. (2000). Antibiosis between ruminal bacteria and ruminal fungi. *Applied and Environmental Microbiology,* **66**, 2921-2927.

Dehority, B. A.and P. A. Tirabasso. (2001). Effect of feeding frequency on bacterial and fungal concentrations, pH, and other paraameters in the rumen. *Journal of Animal Science,* **79**, 2908-2912.

Dehority, B. A. and G. A. Varga. (1991). Bacterial and fungal numbers in ruminal and cecal contents of the blue duiker (*Cephalophus monticola*). *Applied and Environmental Microbiology,* **57**, 469-472.

Dehority, B. A., P. A. Tirabasso and A. P. Grifo, Jr. (1989). Most-probable-number procedures for enumerating ruminal bacteria, including the simultaneous estimation of total and cellulolytic numbers in one medium. *Applied and Environmental Microbiology,* **55**, 2789-2792.

Fonty, G., Ph. Gouet and V. Sante. (1988). Influence d'une bactérie méthanogène sur l'activité cellulolytique et le métabolisme de deux espèces de champignons cellulolytiques du rumen *in vitro.* Résultats preéliminaires. *Reproduction Nutrition Development,* **28**, 133-134.

Gaillard, B., A. Breton and A. Bernalier. (1989). Study of the nuclear cycle of four species of strictly anaerobic rumen fungi by fluorescence microscopy. *Current Microbiology,* **19**, 103-107.

Gaillard-Martinie, B., A. Breton, M. Dusser and V. Julliand. (1995). *Piromyces citronii* sp. nov., a strictly anaerobic fungus from the equine caecum: a morphological, metabolic and ultrastructural study. *FEMS Microbiology Letters*, **130**, 321-326.

Gold, J. J., I. B. Heath and T. Bauchop. (1988). Ultrastructural description of a new chytrid genus of caecum anaerobe, *Caecomyces equi* gen. nov. sp. nov., assigned to the Neocallimasticaceae. *BioSystems*, **21**, 403-415.

Gordon, G.L.R. and M. W. Phillips. (1989). Degradation and utilization of cellulose and straw by three different anaerobic fungi from the ovine rumen. *Applied and Environmental Microbiology*, **55**, 1703-1710.

Gordon, G.L.R. and M. W. Phillips. (1992). Extracellular pectin lyase produced by *Neocallimastix* sp. LM1, a rumen anaerobic fungus. *Letters in Applied Microbiology.* **15**, 113-115.

Grenet, E., G. Fonty, J. Jamot and F. Bonnemoy. (1989). Influence of diet and monensin on development of anaerobic fungi in the rumen, duodenum, cecum and feces of cows. *Applied and Environmental Microbiology*, **55**, 2360-2364.

Hébraud, M. and M. Févre. (1988). Characterization of glycoside and polysaccharide hydrolases secreted by the rumen anaerobic fungi *Neocallimastix frontalis, Sphaeromonas communis* and *Piromonas communis. Journal of General Microbiology*, **134**, 1123-1129.

Heath, I. B., T. Bauchop and R. A. Skipp. (1983). Assignment of the rumen anaerobe *Neocallimastix frontalis* to the Spizellomycetales (Chytridiomycetes) on the basis of its polyflagellate zoospore ultrastructure. *Canadian Journal of Botany*, **71**, 295-307.

Ho, Y. W.and J. S. Barr. (1995). Classification of anaerobic gut fungi from herbivores with emphasis on rumen fungi from Malaysia. *Mycologia*, **87**, 655-677.

Ho, Y. W., N. Abdullah and S. Jalaludin. (1988). Penetrating structures of anaerobic rumen fungi in cattle and swamp buffalo. *Journal of General Microbiology*, **134**, 177-181.

Ho, Y. W., N. Abdullah and S. Jalaludin. (1994). Orpinomyces intercalaris, a new species of polycentric anaerobic rumen fungus from cattle. *Mycotaxon*, **50**, 139-150.

Ho, Y. W., D.J.S. Barr, N. Abdullah, S. Jalaludin and H. Kudo. (1993a). *Neocallimastix variabilis*, a new species of anaerobic fungus from the rumen of cattle. *Mycotaxon*, **46**, 241-258.

Ho, Y. W., D.J.S. Barr, N. Abdullah, S. Jalaludin and H. Kudo. (1993b). A new species of *Piromyces* from the rumen of deer in Malaysia. *Mycotaxon*, **47**, 285-293.

Ho, Y. W., D.J.S. Barr, N. Abdullah, S. Jalaludin and H. Kudo. (1993c). *Piromyces spiralis*, a new species of anaerobic fungus from the rumen of goat. *Mycotaxon*, **48**, 59-68.

Ho, Y. W., T. Bauchop, N. Abdullah and S. Jalaludin. (1990). *Ruminomyces elegans* gen. et sp. nov., A polycentric anaerobic rumen fungus from cattle. *Mycotaxon*, **38**, 397-405.

Joblin, K. N. (1981). Isolation, enumeration, and maintenance of rumen anaerobic fungi in roll tubes. *Applied and Environmental Microbiology*, **42**, 1119-1122.

Joblin, K. N. and G. E. Naylor. (1993). Inhibition of the rumen anaerobic fungus *Neocallimastix frontalis* by fermentation products. *Letters in Applied Microbiology*, **16**, 254-256.

Joblin, K. N. and A. G. Williams. (1991). Effect of cocultivation of ruminal chytrid fungi with *Methanobrevibacter smithii* on lucerne stem degradation and extracellular fungal enzyme activities. *Letters in Applied Microbiology*, **12**, 121-124.

Joblin, K. N., G. P. Campbell, A. J. Richardson and C. S. Stewart. (1989). Fermentation of barley straw by anaerobic rumen bacteria and fungi in axenic culture and in coculture with methanogens. *Letters in Applied Microbiology*, **9**, 195-197.

Joblin, K. N., G. E. Naylor and A. G. Williams. (1990). Effect of *Methanobrevibacter smithii* on xylanolytic activity of anaerobic ruminal fungi. *Applied and Environmental Microbiology*, **56**, 2287-2295.

Kostyukovsky, V. A., O. N. Okunev and B. V. Tarakanov. (1991). Description of two anaerobic fungal strains from the bovine rumen and influence of diet on the fungal population *in vivo*. *Journal of General Microbiology*, **137**, 1759-1764.

Li, J., I. B. Heath, T. Bauchop. (1990). *Piromyces mae* and *Piromyces dumbonica*, two new species of uniflagellate anaerobic chytridiomycete fungi from the hindgut of the horse and elephant. *Canadian Journal of Botany*, **68**, 1021-1033.

Li, J., I. B. Heath and K.-J. Cheng. (1991). The development and zoospore ultrastructure of a polycentric chytridiomycete gut fungus, *Orpinomyces joyonii* comb. nov. *Canadian Journal of Botany*, **69**, 580-589.

Li, J., I. B. Heath and L. Parker. (1993). The phylogenetic relationships of the anaerobic chytridomycetous gut fungi (Neocallimasticaceae) and the Chytridiomycota. II. Cladistic analysis of structural data and description of Neocallimasticales ord. nov. *Canadian Journal of Botany*, **71**, 393-407.

Lowe, S. E., M. K. Theodorou, A.P.J. Trinci and R. B. Hespell. (1985). Growth of anaerobic rumen fungi on defined and semi-defined media lacking rumen fluid. *Journal of General Microbiology*, **131**, 2225-2229.

Lowe, S. E., M. K. Theodorou and A.P.J. Trinci. (1987a). Growth and fermentation of an anaerobic rumen fungus on various carbon sources and effect of temperature or development. *Applied and Environmental Microbiology*, **53**, 1210-1215.

Lowe, S. E., M. K. Theodorou and A.P.J. Trinci. (1987b). Cellulases and xylanase of an anaerobic rumen fungus grown on wheat straw, wheat straw holocellulose, cellulose and xylan. *Applied and Environmental Microbiology*, **53**, 1216-1223.

Lowe, S. E., M. K. Theodorou and A.P.J. Trinci. (1987c). Isolation of anaerobic fungi from saliva and faeces of sheep. *Journal of General Microbiology*, **133**, 1829-1834.

McAllister, T. A., Y. Dong, L. J. Yanke, H. D. Bae, K.-J. Cheng and J. W. Costerton. (1993). Cereal grain digestion by selected strains of ruminal fungi. *Canadian Journal of Microbiology*, **39**, 367-376.

Marvin-Sikkema, F., A. J. Richardson, C. S. Stewart, J. C. Gottschal and R. A. Prins. (1990). Influence of hydrogen-consuming bacteria on cellulose degradation by anaerobic fungi. *Applied and Environmental Microbiology*, **56**, 3793-3797.

Michel, V., G. Fonty, L. Millet, F. Bonnemoy and P. Gouet. (1993). In vitro study of the proteolytic activity of rumen anaerobic fungi. *FEMS Microbiology Letters*, **110**, 5-10.

Milne, A., M. K. Theodorou, M.G.C. Jordan, C. King-Spooner and A.P.J. Trinci. (1989). Survival of anaerobic fungi in feces, saliva and in pure culture. *Experimental Mycology* **13**, 27-37.

Morrison, M., R. I. Mackie and A. Kistner. (1990). Evidence that cellulolysis by an anaerobic ruminal fungus is catabolite regulated by glucose, cellobiose and soluble starch. *Applied and Environmental Microbiology*, **56**, 3227-3229.

Mountfort, D. O. and R. A. Asher. (1983). Role of catabolite regulatory mechanisms in control of carbohydrate utilization by the rumen anaerobic fungus *Neocallimastix frontalis*. *Applied and Environmental Microbiology*, **46**, 1331-1338.

Mountfort, D. O. and R. A. Asher. (1985). Production and regulation of cellulase by two strains of the rumen anaerobic fungus *Neocallimastix frontalis*. *Applied and Environmental Microbiology*, **49**, 1314-1322.

Mountfort, D. O. and R. A. Asher. (1988). Production of α-amylase by the ruminal anaerobic fungus *Neocallimastix frontalis*. *Applied and Environmental Microbiology*, **54**, 2293-2299.

Mountfort, D. O. and R. A. Asher. (1989). Production of xylanase by the ruminal anaerobic fungus *Neocallimastix frontalis*. *Applied and Environmental Microbiology*, **55**, 1016-1022

Mountfort, D. O., R. A. Asher and T. Bauchop. (1982). Fermentation of cellulose to methane and carbon dioxide by a rumen anaerobic fungus in triculture with *Methanobrevibacter* sp. strain RA1 and *Methanosarcina barkeri*. *Applied and Environmental Microbiology*, **44**, 128-134.

Munn, E. A., C. G. Orpin and C. A. Greenwood. (1988). The ultrastructure and possible relationships of four obligate anaerobic chytridiomycete fungi from the rumen of sheep. *BioSystems,* **22**, 67-81.

Obispo, N. E. and B. A. Dehority. (1992). A most probable number method for enumeration of rumen fungi with studies on factors affecting their concentration in the rumen. *Journal of Microbiological Methods*, **16**, 259-270.

Orpin, C. G. (1974). The rumen flagellate *Callimastix frontalis*: does sequestration occur: *Journal of General Microbiology*, **84**, 395-398.

Orpin, C. G. (1975). Studies on the rumen flagellate *Neocallimastix frontalis*. *Journal of General Microbiology*, **91**, 249-262.

Orpin, C. G. (1976). Studies on the rumen flagellate *Sphaeromonas communis*. *Journal of General Microbiology*, **94**, 270-280.

Orpin, C. G. (1977a). Invasion of plant tissue in the rumen by the flagellate *Neocallimastix frontalis*. *Journal of General Microbiology*, **98**, 423-430.

Orpin, C. G. (1977b). The rumen flagellate *Piromonas communis*: Its life-history and invasion of plant material in the rumen. *Journal of General Microbiology*, **99**, 107-117.
Orpin, C. G. (1977c). The occurrence of chitin in the cell walls of the rumen organisms *Neocallimastix frontalis, Piromonas communis* and *Sphaeromonas communis*. *Journal of General Microbiology*, **99**, 215-218.
Orpin, C. G. (1977d). On the induction of zoosporogenesis in the rumen phycomycetes *Neocallimastix frontalis, Piromonas communis* and *Sphaeromonas communis*. *Journal of General Microbiology*, **101**, 181-189.
Orpin, C. G. (1978a). Isolation of phycomycete fungi from the caecum of the horse. *Proceedings of the Society for General Microbiology*, **5**, 46.
Orpin, C. G. (1978b). Induction of zoosporogenesis in the rumen phycomycete *Neocallimastix frontalis* in rumen fluid after the addition of haem-containing compounds. *Proceedings of the Society for General Microbiology*, **7**, 46-47.
Orpin, C. G. (1983/84). The role of ciliate protozoa and fungi in the rumen digestion of plant cell walls. *Animal Feed Science and Technology*, **10**, 121-143.
Orpin, C. G. (1988). Nutrition and biochemistry of anaerobic chytridiomycetes. *BioSystems*, **21**, 365-370.
Orpin, C. G. and L. Bountiff. (1978). Zoospore chemotaxis in the rumen phycomycete *Neocallimastix frontalis*. *Journal of General Microbiology*, **104**, 113-122.
Orpin, C. G. and A. J. Letcher. (1979). Utilization of cellulose, starch, xylan and other hemicelluloses for growth by the rumen phycomycete *Neocallimastix frontalis*. *Current Microbiology*, **3**, 121-124.
Orpin, C. G. and Y. Greenwood. (1986). Nutritional and germination requirements of the rumen chytridiomycete *Neocallimastix patriciarum*. *Transactions of the British Mycological Society*, **86**, 103-109.
Orpin, C. G. and Y. Hart. (1980). Digestion of plant particles by rumen phycomycete fungi. *Journal of Applied Bacteriology*, **49**, x.
Orpin, C. G. and K. N. Joblin. (1988). The rumen anaerobic fungi. IN: *The Rumen Microbial Ecosystem*. Edited by P. N. Hobson. Elsevier Applied Science, London. pp. 129-150.
Orpin, C. G. and E. A. Munn. (1986). *Neocallimastix patriciarum* sp. nov., a new member of the Neocallimasticaceae inhabiting the rumen of sheep. *Transactions of the British Mycological Society*, **86**, 178-181.
Pearce, P. D. and T. Bauchop. (1985). Glycosidases of the rumen anaerobic fungus *Neocallimastix frontalis* grown on cellulosic substrates. *Applied and Environmental Microbiology*, **49**, 1265-1269.
Phillips, M. W. and G.L.R. Gordon. (1988). Sugar and polysaccharide fermentation by rumen anaerobic fungi from Australia, Britain and New Zealand. *BioSystems*, **21**, 377-383.
Phillips, M. W. and G.L.R. Gordon. (1989). Growth characteristics on cellobiose of three different anaerobic fungi isolated from the ovine rumen. *Applied and*

Environmental Microbiology, **55**, 1695-1702.

Richardson, A. J., C. S. Stewart, G. P. Campbell, A. B. Wilson and K. N. Joblin. (1986). Influence of co-culture with rumen bacteria on the lignocellulolytic activity of phycomycetous anaerobic fungi from the rumen. *Abstracts of XIV International Congress of Microbiology*, PG2-24, 233.

Roger, V., A. Bernalier, E. Grenet, G. Fonty, J. Jamot and P. Gouet. (1993). Degradation of wheat straw and maize stem by a monocentric and a polycentric rumen fungi, alone or in association with rumen cellulolytic bacteria. *Animal Feed Science and Technology*, **42**, 69-82.

Stewart, C. S., S. H. Duncan, A. J. Richardson, C. Backwell and R. Begbie. (1992). The inhibition of fungal cellulolysis by cell-free preparations from ruminococci. *FEMS Microbiology Letters*, **97**, 83-88.

Teunissen, M. J., H.J.M. Op den Camp, C. G. Orpin, J.H.S. Huis In't Veld and G. D. Vogels. (1991). Comparisons of growth characteristics of anaerobic fungi isolated from ruminant and non-ruminant herbivores during cultivation in a defined medium. *Journal of General Microbiology*, **137**, 1401-1408.

Theodorou, M. K., S. E. Lowe and A.P.J. Trinci. (1988). The fermentative characteristics of anaerobic rumen fungi. *BioSystems*, **21**, 371-376.

Theodorou, M. K., M. Gill, C. King-Spooner and D. E. Beever. (1990). Enumeration of anaerobic chytridiomycetes as thallus-forming units: novel method for quantification of fibrolytic fungal populations from the digestive tract ecosystem. *Applied and Environmental Microbiology*, **56**, 1073-1078.

Theodorou, M. K., A. C. Longland, M. S. Dhanoa, S. E. Lowe and A.P.J. Trinci. (1989). Growth of *Neocallimastix* sp. strain R1 on Italian ryegrass hay: removal of neutral sugars from plant cell walls. *Applied and Environmental Microbiology*, **55**, 1363-1367.

Ushida, K., H. Tanaka and Y. Kojima. (1989). A simple *in situ* method for estimating fungal population size in the rumen. *Letters in Applied Microbiology*, **9**, 109-111.

Wallace, R. J. and K. N. Joblin. (1985). Proteolytic activity of a rumen anaerobic fungus. *FEMS Microbiology Letters*, **29**, 19-25.

Warner, A.C.I. (1966). Diurnal changes in the concentrations of microorganisms in the rumens of sheep fed limited diets once daily. *Journal of General Microbiology*, **45**, 213-235.

Webb, J. and M. K. Theodorou. (1991). *Neocallimastix hurleyensis* sp. nov., an anaerobic fungus from the ovine rumen. *Canadian Journal of Botany*, **69**, 1220-1224.

Williams A. G. and C. G. Orpin. (1987a). Polysaccharide-degrading enzymes formed by three species of anaerobic rumen fungi grown on a range of carbohydrate substrates. *Canadian Journal of Microbiology*, **33**, 418-426.

Williams, A. G. and C. G. Orpin. (1987b). Glycoside hydrolase enzymes present in the zoospore and vegetative growth stages of the rumen fungi *Neocallimastix patriciarum, Piromonas communis*, and an unidentified isolate, grown on a range of carbohydrates. *Canadian Journal of Microbiology*, **33**, 427-434.

Williams, A. G., S. E. Withers and K. N. Joblin. (1991). Xylanolysis by cocultures of the rumen fungus *Neocallimastix frontalis* and ruminal bacteria. *Letters in Applied Microbiology*, **12**, 232-235.

Windham, W. R. and D. E. Akin. (1984). Rumen fungi and forage fiber digestion. *Applied and Environmental Microbiology*, **48**, 473-476.

Wubah, D. A., M. S. Fuller and D. E. Akin. (1991). Resistant body formation in *Neocallimastix* sp., an anaerobic fungus from the rumen of a cow. *Mycologia*, **83**, 40-47.

CHAPTER 14

ADDITIONAL METABOLIC ACTIVITIES AND INTERACTIONS AMONG RUMEN MICROORGANISMS

In addition to their ability to ferment plant structural carbohydrates, the rumen microorganisms have several other activities or capabilities which contribute to the nutrition of their host. These would include: (1) reproduction or the synthesis of cell protein which becomes available to the host animal; (2) hydrolysis and biohydrogenation of dietary lipids as well as synthesis of microbial lipids; and (3) synthesis of vitamin K and B-complex vitamins.

Composition and nutritive value of microbial protein

Rumen microorganisms and dietary protein are the two sources of protein for the host animal, and microbial protein can be synthesized both from protein and non-protein nitrogen (NPN). It has been estimated that about 40% of the non-ammonia-N entering the small intestine is microbial N when the diet has a high protein level. The percentage increases to 60% with low-protein diets and up to 100% with only NPN as a N source. Cattle can readily grow, reproduce and lactate with NPN as their only nitrogen source (Owens and Zinn, 1988). In general, crude protein content of the microorganisms averages around 50% for bacteria, 40% for protozoa and 43% for fungi (Kemp *et al.*, 1985; Owens and Zinn, 1988).

Digestibility and biological value of bacteria has been determined by a number of investigators, using chemical, biological and enzymatic procedures (McNaught *et al.*, 1954; Weller, 1957; Purser and Buechler, 1966; Bergen *et al.*, 1968). Table 14.1 lists reported ranges for biological value, true digestibility and net protein utilization (biological value times digestibility) for rumen bacteria and protozoa (Owens and Zinn, 1988).

Table 14.1 ESTIMATES OF THE NUTRITIVE VALUE OF RUMEN MICROBIAL PROTEIN

	Biological value	*True digestibility*	*Net protein utilization*
Rumen bacteria	66-87	74-79	63
Rumen protozoa	82	87-91	71

Purser and Buechler (1966) determined the amino acid composition of 22 pure cultures of rumen bacteria and calculated their biological value using the essential amino acid index method (Oser, 1951). Values ranged from 59 to 73 with an overall mean of 69. This compares quite closely to the mean value of 70 determined by Weller (1957) on bacterial preparations obtained from rumen contents of sheep fed four different rations. It appears that amino acid composition of rumen bacteria is fairly constant and thus the bulk amino acid composition of rumen bacterial preparations is not markedly affected by diet. This was confirmed in a subsequent study by Bergen *et al.* (1968). Amino acid analysis of protozoal preparations by Weller (1957) and Purser and Buechler (1966) both calculated out to the same biological value, 69. Church (1976) concluded from the information available that biological value of the bacteria and protozoa are very similar; however, digestibility of the protozoa is higher and thus net protein utilization is higher for the protozoa. Unfortunately there is very little information available on biological value and digestibility of fungal protein. Kemp *et al.* (1985) determined the amino acid profiles for *N. patriciarum* and *P. communis* and found they were similar to each other and compared favorably with the profile of casein, suggesting a rather high biological value.

The contribution of microbial protein to the host is obviously dependent upon its passage on down the digestive tract. The quantity of total protein reaching the small intestine is primarily a balance between the level of dietary protein intake, microbial protein synthesis and extent of degradation in the rumen. Feed protein with a low biological value can be improved by digestion and conversion to microbial protein, while conversely, biological value can be lowered when a high biological value protein is fed. For diets high in protein, the concentration is generally reduced in the rumen, while concentration increases with low protein diets. In general, when crude protein levels are below 13-15%, output from the rumen is greater than input. At higher intake levels, output is lower than input (Owens and Zinn, 1988).

Quantification of microbial passage to the hindgut

Several methods have been used to estimate the amount of microbial protein flowing into the small intestine; unfortunately, all of them have drawbacks which effect the accuracy of the determination. Most methods are based on the use of markers, i.e., a given component of the microorganism which is proportional to cell numbers or weight. Microbial markers can be internal (normal component of the microbial cell) or external (a label which is uniformly incorporated into new cells). The ideal microbial marker should meet the following criteria: (1) not present in the feed; (2) not absorbed; (3) biologically stable (not affected by digestive tract enzymes or microbes); (4) have a simple, specific and sensitive assay procedure; (5) be a constant percentage of the intact cell in all stages of growth; and (6) all cellular forms should flow at a similar rate, i.e., whether free, bound in a cellular fraction of a ruptured cell or within an intact cell. At present no marker has been found which will satisfy even a majority of these criteria.

Additional metabolic activities and interactions

In addition, it must also be remembered that no marker technique can be any better than our ability to isolate a specific microbial fraction from the rumen to serve as a reference standard. This fraction obviously needs to be representative of the microbial population which we wish to estimate.

Protein flow per day to the duodenum can be calculated by measuring microbial nitrogen in duodenal digesta and multiplying by grams (g) digesta flow per day. (Owens and Hanson, 1992; Broderick and Merchen, 1992; Stern et al., 1994). The ratio of marker to nitrogen (N) is determined both in a reference bacterial or protozoal fraction which is physically isolated from rumen contents and in duodenal digesta.

Protein flow per day to the duodenum is calculated as shown below:

1. $$\frac{\text{marker:N ratio (duodenal digesta)}}{\text{marker: N ratio (reference)}} \times 100 = \% \text{ microbial N in total duodenal digesta N}$$

2. $$\frac{\text{g inert passage marker fed / d}}{\text{g inert passage marker / g digesta}} = \text{g digesta flow / d}$$

3. Total g N flow / d × % microbial N in total digesta N = g microbial N / d

4. g microbial N / d × g protein / g N = g protein flow / d

Many of the studies reported in the literature have used an average value of 16% N for microbial proteins, or 1.00/.16 = 6.25 g protein per g N factor. However, about 30% of total microbial N occurs as NPN in the indigestible cell wall. True microbial protein has been found to contain only about 15% N, which gives a correction factor of 1.00/.15 or 6.67 (Hespell and Bryant, 1979; Van Soest, 1994). If 100 g of mixed ruminal bacteria contained 10 g of N, 3 g would be NPN and 7 g would be true microbial protein N. Multiplying 7 g times 6.67 gives a total of 46.7 g of true microbial protein. As generally calculated, the 10 g of N would be multiplied by 6.25, giving a value of 62.5 g microbial protein per 100 g of mixed ruminal bacteria, which overestimates true microbial protein by 34%. Therefore, multiplying the g microbial N / d times 0.7 times 6.67 (equation 4 above) will give the g true microbial protein flow / d.

Nitrogen content per unit of dry matter for protozoa and fungi is less than found in bacteria. Most values reported in the literature for these organisms fall between 4 and 8% (Weller, 1957; Kemp et al., 1985; Gulati et al., 1989), compared to 15% for bacteria. This would give a conversion factor for N to protein between 12.5 and 25. In addition, if the percentage bacteria, protozoa and fungi in the reference standard isolated from rumen contents differs from that found in duodenal contents, considerable error would be introduced into estimates of microbial protein passage to the small intestine. Essentially these two factors cast considerable doubt on the validity of using a single marker to estimate passage of total microbial protein.

Some of the more commonly used internal and external markers for rumen microbes are listed in Tables 14.2 and 14.3. Their principal deficiencies from the ideal marker are also listed. Almost all of the internal markers listed in Table 14.2 are associated with or are part of the cell wall, which is more resistant to digestion than the cell contents. Because of this, the duodenal digesta may become enriched with cell wall components which could overestimate the outflow of microorganisms (Owens and Goetsch, 1988). In addition to the drawbacks listed for the external markers, there are also some other disadvantages, i.e., using either ^{15}N or ^{35}S as markers involves complicated and costly assay procedures (Stern and Hoover, 1979; Broderick and Merchen, 1992). Using ^{35}S or ^{32}P also requires adherence to all of the precautions mandated for conducting animal trials with radioactive isotopes.

Broderick and Merchen (1992) and more recently, Stern et al. (1994) have recommended the simultaneous use of two microbial marker systems. The total purine method of Zinn and Owens (1986) is a simple procedure for quantifying microbial protein yields under practical conditions. However, in a recent study by Obispo and Dehority (1999), the purine:protein ratio for ten pure cultures of rumen bacteria was 0.0883 compared to 0.0306 for mixed bacterial samples isolated from rumen contents. Using the value from the mixed bacterial sample would give a threefold overestimate of microbial protein. It appeared that this discrepancy resulted from contamination of the mixed bacterial sample with protein containing feed particles. Although the ^{15}NH$_3$ method is more laborious and expensive, it appears to be somewhat superior in measuring the different microbial pools, i.e., fluid associated bacteria, particle associated bacteria and protozoa. Using the modifications of Obispo and Dehority (1999) a direct comparison of the results between these two methods should determine if the purine:protein procedure is a reliable estimate of microbial protein for routine use.

To date, the fungi have been almost completely ignored with regard to their contribution of protein to the host animal. Since fungi are the only rumen organisms known to contain chitin, it has been suggested as a possible marker. However, considerable variation has been found in chitin concentration both between different fungal species and strains (Orpin, 1977; Phillips and Gordon, 1989). Most feedstuffs also contain some chitin as a result of aerobic fungal growth prior to consumption by the animal. Gay et al. (1988) found a linear relationship between chitin synthase concentration and protein content of fungal cultures; however, no verification of the procedure has been reported. Akin (1987) used loss of weight after treatment with chitinase to estimate fungal biomass in fibrous residues from in vitro digestion trials. Tetrahymanol, a triterpenol, was found to occur in two species of fungi, and suggested as a possible fungal marker (Kemp et al. 1984). However, to date, no follow-up studies have been reported for any of these suggested fungal markers.

Table 14.2 MOST COMMON INTERNAL MARKERS USED FOR ESTIMATING MICROBIAL PROTEINS IN DUODENAL DIGESTA AND THEIR DEFICIENCIES

Marker[a]	Microbial organism(s) identified	Principal deficiencies of marker	References[b]
DAP	Bacteria	% varies between species	1
		Also occurs in protozoa and feedstuffs	2,3
		% composition of free, bound and cell associated DAP varies with time after feeding	4
D-Alanine	Bacteria	Similar deviations as listed for DAP, except it does not occur in feedstuffs	5,6,7
		Analysis not very precise	8
AEP	Protozoa	% composition varies between genera	9
		Also occurs in bacteria and feedstuffs	10,11
Nucleic acids	Bacteria and protozoa	Occurs in feedstuffs	12,13
		% composition varies between bacteria, protozoa, different bacterial pools and time after feeding	14,15,16,17
ATP	Bacteria and protozoa	Different distribution between bacteria and protozoa	18,19
Total purines	Bacteria and protozoa	Similar deviations as those listed for nucleic acids, but differences are less.	14,15,16,20,21,22

[a] DAP = diaminopimelic acid; AEP = aminoethylphosphonic acid; Nucleic acids = RNA and DNA; ATP = adenosine triphosphate.
[b] (1) Purser and Buechler, 1966; (2) Czerkawski, 1974; (3) Rahnema and Theurer, 1986; (4) Masson et al., 1991; (5) Garret et al., 1982; (6) Garret et al., 1986; (7) Ling, 1990; (8) Quigley and Schwab, 1988; (9) Whitelaw et al., 1983; (10) Horigane and Horiguchi, 1990; (11) Ankrah et al., 1989; (12) Schelling et al., 1982; (13) Titgemeyer et al., 1989; (14) Cecava et al., 1990; (15) Craig et al., 1987; (16) Firkins et al., 1987; (17) Smith and McAllan, 1974; (18) Wallace and West, 1982; (19) Wolstrup and Jensen, 1978; (20) Zinn and Owens, 1986; (21) Clarke et al., 1992; (22) Obispo and Dehority, 1999.

Table 14.3 EXTERNAL MARKERS FOR ESTIMATING MICROBIAL PROTEINS IN DUODENAL DIGESTA AND THEIR DEFICIENCIES

Marker	Microbial organism(s) identified	Principal deficiencies of marker	Reference[a]
^{15}N	Bacteria and protozoa	Bacterial and protozoal pools are not equally enriched	1
^{35}S	Bacteria and protozoa	Sulfur in microbial amino acids does not all come from sulfate or sulfide	2,3
^{32}P	Bacteria and protozoa	Cell composition of P changes during growth	4

[a] (1) Firkins et al., 1987; (2) Gawthorne and Nader, 1976; (3) Stern and Hoover, 1979; (4) Van Nevel and Demeyer, 1977.

One of the more promising future possibilities for estimating microbial protein in the small intestine is the use of oligonucleotide probes. Bacteria (prokaryotes) can be identified using 16S rRNA oligonucleotide probes, while 18S rRNA probes are used for the protozoa and fungi (eukaryotes). Numerous studies have been conducted in which certain species or groups of bacteria are monitored in complex microbial communities (Stahl et al., 1988; Amann et al., 1990; Briesacher et al., 1992; Odenyo et al., 1994a, b; Forster et al., 1997; Wood et al.,1998; Krause et al., 2000; Michalet-Doreau et al., 2002). Recent studies with protozoa have shown progress in the development of a protozoa-specific primer which should allow assessment of the overall composition (Karnati et al., 2003) as well as using PCR-RFLP methods to quantify the flow of different groups of protozoa into the small intestine (Newbold et al., 2002). Similar techniques have been developed for the rumen fungi (Dore and Stahl, 1991; Dore et al., 1993; Faichney et al., 1997). At present, these techniques may be more qualitative than quantitative because of primer specificity and bias in DNA amplification by PCR. An excellent review on this subject has been published by Wintzingerode et al., (1997). They list several areas as "pitfalls" of PCR-based rRNA analysis. These are: (1) Sample collection, always a critical step; (2) Cell lysis and extraction of DNA can be a problem in that the rigorous conditions required for lysis of Gram-positive cells may result in highly fragmented nucleic acids from Gram-negative cells. The fragmented nucleic acids are sources of artifacts in PCR amplification experiments; (3) Cell lysis and extraction of RNA, can be a problem in that RNAs are easily degraded by cellular Rnases during extraction; (4) PCR amplification. The authors list five sources of potential error under this category, i.e., inhibition by humic substances co-extracted with nucleic acids, differential PCR amplification, formation of PCR artifacts, contaminating DNA and 16S rRNA sequence variations due to *rrn* operon heterogeneity. Thus, considerable care is needed in using these methods for estimating microbial protein in duodenal contents.

Role of rumen microorganisms in lipid metabolism

The principal effects of the rumen microorganisms (primarily bacteria) upon dietary lipids are hydrolysis and biohydrogenation (Garton, 1958,1965). Triglycerides are hydrolyzed by the rumen microbes releasing free fatty acids and glycerol. In addition, galactose is released from galactoglycerides, which are the main lipids in green leaves. Glycerol is readily fermented by several species of rumen bacteria, *Selenomonas ruminantium* var. *lactolytica* and *Anaerovibrio lipolytica,* producing propionic acid as the main end product (Hobson and Mann, 1961; Hungate, 1966). Galactose, a simple sugar, is readily fermented by a large number of rumen bacteria as well as the protozoan, *Dasytricha ruminantium* (Howard, 1959; Hungate, 1966). The free fatty acids produced by hydrolysis of triglycerides are rapidly hydrogenated, and neither mono- nor diglycerides were found to be present as intermediates (Garton *et al.*, 1961)

HYDROLYSIS

Lipase and phospholipase activity are found in only a small proportion of rumen bacteria. However, numerous investigators have been successful in isolating lipid hydrolyzing organisms from rumen contents, using anaerobic techniques with both differential and selective media (Harfoot and Hazelwood, 1997). In general, two species have been found, *Anaerovibrio lipolytica* and various strains of *Butyrivibrio fibrosolvens*. Henderson (1971) found that the lipase of *A. lipolytica* was entirely extracellular and associated with the cell surface. It attacked diglycerides more readily than triglycerides and did not hydrolyze phospholipids or galactolipids. The organism occurred in rumen contents at concentrations around 10^7/ml (Prins *et al.*, 1975). Most of the *B. fibrosolvens* strains readily hydrolyze phospholipid substrates and activity was initially cell associated (Latham *et al.*, 1972; Hazelwood and Dawson, 1975, 1979).

There are some reports suggesting that rumen ciliate protozoa are capable of hydrolyzing dietary lipids; however, the evidence is rather limited (Wright, 1961; Bailey and Howard, 1963; Latham *et al.*, 1972). At this time, the rumen fungi have not been shown to have any role in hydrolysis of dietary lipids.

BIOHYDROGENATION

Polyunsaturated fatty acids or lipid-rich forages are biohydrogenated when incubated with whole rumen contents (Reiser, 1951; Shorland et al., 1955; Ward et al., 1964). Wright (1959, 1960) observed biohydrogenation of lipids by both bacterial and protozoal fractions of rumen contents and concluded that both were capable of this activity. Dawson and Kemp (1969) questioned whether this activity in the protozoal fraction might be attributed to ingested bacteria and proceeded to measure biohydrogenation rates in normal and defaunated sheep. They found no differences and concluded that the protozoa were not essential. Results of subsequent studies by Girard and Hawke (1978) and Singh and Hawke (1979), using ^{14}C labeled substrates, indicated that the protozoa have limited if any capability to biohydrogenate lipids.

It appears that the rumen bacteria are responsible for the major portion of biohydrogenation in the rumen, and this activity is primarily associated with those bacteria attached to the particulate matter. The suggested mechanism for this is that ingested or added triglycerides are hydrolyzed and the resulting free fatty acids are absorbed onto the plant particles where it is hydrogenated by the attached bacteria (Harfoot, 1975; Gerson et al., 1988; Legay-Carmier, 1989; Bauchart et al., 1990). *Butyrivibrio fibrosolvens* was the first bacterial species identified as capable of biohydrogenation (Polan et al., 1964; Kepler et al., 1966). Harfoot and Hazelwood (1997) have compiled a list of the more recent bacterial isolates capable of biohydrogenation and their ability to hydrogenate linolenic, linoleic and oleic acids. The species included are in the genera *Butyrivibrio, Treponema, Micrococcus, Ruminococcus, Eubacterium, Fusocillus* and several other organisms not classified. As pointed out by these authors, although only a small number of species have been isolated, this is a function of the fact that enrichment cultures or selective media cannot be used to identify and isolate these organisms. Essentially a large number of organisms must be isolated on a non-selective medium and then screened for biohydrogenation activity.

The major dietary unsaturated fatty acids of the ruminant are linolenic acid, either present in glycolipids or phospholipids of forage or linoleic acid, present as a triglyceride in a dietary supplement. Before hydrogenation can take place, these lipids must be hydrolyzed since only fatty acids with a free carboxyl group can be biohydrogenated (Hazelwood et al., 1976). In general, α- and γ- linolenic acids undergo isomerization to form octadecatrienoic acids which are hydrogenated to octadecadienoic acids and then further hydrogenated to vaccenic acid and finally stearic acid. Linoleic acid undergoes isomerization and hydrogenation to vaccenic acid and then stearic acid (Harfoot and Hazelwood, 1997).

In recent years, the conjugated linoleic acids (CLA) have been shown to have several health benefits, particularly in the prevention of carcinogenesis, cardiovascular diseases and obesity. The major dietary sources of CLA are the meat and milk of ruminants, a portion of which are presumed to be of rumen origin. However, just recently it was found that mammalian tissues can also convert vaccenic acid (*trans*-$C_{18:1}$) to *cis*-9, *trans*-11 CLA (Griinari and Bauman, 1999). Martin and Jenkins (2002) have reported that growth of mixed rumen bacteria in continuous culture at a pH below 6.0 markedly reduces the production of *trans*-$C_{18:1}$ and CLA isomers. Since the *trans*-$C_{18:1}$ monoenes apparently serve as the precursor of CLA at the tissue level (i.e., mammary gland), diets which promote low rumen pH should be avoided.

Although there are 15 isomers of CLA, only the *cis*-9, *trans*-11 and *trans*-10, *cis*-12 isomers are produced in significant quantities. *Butyrivibrio fibrisolvens* A38 produces the *cis*-9, *trans* -11 isomer but not the *trans*-10, *cis*-12 isomer (Kim *et al.*, 2000). Just recently, Kim *et al.* (2002) isolated a strain of *Megasphaera elsdenii*, YJ-4, that produces only the *trans*-10, *cis*-12 isomer.

MICROBIAL LIPIDS

The microbial cellular lipids may be synthesized *de novo* by the microorganisms or be directly incorporated into their cell from dietary sources. It has been estimated that in sheep, bacterial and protozoal lipids account for 10-20 % of the total lipids present in the rumen (Keeny, 1970). Garton and Oxford (1955) analyzed a sample of mixed rumen bacteria and found that 9% of the dry weight was lipid. They broke this down further into 39% phospholipids, 38% neutral lipids, 12% steam-volatile fatty acids and 10% non-saponifiable material. Harfoot and Hazelwood (1997) have summarized the data on composition from a number of studies. Although the membrane lipids of the bacteria may contain small quantities of rare or unusual lipids, they primarily contain saturated C_{15}, C_{16} and C_{18} fatty acids. In contrast, mixed protozoa lipids were found to contain about 86% phospholipids and very low amounts of mono-, di- and triglycerides (Harfoot, 1978). The fatty acids in protozoa were also less saturated than in bacteria. Data on lipid composition of fungi is based on analyses from two species: *Piromonas communis* contains about 87% phospholipid (Kemp *et al.*, 1984); and *Neocallimastix frontalis is* reported to contain only 56% polar lipids (Body and Bauchop, 1985).

Vitamin synthesis

The ruminant animal itself requires all the vitamins of other mammals; however, it is aided by the fact that the rumen microorganisms, principally the bacteria, synthesize vitamin K and the water-soluble B-vitamins. Synthesis of the B-vitamins was first demonstrated during *in vitro* incubations with rumen contents (Bechdel *et al.*, 1928). Vitamin K synthesis was later observed by McElroy and Goss (1940). Virtanen (1963) fed milking cows a vitamin-free ration and found that the rumen concentrations of thiamine, riboflavin, nicotinic acid, pyridoxine, folic acid, biotin and pantothenic acid were similar to those in the control cows fed a conventional diet. *In vitro* synthesis of vitamin B_{12} by mixed cultures of rumen bacteria was reported by Hunt *et al.*, in 1954.

Table 14.4 lists the concentrations of the B-vitamins in rumen contents of steers fed several different diets. As can be seen, including penicillin in the diet only had an effect on production of thiamine, pantothenic acid and folic acid.

Table 14.4 CONCENTRATION OF B VITAMINS IN RUMEN CONTENTS OF STEERS FED DIFFERENT DIETS[a]

Vitamin	Concentration (µg per gram of dry rumen contents)		
	Hay	Hay + concentrate	Hay + conc. + penicillin
Thiamine	2.1	3.0	-
Riboflavin	11.0	13.0	20.0
Nicotinic acid	50.0	60.0	63.0
Pantothenic acid	10.0	28.0	-
Pyridoxine	2.8	2.5	3.0
Biotin	0.16	0.22	0.16
Folic acid	1.7	2.3	-
B_{12} (all forms)	5.0	6.5	5.0

[a] Kon and Porter (1953).

In addition to the host, most of the rumen microorganisms themselves require one or more of the B vitamins. Considerable data is available on vitamin requirements of the rumen bacteria, primarily because it is relatively easy to determine their requirement in defined media. Wolin, *et al*. (1997) compiled data on bacterial B vitamin requirements for nine different species (Table 14.5). Data from Bryant *et al*. (1958) and Scott and Dehority (1965) has also been included.

Growth of the protozoa in axenic culture has not been achieved to date, which prevents assessment of either their vitamin production or utilization. However, production of several of the B-vitamins with diets containing penicillin may suggest that they have some ability to do so (Table 14.4). Kandatsu and Takehashi (1955a,b, 1956) and Bonhomme *et al*. (1982) have reported a marked stimulation in the growth of *Entodinium* spp. in the presence of vitamin B_{12}.

To date, vitamin requirements have only been determined for one species of rumen fungi, *Neocallimastix patriciarum* (Orpin and Greenwod, 1986). They found this species to require biotin and thiamine (or its precursors) for growth in a minimal medium. However, growth was stimulated by the addition of a number of the other vitamins.

Interactions among the rumen microorganisms

Interactions among the rumen microorganisms can be either positive or negative, occurring both within and between the different microbial types. Associations between microorganisms can be described as follows: mutualism, an association which is beneficial to both; commensalism, an association which is beneficial to one of the partners but without effect on the other; and parasitism, an association in which one of the partners gains at the expense of the other (Prins and Vorstenbosch, 1975). The various interactions

Additional metabolic activities and interactions 331

Table 14.5 VITAMIN REQUIREMENTS OF RUMEN BACTERIA[a]

Organism	Biotin	Folic acid	PABA	Pyridoxine	Pantothenic acid	Thiamine	Riboflavin	Niacin	B_{12}	Vitamin K
Fibrobacter succinogenes	+	–	+	–	–	–	–	–	–	–
Ruminobacter amylophilus	+	–	–	–	–	–	–	–	–	–
Ruminococcus flavefaciens	+	+[b]	+[b]	+	–	+	+	–	+[c]	–
Ruminococcus albus	+	–	+	+	–	–	–	–	–	–
Butyrivibrio fibrisolvens	+	+	–	+	–	–	–	–	–	–
Streptococcus bovis	+	–	–	–	+	+	–	+	–	–
Selenomonas ruminantium	+	–	+	–	–	–	–	–	–	–
Succinovibrio dextrinosolvens	–	–	+	–	–	–	–	–	–	+[d]
Megasphera elsdeni	+	–	–	+	+	–	–	–	–	–
Prevotella ruminocola	+	–	+	–	–	–	–	–	–	–

+ = required or stimulatory; – = not required.
[a] Data from Bryant *et al.*, 1958; Scott and Dehority, 1965; and Wolin, *et al.* (1997).
[b] Some strains require tetrahydrofolate, some can use either folic acid or PABA and some can only use PABA (Slyter and Weaver, 1977).
[c] Required by only one strain (C1a).
[d] Gomez-Alarcon *et al.* (1982).

which have been observed among rumen microorganisms are shown in Table 14.6 (Dehority, 1998). The positive interactions are shown in bold print. Synergism would best fit under the category of mutualism while cross feeding and serving as an essential nutrient source would be described as commensalism. All other effects listed are negative in nature and would be classified as parasitism. Several of these interactions, particularly within the same microbial type, have been discussed in earlier Chapters and will not be presented in detail.

Table 14.6 INTERACTIONS BETWEEN RUMEN MICROORGANISMS[a]

	Bacteria	*Protozoa*	*Fungi*
Bacteria	**Synergism** **Cross feeding** Inhibition between species	**Provide nutrients**	**Increased biomass and activity** Growth inhibition
Protozoa	Predation	Specific and accidental predation Cannibalism Nutrient competition	Predation
Fungi	**Synergism**	No direct effect	No direct effect

[a] Dehority (1998).

BACTERIAL INTERACTIONS

Between bacteria. Both synergism between bacteria in the digestion of plant structural carbohydrates and inhibition between species has been presented earlier. Cross feeding of hydrolysis products, utilization of end-products or production of an essential nutrient are positive interactions which can occur between bacterial species. For example, non-cellulolytic bacteria can utilize the cellodextrins produced by the cellulolytic species (Russell, 1985). Rumen methanogens obtain energy by converting the metabolic end-products produced by carbohydrate-fermenting species, hydrogen and carbon dioxide, to methane (Russell and Wallace, 1988, Wolin and Miller, 1988). Another example of synergism between species is the conversion of succinate, a normal end product of several cellulolytic and amylolytic bacteria, to propionate (Scheifinger and Wolin, 1973; Wolin and Miller, 1988). Production of nutrients such as vitamins (mentioned previously), amino acids or branched-chain fatty acids by one bacterial species, which are essential for the growth of a second species, also occurs in the rumen (Miura *et al*. 1980; Wallace, 1985; Wolin and Miller, 1988).

The synergism which results when one bacterial species "unmasks" or makes a substrate available to a second organism, cross feeding, use of end products and nutrient production, can all be classified under commensalism. That is, the second species benefits from the action of the first, without any detrimental effect on the first organism.

Inhibition between species with regard to intact forage cellulose digestion was shown in Table 8.6. While studying synergism between bacterial species in the digestion of forage structural carbohydrates, it was noted that some combinations of organisms reduced the extent of digestion. For example, forage cellulose digestion was decreased by combining *F. succinogenes* A3c with *R. flavefaciens* B34b, or *R. albus* 7 with either *R. flavefaciens* B1a or *B. fibrisolvens* H10b. Similar decreases in intact forage cellulose digestion have been observed with other strains of these same species, i.e., between *F. succinogenes* and *R. flavefaciens* (Saluzzi et al., 1993) and between *R. albus* and *R. flavefaciens* (Odenyo et al., 1994b). One possible explanation for these negative responses would be that the two organisms produce different depolymerases and the resulting oligosaccharides cannot be further metabolized by the available glycosidases. Another possibility would be the production of bacterocin-like substances by one organism, which are inhibitory to the second organism. Odenyo et al. (1994) observed that *R. albus* 8 produced proteinaceous factors which inhibited growth of *R. flavefaciens* FD-1; but not *F. succinogenes* S85. Subsequently, Chan and Dehority (1999) found that *R. albus* 7, plus two additional strains of *R. albus*, all produced inhibitory activity against a number of *R. flavefaciens* strains, but not against *F. succinogenes*, *B. fibrisolvens* or *P. ruminicola*. The inhibitory substance(s) was present in cell-free culture filtrates, was heat-labile and could be destroyed by a proteolytic enzyme. Kalmokoff and Teather (1997) screened 49 *Butyrivibrio fibrisolvens* isolates for possible bacteriocin production. Twenty five strains produced products which showed varying degrees of inhibition to the other isolates plus some unrelated Gram-positive rumen bacteria. .

The antagonism between *R. flavefaciens* B34b and *F. succinogenes* A3c, shown in Table 8.6, did not appear to be caused by a bacterocin (Fondevila and Dehority, 1996). When the two cultures were added sequentially, regardless of the order in which they were added, cellulose digestion from the forage was not different from A3c alone,. In additional experiments, the authors found that *R. flavefaciens* only suppresses the cellulolytic activity or growth of *F. succinogenes* when the organisms are present simultaneously in the fermentation medium. In other words, the inhibitory substance(s) is only produced by *R. flavefaciens* when it is cocultured with *F. succinogenes*. The inhibitory material was stable to autoclaving at 121°C for 20 min.

Between bacteria and protozoa. Since the protozoa cannot be grown in axenic culture, the bacteria obviously provide nutrients essential for their growth.

Between bacteria and fungi. Both the positive increase in fungal biomass and activity and inhibitory effects observed between bacteria and fungi have been discussed in detail in Chapter 13. The fungi themselves also depend on the bacteria to supply their nutritional requirements of B vitamins, heme, amino acids, etc. (Williams et al., 1994).

PROTOZOAL INTERACTIONS

Between protozoa and bacteria. Primarily predation, i.e., bacterial concentrations are generally lower in rumen contents of faunated animals and increase when the animal is defaunated. Presumably this is a result of predation by the protozoa (Williams and Coleman, 1988) which should result in an increase in both the rate and efficiency of bacterial growth, since more food and nutrients should be available (Prins, 1991). Protozoal predation appears to be random and not species-specific, probably more a function of bacterial concentration. A possible exception would be that those bacteria attached to particulate matter would be less likely to be ingested.

At this time, the protozoa must be considered to be parasitic, since we are unable to grow them in the absence of bacteria. In contrast, the bacteria are able to carry out the normal digestive activities in the rumen by themselves.

Between protozoa. Predation and competition for nutrients are the two major interactions occurring between rumen protozoa. Predation can be specific as described in Chapter 4 or accidental, as described by Lubinsky (1957). Williams and Coleman (1992) have summarized the examples of protozoal predation reported by various authors. In general specific predation seems to be the most important, since it can lead to removal of the "prey" from the population.

Between protozoa and fungi. Predation of fungi by the protozoa is mostly based on circumstantial evidence, i.e., the increase in fungal concentrations when animals are defaunated (Orpin, 1977; Soetanto *et al.*, 1985; Romulo *et al.*, 1986). However, contradictory findings have been reported by Ushida *et al.* (1989), Newbold and Hillman (1990) and Williams and Withers (1993). Fungal concentrations were measured in whole rumen contents of three sheep before and after defaunation, and no effect was observed in two of the sheep while a 10-fold increase in fungal concentrations occurred in the third animal (Bond, 1994). Scanning electron micrographs clearly show protozoa ingesting fungal rhizoids and sporangia, and a marked increase in the release of ^{14}C occurred *in vitro* when protozoa were incubated with ^{14}C-labeled fungi (Williams and Coleman, 1992; Williams *et al.*, 1994). The evidence for predation of fungi by protozoa is somewhat variable; however, it does suggest that predation occurs, but probably to a lesser extent than with the bacteria.

FUNGAL INTERACTIONS

Between fungi and bacteria, protozoa or other species of fungi. The interactions of fungi with bacteria were presented in Chapter 13. There are no reported direct interactions of fungi upon the growth of protozoa or other species of fungi.

In summary, most of the interactions between rumen organisms are based on *in vitro* experiments, both with pure and mixed cultures. Whether these same interactions occur *in vivo* is not known. Since the metabolic capabilities of all three types of rumen microorganisms are similar, it might be expected that another organism could take over any activity specifically reduced by inhibition of a particular organism. Other factors such as the type of forage or feed and its potential digestibility as well as its rate of passage through the rumen would also have an influence. How these interactions could effect *in vivo* digestibilities is illustrated in Table 14.7. The greatest amount of cellulose is digested *in vitro* by combining *F. succinogenes* A3c with *P. ruminicola* H8a. However, combining A3c with *R. flavefaciens* B34b reduces cellulose digestion. These three cultures combined with three additional cultures (*R. albus* 7, *R. flavefaciens* B1a and *Butyrivibrio fibrisolvens* H10b) does not digest as much cellulose as A3c alone.

Table 14.7 CELLULOSE DIGESTION FOR 12 FORAGES DETERMINED *IN VITRO* WITH PURE CULTURES (SINGLY AND IN VARIOUS COMBINATIONS) AND *IN VIVO* BY SHEEP DIGESTIBILITY TRIALS[a]

Inoculum	Cellulose digestion, %
Fibrobacter succinogenes A3c	61.9[w]
Ruminococcus flavefaciens B34b	44.1[x]
F. succinogenes A3c + *R. flavefaciens* B34b	44.7[x]
F. succinogenes A3c + *Prevotella ruminicola* H8a	66.2[y]
Combination of 6 cultures[b]	54.6[z]
In vivo digestibility trials	59.8[w]

[a]Data from Dehority and Scott (1967) and Dehority (1991).
[b]*F. succinogenes* A3c; *R. flavefaciens* B1a and B34b; *R. albus* 7; *P. ruminicola* H8a; and *Butyrivibrio fibrisolvens* H10b.
[w,x,y,z]Means in the column followed by different superscripts differ at $P < 0.05$.

In vivo digestibility for these forages, as measured by sheep digestion trials, is less than A3c + H8a combined, similar to A3c alone and greater than all the others. The inhibition which occurs by combining A3c and B34b is partially alleviated with addition of the four additional cultures and almost completely disappears *in vivo*. A slightly lower extent of cellulose digestion *in vivo* would be expected as a result of passage rate through the rumen. Although the microbial interactions described are demonstrable *in vitro*, their importance *in vivo* may be extremely limited.

References

Akin, D. E. (1987). Use of chitinase to assess ruminal fungi associated with plant residues in vitro. *Applied and Environmental Microbiology*, **53**, 1955-1958.

Amann, R. I., L. Krumholz, and D. A. Stahl. (1990). Fluorescent-oligonucleotide probing of whole cells for determinative, phylogenetic, and environmental studies in microbiology. *Journal of Bacteriology*, **172**, 762-770.

Ankrah, P., S. C. Loerch, and B. A. Dehority. (1989). Occurrence of 2-aminoethylphosphonic acid in feeds, ruminal bacteria and duodenal digesta from defaunated sheep. *Journal of Animal Science*, **67**, 1061-1069.

Bailey, R. W. and B. H. Howard. (1963). Carbohydrases of the rumen ciliate *Epidinium ecaudatum* (Crawley). 2. α-Galactosidase and isomaltase. *Biochemical Journal*, **87**, 146-151.

Bauchart, D., F. Legay-Carmier, M. Doreau, and B. Gaillard. (1990). Lipid metabolism of liquid-associated and solid-adherent bacteria in rumen contents of dairy cows offered lipid-supplemented diets. *British Journal of Nutrition*, **63**, 563-578.

Bechdel, S. I., H. E. Honeywell, R. A. Dutcher, and M. H. Knutsen. (1928). Synthesis of vitamin B by bacteria in the rumen of cattle. *Journal of Biological Chemistry*, **80**, 231-238.

Bergen, W. G., D. B. Purser and J. H. Cline. (1968). Effect of ration on the nutritive quality of rumen microbial protein. *Journal of Animal Science,* **27**, 1497-1501.

Body, D. R. and T. Bauchop. (1985). Lipid composition of an obligatory anaerobic fungus, *Neocallimastix frontalis*, isolated from a bovine rumen. *Canadian Journal of Microbiology*, **31**, 463-466.

Bond, D. R. (1994). The effects of fiber source, defaunation, and antibiotic treatment on the anaerobic fungi population in vivo. M.S. Thesis. The Ohio State University, Columbus.

Bonhomme, A., G. Fonty and J. Senaud. (1982). Obtention de *Polyplastron multivesiculatum* (cilié entodiniomorphe du rumen) en condition axenique. *Journal of Protozoology*, **29**, 231-233.

Briesacher, S. L., T. May, K. N. Grigsby, M. S. Kerley, R. V. Anthony, and J. A. Paterson. (1992). Use of DNA probes to monitor nutritional effects on ruminal prokaryotes and *Fibrobacter succinogenes* S85. *Journal of Animal Science*, **70**, 289-295.

Broderick, G. A. and N. R. Merchen. (1992). Markers for quantifying microbial protein synthesis in the rumen. *Journal of Dairy Science*, **75**, 2618-2632.

Bryant, M. P., N. Small, C. Bouma, and H. Chu. (1958). *Bacteroides ruminicola* n. sp. and *Succinimonas amylolytica* the new genus and species. *Journal of Bacteriology,* **76**, 15-23.

Cecava, M. J., N. R. Merchen, L. L. Berger, and D. R. Nelson. (1990). Effect of energy level and feeding frequency on site of digestion and postruminal nutrient flows in steers. *Journal of Dairy Science*, **73**, 2470-2479.

Chan, W. W. and B. A. Dehority. 1999. Production of *Ruminococcus flavefaciens* growth inhibitor(s) by *Ruminococcus albus*. *Animal Feed Science and Technology*, **77**, 61-71.

Church, D. C. (1976). *Digestive Physiology and Nutrition of Ruminants.* Vol. 1. OSU Book Stores Inc., Corvallis, OR. USA.

Clarke, J. H., T. H. Klusmeyer, and M. K. Cameron. (1992). Microbial protein synthesis and flows of nitrogen fractions to the duodenum of dairy cows. *Journal of Dairy Science*, **75**, 2304-2323.

Craig, W. M., D. R. Brown, G. A. Broderick, and D. B. Ricker. (1987). Post-prandial composition changes of fluid- and particle-associated ruminal microorganisms. *Journal of Animal Science*, **65**, 1042-1048.

Czerkawski, J. W. (1974). Methods for determining 2, 6-diaminopimelic acid and 2-aminoethylphosphonic acid in gut contents. *Journal of Science and Food Agriculture*, **25**, 45-55.

Dawson, R.C.M. and P. Kemp. (1969). The effect of defaunation on the phospholipids and on the hydrogenation of unsaturated fatty acids in the rumen. *Biochemical Journal*, **115**, 351-352.

Dehority, B. A. (1991). Effects of microbial synergism on fibre digestion in the rumen. *Proceedings of The Nutrition Society*, **50**, 149-159.

Dehority, B. A. (1998). Microbial interactions in the rumen. *Revista de la Facultad de Agronomia* (Universidad del Zulia, Maracaibo, Venezuela), **15**, 69-86.

Dehority, B. A. and H. W. Scott. (1967). Extent of cellulose and hemicellulose digestion in various forages by pure cultures of rumen bacteria. *Journal of Dairy Science*, **50**, 1136-1141.

Doré, J. and D. A. Stahl. (1991). Phylogeny of anaerobic rumen Chytridiomycetes inferred from small subunit ribosomal RNA sequence comparisons. *Canadian Journal of Botany*, **69**, 1964-1971.

Doré, J., A. G. Brownlee, L. Millet, I. Virlogeux, M. Saigne, G. Fonty, and P. Gouet. (1993). Ribosomal DNA-targeted hybridization probes for the detection, identification and quantitation of anaerobic rumen fungi. *Proceedings of The Nutrition Society*, **52**, 176A.

Faichney, G. J., C. Poncet, B. Lassalas, J. P. Jouany, L. Millet, J. Doré, and A. G. Brownlee. (1997). Effect of concentrates in a hay diet on the contribution of anaerobic fungi, protozoa and bacteria to nitrogen in rumen and duodenal digesta in sheep. *Animal Feed Science and Technology*, **64**,193-213.

Firkins, J. L., L. L. Berger, N. R. Merchen, G. C. Fahey, Jr., and R. L. Mulvaney. (1987). Ruminal nitrogen metabolism in steers as affected by feed intake and dietary urea concentration. *Journal of Dairy Science*, **70**, 2302-2311.

Fondevila, M. and B. A. Dehority. (1996). Interactions between *Fibrobacter succinogenes, Prevotella ruminicola* and *Ruminococcus flavefaciens* in the digestion of cellulose from forages. *Journal of Animal Science*, **74**, 678-684.

Forster, R. J., J. Gong, and R. M. Teather. (1997). Group-specific 16S rRNA hybridization probes for determinative and community structure studies of *Butyrivibrio fibrisolvens* in the rumen. *Applied and Environmental Microbiology*, **63**, 1256-1260.

Garrett, J. E., R. D. Goodrich, and J. C. Meiske. (1982). Measurement of bacterial nitrogen using D-alanine. In: Protein Requirements for Cattle: Symposium. p 23. F. N. Owens (Ed.) Oklahoma State Univ., Stillwater.

Garrett, J. E., R. D. Goodrich, J. C. Meiske, and M. D. Stern. (1986). Influence of supplemental nitrogen source on digestion of nitrogen, dry matter and organic matter and on in vivo rate of ruminal protein degradation. *Journal of Animal Science,* **64**, 1801-1812.

Garton, G. A. (1958). Lipolysis in the rumen. *Nature,* **182**, 1511-1512.

Garton, G. A. (1965). The digestion and assimilation of lipids. In: *Physiology of Digestion in the Ruminant.* Edited by R. W. Dougherty. Butterworth Inc., Washington, D. C. USA. pp.390-398.

Garton, G. A. and A. E. Oxford. (1955). The nature of bacterial lipids in the rumen of hay-fed sheep. *Journal of the Science of Food and Agriculture,* **3**, 142-148.

Garton, G. A., A. K. Lough, and E. Vioque. (1961). Glyceride hydrolysis and glycerol fermentation by sheep rumen contents. *Journal of General Microbiology,* **25**, 215-225.

Gawthorne, J. W. and C. J. Nader. (1976). The effect of molybdenum on the conversion of sulphate to sulphide and microbial-protein-sulphur in the rumen of sheep. *British Journal of Nutrition,* **35**, 11-23.

Gay, L., M. Hebraud, V. Girard, and M. Fevre. (1988). La chitine synthase de *Neocallimastix frontalis* un marquer enzymatique de la biomasse fongique. *Reproduction Nutrition Development,* **28**, 69-70.

Gerson, T., A.S.D. King, K. E. Kelly, and W. J. Kelly. (1988). Influence of particle size and surface area on *in vitro* rates of gas production, lipolysis of triacylglycerol and hydrogenation of linoleic acid by sheep rumen digesta or *Ruminococcus flavefaciens. Journal of Agricultural Science,* Cambridge, **110**, 31-37.

Girard, V. and J. C. Hawke. (1978). The role of holotrichs in the metabolism of dietary linoleic acid in the rumen. *Biochemical Biophysical Acta,* **528**, 17-27.

Gomez-Alarcon, R. A., C. O'Dowd, J.A.Z. Leedle, and M. P. Bryant. (1982). 1,4-naphthoquinone and other nutrient requirements of *Succinivibrio dextrinosolvens. Applied and Environmental Microbiology,* **44**, 346-350.

Griinari, J. M. and D. E. Bauman. (1999). Biosynthesis of conjugated linoleic acid and its incorporation into meat and milk in ruminants. In *Advances in Conjugated Linoleic Acid Research,* Vol. 1. Edited by P. Yurawez, M.M. Mossoba, J.K.G. Kramer, G. Nelson and M.W. Pariza. American Oil Chemists Society Press. Champaign, IL, USA. pp. 180-200.

Gulati, S. K., J. R. Ashes, and G.L.R. Gordon. (1989). Nutritional availability of amino acids from the rumen anaerobic fungus *Neocallimastix* sp. LM1 in sheep. *Journal of Agricultural Science,* Cambridge, **113**, 383-387.

Harfoot, C. G. (1978). Lipid metabolism in the rumen. *Progress in Lipid Research,* **17**, 21-54.

Harfoot, C. G. and G. P. Hazelwood. (1997). Lipid metabolism in the rumen. In: *The Rumen Microbial Ecosystem.* Second edition. Blackie Academic & Professional, Chapman and Hall, London, UK. pp. 382-426.

Harfoot, C. G., R. C. Noble and J. H. Moore. (1975). The role of plant particles, bacteria and cell-free supernatant fractions of rumen contents in the hydrolysis of trilinolein and subsequent hydrogenation of linoleic acid. *Antonie van Leeuwenhoek*, **41**, 533-542.

Hazelwood, G. P. and R. M.C. Dawson. (1975). Isolation and properties of a phospholipid-hydrolysing bacterium from ovine rumen fluid. *Journal of General Microbiology*, **89**, 163-174.

Hazlewood, G. P. and R.M.C. Dawson. (1979). Characteristics of a lipolytic and fatty acid-requiring *Butyrivibrio* sp. isolated from the ovine rumen. *Journal of General Microbiology*, **112**, 15-27.

Hazlewood, G. P., P. Kemp, D. Lander, and R.M.C. Dawson. (1976). C_{18} unsaturated fatty acid hydrogenation patterns of some rumen bacteria and their ability to hydrolyse exogenous phospholipid. *British Journal of Nutrition*, **35**, 293-297.

Henderson, C. (1971). A study of the lipase produced by *Anaerovibrio lipolytica*, a rumen bacterium. *Journal of General Microbiology*, **65**, 81-89.

Hespell, R. B. and M. P. Bryant. (1979). Efficiency of rumen microbial growth: influence of some theoretical and experimental factors on Y_{ATP}. *Journal of Animal Science*, **49**, 1640-1659.

Hobson, P. N. and S. O. Mann. (1961). The isolation of glycerol-fermenting and lipolytic bacteria from the rumen of the sheep. *Journal of General Microbiology*, **25**, 227-240.

Horigane, A. and M. Horiguchi. (1990). Nutritional aspects and metabolism of aminophosphonic acids in ruminants. In: *The Rumen Ecosystem. The Microbial Metabolism and Its Regulation.* Edited by S. Hoshino, R. Onodera, H. Minato and H. Itabashi. Springer-Verlag, New York, NY. pp. 51-60.

Howard, B. H. (1959). The biochemistry of rumen protozoa. 1. Carbohydrate fermentation by *Dasytricha* and *Isotricha*. *Biochemical Journal*, **71**, 671-675.

Hungate, R. E. (1966). *The Rumen and its Microbes.* Academic Press. New York, N.Y.

Hunt, C. H., O. G. Bentley, T. V. Hershberger and J. H. Cline. (1954). The effect of carbohydrates and sulfur on B-vitamins synthesis, cellulose digestion, and urea utilization by rumen microorganisms *in vitro*. *Journal of Animal Science*, **13**, 570-580.

Kalmokoff, M. L. and R. M. Teather. (1997). Isolation and characterization of a bacteriocin (Butyrivibriocin AR10) from the ruminal anaerobe *Butyrivibrio fibrisolvens* AR10: evidence in support of the widespread occurrence of bacteriocin-like activity among rumen isolates of *B. fibrisolvens*. *Applied and Environmental Microbiology*, **63**, 394-402.

Kandatsu, M. and N. Takahashi. (1955a). Studies on reticulo-rumen digestion. Part 2. On the artificial culture of some *Entodina* I. *Journal of the Agricultural Chemistry Society, Japan*, **29**, 883-839.

Kandatsu, M. and N. Takahashi. (1955b). Studies on reticulo-rumen digestion. Part 3. On the artificial culture of some *Entodina* II. *Journal of the Agricultural Chemistry Society, Japan*, **29**, 915-920.

Kandatsu, M. and N. Takahashi. (1956). Studies on reticulo-rumen digestion. Part 4. On the artificial culture of some *Entodina* III. *Journal of the Agricultural Chemistry Society, Japan*, **30**, 96-101.

Karnati, S.K.R., Z. Yu, J. T. Sylvester, B. A. Dehority, M. Morrison and J. L. Firkins. (2003). Specific PCR amplification of protozoal 18S rDNA sequences from DNA extracted from rumen samples of cows for ecological analysis of ruminal protozoa. *Journal of Animal Science*, **81**, 812-815.

Keeny, M. (1970). Lipid metabolism in the rumen. In: *Physiology of Digestion and Metabolism in the Ruminant.* Edited by A. T. Phillipson. Oriel Press, Newcastle-upon-Tyne, pp. 489-503.

Kemp, P., D. J. Lander, and C. G. Orpin. (1984). The lipids of the rumen fungus *Piromonas communis*. *Journal of General Microbiology*, **130**, 27-37.

Kemp, P., D. J. Jordan and C. G. Orpin. (1985). The free and protein amino acids of the rumen phycomycete fungi *Neocallimastix frontalis* and *Piromyces communis*. *Journal of Agricultural Science*, **105**, 523-526.

Kepler, C. R., K. P. Hirons, J. J. McNeill, and S. B. Tove. (1966). Intermediates and products of the biohydrogenation of linoleic acid by *Butyrivibrio fibrisolvens*. *Journal of Biological Chemistry*, **241**, 1350-1354.

Kim, Y. J., R. H. Liu, D. R. Bond, and J. B. Russell. (2000). Effect of linoleic acid concentration on conjugated linoleic acid production by *Butyrivibrio fibrisolvens* A38. *Applied and Environmental Microbiology*, **66**, 5226-5230.

Kim, Y. J., R. H. Liu, J. L. Rychlik, and J. B. Russell. (2002). The enrichment of a ruminal bacterium (*Megasphaera elsdenii* YJ-4) that produces the *trans*-10, *cis*-12 isomer of conjugated linoleic acid. *Journal of Applied Microbiology*, **92**, 976-982.

Kon, S. K. and J.W.G. Porter. (1953). The B vitamin content of the rumen of steers given various diets. *Proceedings of the Nutrition Society*, **12**, xii.

Krause, D. O., W.J.M. Smith, F.M.E. Ryan, R. I. Mackie, and C.S. McSweeney. (2000). Use of 16S-rRNA based techniques to investigate the ecological succession of microbial populations in the immature lamb rumen: Tracking of a specific strain of inoculated *Ruminococcus* and interactions with other microbial populations *in vivo*. *Microbial Ecology*, **38**, 365-376.

Latham, M. J., J. E. Storry, and M. E. Sharpe. (1972). Effect of low-roughage diets on the microflora and lipid metabolism in the rumen. *Applied Microbiology*, **24**, 871-877.

Legay-Carmier, F., D. Bauchart, and M. Doreau. (1989). Distribution of bacteria in the rumen contents of dairy cows given a diet supplemented with soybean oil. *British Journal of Nutrition*, **61**, 725-740.

Ling, J. R. (1990). Digestion of bacterial cell walls in the rumen. In: *The Rumen Ecosystem. The Microbial Metabolism and Its Regulation.* Edited by S. Hoshino, R. Onodera, H. Minato, and H. Itabashi. Springer-Verlag, New York, NY. pp. 83-90.

Lubinsky, G. (1957). Note on the phylogenetic significance of predatory habits in the Ophryoscolecidae (Cilata:Oligotricha). *Canadian Journal of Zoology*, **35**, 579-580.

Martin, S. A., and T. C. Jenkins. (2002). Factors affecting conjugated linoleic acid and *trans*-$C_{18:1}$ fatty acid production by mixed ruminal bacteria. *Journal of Animal Science*, **80**, 3347-3352.

Masson, H. A., A. M. Denholm, and J. R. Ling. (1991). In vivo metabolism of 2, 2'-diaminopimelic acid from Gram-positive and Gram-negative bacterial cells by ruminal microorganisms and ruminants and its use as a marker of bacterial biomass. *Applied and Environmental Microbiology*, **57**, 1714-1720.

McElroy, L. W., and H. Goss. (1940). A quantitative study of vitamins in the rumen contents of sheep and cows fed vitamin-low diets. I. Riboflavin and vitamin K. *Journal of Nutrition*, **20**, 527-541.

McNaught, M. L., E. C. Owens, K. M. Henry and S. K. Kon. (1954). The utilization of nonprotein nitrogen in the bovine rumen. 8. The nutritive value of the proteins of preparations of dried rumen bacteria, rumen protozoa and brewer's yeast for rats. *Biochemical Journal,* **56,** 151-156.

Michalet-Doreau, B., I. Fernandez, and G. Fonty. (2002). A comparison of enzymatic and molecular approaches to characterize the cellulolytic microbial ecosystems of the rumen and the cecum. *Journal of Animal Science*, **80**, 790-796.

Miura, H., M. Horiguchi, and T. Matsumoto. (1980). Nutritional interdependence among rumen bacteria, *Bacteroides amylophilus, Megasphaera elsdenii,* and *Ruminococcus albus*. *Applied and Environmental Microbiology*, **40**, 294-300.

Newbold, C. J., and K. Hillman. 1990. The effect of ciliate protozoa on the turnover of bacterial and fungal protein in the rumen of sheep. *Letters in Applied Microbiology*, **11,** 100-102.

Newbold, C. J., B. A. Dehority, J. Sylvester, J. Firkins, M. Morrison, Z. Yu, G. Van der Staay, J.H.P. Hackstein, P. Pristaš, K. Kišidayová, J. -P. Jouany, T. Michaowski, and N. R. McEwan. (2002). Identification of rumen protozoa by PCR-RFLP. *Reproduction Nutrition Development*, **42** (Suppl. 1),S82.

Obispo, N. E., and B. A. Dehority. (1999). Feasibility of using total purines as a marker for ruminal bacteria. *Journal of Animal Science*, **77**, 3084-3095.

Odenyo, A. A., R. I. Mackie, D. A. Stahl, and B. A. White. (1994a). The use of 16S rDNA-targeted oligonucleotide probes to study competition between ruminal fibrolytic bacteria: development of probes for *Ruminococcus* species and evidence for bacteriocin production. *Applied and Environmental Microbiology*, **60**, 3688-3696.

Odenyo, A. A., R. I. Mackie, D. A. Stahl, and B. A. White. (1994b). The use of 16S rRNA-targeted oligonucleotide probes to study competition between ruminal fibrolytic bacteria: pure-culture studies with cellulose and alkaline peroxide-treated wheat straw. *Applied and Environmental Microbiology*, **60**, 3697-3793.

Orpin, C. G. (1977). Studies on the defaunation of the ovine rumen using dioctyl sodium sulphosuccinate. *Journal of Applied Bacteriology*, **43**, 309-318.

Orpin, C. G. (1977). The occurrence of chitin in the cell walls of the rumen organisms *Neocallimastix frontalis, Piromonas communis* and *Sphaeromonas communis*. *Journal of General Microbiology,* **99**, 215-218.

Orpin, C. G. and Y. Greenwood. (1986). Nutrition and germination requirements of the rumen phycomycete *Neocallimastix patriciarum*. *Transactions of the British Mycological Society*, **86**, 103-109.

Oser, B. L. (1951). Method of integrating essential amino acid content in the nutritional evaluation of protein. *Journal of the American Dietetic Association*, **27**, 396-402.

Owens, F. N. and A. L. Goetsch. (1988). Ruminal fermentation. In: *The Ruminant Animal. Digestive Physiology and Nutrition*. Edited by D. C. Church. Waveland Press, Inc., Prospect Heights, IL, USA. pp. 145-171.

Owens, F. N. and C. F. Hanson. (1992). External and internal markers for appraising site and extent of digestion in ruminants. *Journal of Dairy Science*, **75**, 2605-2617.

Owens, F. N. and R. Zinn. (1988). Protein metabolism of ruminant animals. In: *The Ruminant Animal, Digestive Physiology and Nutrition.* Edited by D. C. Church. Waveland Press, Inc. Prospect Heights, IL, USA. pp.227-249.

Phillips, M. W. and G.L.R. Gordon. (1989). Growth characteristics on cellobiose of three different anaerobic fungi isolated from the ovine rumen. *Applied and Environmental Microbiology*, **55**, 1695-1702.

Polan, C. E., J. J. McNeill, and S. B. Tove. (1964). Biohydrogenation of unsaturated fatty acids by rumen bacteria. *Journal of Bacteriology*, **88**, 1056-1064.

Prins, R. A. (1991) The rumen cilaites and their functions. In: *Rumen Microbial Meatbolism and Ruminant Digestion*. Edited by J. P. Jouany. INRA Editions, Paris. pp. 39-52.

Prins, R. A., and C.J.A.H.V. van den Vorstenbosch. (1975). Interrelationships between rumen microorganisms. In: Miscellaneous Papers, Landbouwhogeschool Wageningen. pp. 15.

Prins, R. A., A. Lankhorst, P. Van der Meer, and C. J. Van Nevel. (1975). Some characteristics of *Anaerovibrio lipolytica*, a rumen lipolytic organism. *Antonie van Leeuwenhoek,* **41**, 1-11.

Purser, D. B. and S. M. Buechler. (1966). Amino acid composition of rumen organisms.

Journal of Dairy Science, **49**, 81-84.

Quigley, J.D. III and C. G. Schwab. (1988). Comparison of D-alanine and diaminopimelic acid as bacterial markers in young calves. *Journal of Animal Science*, **66**, 758-763.

Rahnema, S. H., and B. Theurer. (1986). Comparison of various amino acids for estimation of microbial nitrogen in digesta. *Journal of Animal Science*, **63**, 603-612.

Reiser, R. (1951). Hydrogenation of polyunsaturated fatty acids by the ruminant. *Federation Proceedings*, **10**, 236.

Romulo, B. H., S. H. Bird, and R. A. Leng. (1986). The effects of defaunation on digestibility and rumen fungi counts in sheep fed high-fibre diets. *Proceedings of the Australian Society of Animal Production*, **16**, 327-330.

Russell, J. B. (1985). Fermentaion of cellodextrins by cellulolytic and noncellulolytic rumen bacteria. *Applied and Environmental Microbiology*, **49**, 572-576.

Russell, J. B. and R. J. Wallace. (1988). Energy yielding and consuming reactions. In: *The Rumen Microbial Ecosystem.* Edited by P. N. Hobson. Elsevier Science Publications, London. pp. 185-216.

Saluzzi, L., A. Smith, and C. S. Stewart. (1993). Analysis of bacterial phospholipid markers and plant monosaccharides during forage degradation by *Ruminococcus flavefaciens* and *Fibrobacter succinogenes* in co-culture. *Journal of General Microbiology*, **139**, 2865-2873.

Scheifinger, C.C. and M. J. Wolin. (1973). Propionate formation from cellulose and soluble sugars by combined cultures of *Bacteriodes succinogenes* and *Selenomonas ruminantium*. *Journal of Applied Microbiology*, **25**, 789-795.

Schelling, G. T., S. E. Koenig, and T. C. Jackson, Jr. (1982). Nucleic acids and purine or pyrimidine bases as markers for protein synthesis in the rumen. In: *Protein Requirements for Cattle*: Symposium. Edited by F.N. Owens. Oklahoma State Univ., Stillwater. pp. 1-9.

Scott, H. W. and B. A. Dehority. (1965). Vitamin requirements of several cellulolytic rumen bacteria. *Journal of Bacteriology*, **89**, 1169-1175.

Shorland, F. B., R. O. Weenink, and A. T. Johns. (1955). Effect of the rumen on dietary fat. *Nature, (London)*, **175**, 1129.

Singh, S. and J. C. Hawke. (1979). The *in vitro* lipolysis and biohydrogenation of monogalactosyldiglyceride by whole rumen contents and its fractions. *Journal of Science and Food Agriculture*, **30**, 603-612.

Slyter, L. L. and J. M. Weaver. (1977). Tetrahydrofolate and other growth requirements of certain strains of *Ruminococcus flavefaciens*. *Applied and Environmental Microbiology*, **33**, 363-369.

Smith, R. H. and A. B. McAllan. (1974). Some factors influencing the chemical composition of mixed rumen bacteria. *British Journal of Nutrition*, **31**, 27-34.

Soetanto, H., G.L.R. Gordon, I. D. Hume, and R. A. Leng. 1985. The role of protozoa and fungi in fibre digestion in the rumen of sheep. *Proceedings of the 3rd AAAP*

Animal Science Congress, **2**, 805-807.

Stahl, D. A., B. A, Flesher, H. R. Mansfield and L. A. Montgomery. (1988). Use of phylogenetically based hybridization probes for studies of ruminal microbial ecology. *Applied and Environmental Microbiology*, **54**, 1079-1084.

Stern, M. D. and W. H. Hoover. (1979). Methods for determining and factors affecting rumen microbial protein synthesis: A review. *Journal of Animal Science*, **49**, 1590-1603.

Stern, M. D., G. A. Varga, J. H. Clark, J. L. Firkins, J. T. Huber, and D. L. Palmquist. (1994). Evaluation of chemical and physical properties of feeds that affect protein metabolism in the rumen. *Journal of Dairy Science*, **77**, 2762-2786.

Titgemeyer, E. C., N. R. Merchen, and L. L. Berger. (1989). Evaluation of soybean meal, corn gluten meal, blood meal and fish meal as sources of nitrogen and amino acids disappearing from the small intestine of steers. *Journal of Animal Science*, **67**, 262-275.

Ushida, K., H. Tanaka, and Y. Kojima. (1989). A simple in situ method for estimating fungal population size in the rumen. *Letters in Applied Microbiology*, **9**, 109-111.

Van Nevel, C. and D. I. Demeyer. (1977). Determination of rumen microbial growth in vitro from ^{32}P labelled phosphate incorporation. *British Journal of Nutrition*, **38**, 101-114.

Van Soest, P. J. (1994). *Nutritional Ecology of the Ruminant*. Cornell University Press, Ithaca, NY.

Virtanen, A. I. (1963). Production of cow milk without [feeding] protein, with urea and ammonium salts as nitrogen source and purified carbohydrates as energy source. *Biochemische Zeitschrift*, **338**, 443-453.

Wallace, R. J. (1985). Synergism between different species of proteolytic rumen bacteria. *Current Microbiology*, **12**, 59-64.

Wallace, R. J. and A. A. West. (1982). Adenosine 5'-triphosphate and adenylate energy charge in sheep digesta. *Journal of Agricultural Science* (Cambridge) **98**, 523-528.

Ward, P.F.V., T. W. Scott, and R.M.C. Dawson. (1964). The hydrogenation of unsaturated fatty acids in the ovine digestive tract. *Biochemistry Journal*, **92**, 60-68.

Weller, R. A. (1957). The amino acid composition of hydrolysates of microbial preparations from the rumen of sheep. *Australian Journal of Biological Science*, **10**, 384-389.

Whitelaw, F. G., L. A. Bruce, J. M. Eadie, and W. J. Shand. (1983). 2-Aminoethylphosphonic acid concentrations in some rumen ciliate protozoa. *Applied and Environmental Microbiology*, **46**, 951-953.

Williams, A. G. and G. S. Coleman. (1988). The rumen protozoa. In: *The Rumen Microbial Ecosystem*. Edited by P. N. Hobson. Elsevier Applied Science, London. pp. 77-182.

Williams, A. G. and G. S. Coleman. (1992). The rumen protozoa. Springer-Verlag New York, Inc., New York, N.Y.
Williams, A. G.. and S. E. Withers. (1993). Changes in the rumen microbial populations and its activities during the refaunation period after the reintroduction of ciliate protozoa into the rumen of defaunated sheep. *Canadian Journal of Microbiology*, **31**, 61-69.
Williams, A. G., K. N. Joblin, and G. Fonty. (1994). Interactions between the rumen chytrid fungi and other microorganisms. In: *Anaerobic Fungi*. Edited by D. O. Mountford and C. G. Orpin. Marcel Dekker, Inc., New York. pp. 191-228.
Wintzingerode, F. V., U. B. Göbel, and E. Stackebrandt. (1997). Determination of microbial diversity in environmental samples: pitfalls of PCR-based rRNA analysis. *FEMS Microbiology Reviews*, **21**, 213-229.
Wolin, M. J. and T. L. Miller. (1988). Microbe-microbe interactions. In: *The Rumen Microbial Ecosystem*. Edited by P. N. Hobson. Elsevier Scientific Publication Ltd., London. pp. 343-359.
Wolin, M. J., T. L. Miller, and C. S. Stewart. (1997). Microbe-microbe interactions. In: *The Rumen Microbial Ecosystem*, 2nd Edition. Edited by P. N. Hobson and C. S. Stewart. Blackie Academic & Professional, London, UK. pp. 467-491.
Wolstrup, J. and K. Jensen. (1978). Adenosine triphosphate and deoxyribonucleic acid in the alimentary tract of cattle fed different nitrogen sources. *Journal of Applied Bacteriology*, **45**, 49-56.
Wood, J., K. P. Scott, G. Avguštin, C. J. Newbold, and H. J. Flint. (1998). Estimation of the relative abundance of different *Bacteroides* and *Prevotella* ribotypes in gut samples by restriction enzyme profiling of PCR-amplified 16S rRNA gene sequences. *Applied and Environmental Microbiology*, **64**, 3683-3689.
Wright, D. E. (1959). Hydrogenation of lipids by rumen protozoa. *Nature (London)*, **184**, 875-876.
Wright, D. E. (1960). Hydrogenation of chloroplast lipids by rumen bacteria. *Nature (London)*, **185**, 546-547.
Wright, D. E. (1961). Bloat in cattle. XX. Lipase activity of rumen microorganisms. *New Zealand Journal of Agricultural Research*, **4**, 216-223.
Zinn, R. A. and F. N. Owens. (1986). A rapid procedure for purine measurement and its use for estimating net ruminal protein synthesis. *Canadian Journal of Animal Science*, **66**, 157-166.

APPENDIX

The subject material included in this book has been used as the major source of information presented to students in the Rumen Microbiology course at The Ohio State University. As mentioned in the Preface, this course included a laboratory. Although there were variations over the years, the primary Experiments included were as follows:

Experiment No.1. Gastrointestinal anatomy of the ruminant animal and procedures used for sampling rumen contents.

OBJECTIVES

1. Surgical removal of the gastrointestinal (GI) tract from a sheep and observation of the structure and linings of the various compartments.
2. Demonstrate the procedure used to determine total weight of rumen-reticulum contents and to obtain a subsample of rumen contents from the sacrificed sheep.
3. Demonstrate methods used for obtaining samples of rumen contents through a fistula and by stomach tube (sheep and cattle).
4. Demonstration of the procedures used for subsampling rumen contents and preserving in formalin.
5. Observation of protozoa in live mounts of rumen contents.

EXPERIMENTAL PROCEDURES

1. A small plastic container (10-50 ml capacity, depending upon the size of particulate matter in the sample), is filled with a subsample of rumen contents which are transferred to a beaker and preserved by adding an equal volume (use the same container) of 50% formalin (18.5% formaldehyde).
2. After the sample has been preserved, filter some of the remaining rumen contents through a small square of cheesecloth and place several drops of the fluid on a slide. Use a cover slip and observe the live mounts microscopically.
3. Duplicate one ml aliquots of the preserved sample are pipetted into 16 x 150 mm test tubes using a wide-bore pipette. Two drops of Brilliant green dye are added, the tubes mixed and allowed to stand at least 4 hours (overnight is preferable).

REAGENTS

1. 50% formalin (Commercial 37% formaldehyde solution is diluted with an equal quantity of distilled H_2O).

2.   Brilliant green dye: 2.0 g Brilliant green
2.0 ml Glacial acetic acid
Dilute to 100 ml with distilled H_2O.

REFERENCES

Dehority, B. A. 1984. Evaluation of subsampling and fixation procedures used for counting rumen protozoa. *Applied and Environmental Microbiology*, **48**, 182-185.

Experiment No. 2. Diurnal changes in rumen pH and protozoal numbers.

OBJECTIVES

1. Demonstrate procedures for diluting the stained protozoal sample from Expt. 1 and filling the Sedgewick-Rafter chamber used for counting protozoa. Work with each student individually to explain how to determine size of counting grid, how to use grid for counting, how to recognize protozoa genera and how to calculate protozoal concentration.
2. Using a fistulated animal, measure pH and concentration of rumen protozoa in rumen contents at various times after feeding in an animal fed once daily (0, 0.5, 1.5, 3, 6, 9 and 24 hours).
3. Identify protozoa to the subfamily or generic level.

EXPERIMENTAL PROCEDURE

1. Remove samples of rumen contents from the animal at the required times, return to laboratory and measure pH as quickly as possible.
2. Subsample and fix the rumen contents for subsequent counting.
3. Nine ml of 30% glycerol are added to the one ml stained sample, giving a 1:20 dilution of the original rumen contents. A 30% glycerol solution is used because it has a high enough viscosity to prevent rapid settling of the protozoa during the process of pipetting subsamples for counting or further dilution. However, the protozoan cells will settle to the bottom of the counting chamber in a short time, i.e., 5 to 10 minutes.
4. Using a wide-bore pipet, a one ml aliquot of the stained 1:20 dilution is pipetted into a Sedgewick-Rafter chamber. Counts are made microscopically using a l0x eyepiece and l0x objective for a total magnification of 100x. A counting grid measuring 0.5 mm square is used in the eyepiece. A diagram of the grid is shown below.

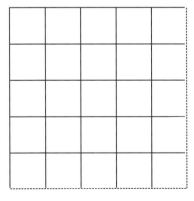

As a standard practice, any protozoan cells touching the two solid outside lines (top and left side) are counted, while any cells touching the dotted outside lines (bottom and right side) are not counted. Two to five grids are quickly counted and the approximate total number of protozoa that would be counted in 50 fields is calculated. If required, a further dilution is made to bring the total count for 50 grids into the range of 100 to 200 protozoa. For example, if there are 43 protozoa in five grids, the total would be about 430 in 50 grids. Diluting 1:3 with 30% glycerol would bring the total count down to approximately 143. The final dilution is then 1:20 x 1:3 = 1:60.

5. Concentration of protozoa per ml of original rumen contents is calculated as follows:

No. in 50 grids × volume of cell/volume of 50 grids × dilution

Volume of cell = 20mm × 50 mm × 1mm = 1000 mm^3.
Volume of 50 grids = 0.5 mm × 0.5 mm × 1 mm × 50 = 12.5 mm^3.

or:

No. in 50 grids × 1000/12.5 × dilution = concentration/ ml

REFERENCES

Dehority, B. A. 1984. Evaluation of subsampling and fixation procedures used for counting rumen protozoa. *Applied and Environmental Microbiology*, **48**, 182-185.

Dehority, B. A. 1993. *Laboratory Manual for Classification and Morphology of Rumen Ciliate Protozoa*. CRC Press, Inc., Boca Raton, FL.

Experiment No. 3. Comparison of the generic distribution of protozoa in a single sheep sequentially fed an all forage diet and a 60% corn-40% forage diet.

OBJECTIVES

1. Determine total concentration and the subfamily and generic composition of protozoa in the same sheep when switched from all forage to a 60% corn-40% forage diet.
2. Demonstrate the methodology for staining the nucleus and skeletal plates.
3. Identify and make drawings of at least one species of *Entodinium* and Diplodiniinae from each diet.

EXPERIMENTAL PROCEDURE

1. Obtain samples of rumen contents from the sheep prior to the morning feeding and preserve as in Expt. 1. Allow two weeks on 60-40 diet before sampling.
2. Using the key for identifying genera of rumen protozoa (Dehority, 1993), make a total count while simultaneously classifying protozoa into the following subfamily and genera:
   Isotricha
   Dasytricha
   Entodinium
   Diplodiniinae (contains the genera *Diplodinium, Eudiplodinium, Ostracodinium, Metadinium, Enoploplastron, Elytroplastron,* and *Polyplastron*) NOTE: It is extremely difficult to identify these to the generic level at the maximum magnification of 100x usable with the Sedgewick-Rafter chamber.
   Epidinium
   Ophryoscolex
3. For species identification the following procedures are used:
   a. Filter the preserved sample through a single layer of cheese cloth to remove particulate matter.
   b. Two to three drops of acidified methylene blue are added to one ml of the filtered sample. The sample is mixed and allowed to stand 4-6h or overnight. The sample is then examined microscopically on a slide with cover slip, either at 450x or 1000x. Cell measurements (length, width, length of macronucleus, etc.) should be made using the calibrated ocular scale. Methylene blue stains the macronucleus and micronucleus a dark blue.
   c. Approximately one-half ml of Lugol's iodine is added to one ml of the filtered sample. The sample should be examined as described above about 15-30 minutes after the addition of Lugol's iodine. If present, skeletal plates are stained a deep reddish-brown.

REAGENTS

1. Acidified methylene blue:

    Methylene blue - 0.5 g
    Acetic acid   - 2.0 ml
    Distilled H_2O - to 100 ml volume

2. Lugol's iodine:

    Iodine   - 1.0 g
    KI   - 2.0 g
    Distilled H_2O - 300.0 ml

    Dissolve KI in distilled water and then add the iodine.

REFERENCES

Dehority, B. A. 1978. Specificity of rumen ciliate protozoa in cattle and sheep. *Journal of Protozoology*, **25**, 509-513.

Dehority, B. A. 1993. *Laboratory Manual for Classification and Morphology of Rumen Ciliate Protozoa.* CRC Press, Inc., Boca Raton, Fl.

Experiment No. 4. Most-probable-number procedures for enumeration of total and cellulolytic rumen bacterial numbers.

OBJECTIVES

1. Observe the laboratory procedures used to prepare anaerobic dilution solution (ADS) and most-probable-number (MPN) broth.
2. Observe the procedures used in diluting rumen contents and inoculating a three tube MPN assay.
3. Preparation of ADS and MPN broth by each student for subsequent use.

EXPERIMENTAL PROCEDURES

1. Class will meet in the laboratory for a demonstration of anaerobic techniques used in rumen microbiology. ADS and MPN broth will be prepared by the instructor.
2. Using the ADS and MPN broth prepared under step 1, rumen contents will be diluted and an MPN assay inoculated.
3. Each student will prepare their own ADS and MPN broth for use in Expt. 5.

DILUTION SOLUTION AND MEDIA

1. Anaerobic dilution solution (ADS) - 300 ml:
    - 45.0 ml Mineral solution I*
    - 45.0 ml Mineral solution II*
    - 0.3 ml of 0.1 % Resazurin solution
    - 197.0 ml distilled water

    *See MPN medium for composition

    Heat flask carefully over burner and gas with O_2 free CO_2. When solution is fairly well reduced (changes from pink to colorless), add:
    - 7.5 ml of 12% Na_2CO_3
    - 5.0 ml of 3% cysteine-HCl

    Tube 9.0 ml aliquots anaerobically under CO_2 into 13 culture tubes. Pipet an additional 3 ml of ADS from the flask and discard. Seal the flask (containing 180 ml ADS) with a rubber stopper and wire in place. Autoclave tubes in racks and the flask for 20 min at 15# pressure.

2. MPN broth - 300 ml:
   - 45.0 ml Mineral solution I*
   - 45.0 ml Mineral solution II**
   - 0.3 ml of 0.1% Resazurin solution
   - 0.3 g glucose
   - 0.3 g cellobiose
   - 0.3 g maltose
   - 0.3 g xylose
   - 75.0 ml of a 3% suspension of ball-milled cellulose (Sigmacell-20)
   - 120.0 ml of Rumen Fluid (Supernatant from centrifugation at 1000 x g for 10 min)

Gas with CO_2 and heat carefully over burner. When medium is fairly well reduced, add:
   - 10.0 ml of 12% Na_2CO_3

Continue gassing for about 20 min, then add:
   - 5.0 ml of 3% cysteine-HCl

Gas for an additional 10-15 min and check pH. If pH is outside the range of 6.6 to 6.9, adjust as required with NaOH or H_3PO_4. Tube anaerobically in 8.0 ml aliquots into 16 x 150 mm tubes. Autoclave in tubes at 15# for 20 min.

*Mineral solution I:
3.0 g K_2HPO_4 / liter

**Mineral solution II:
3.0 g KH_2PO_4 / liter
6.0 g $(NH_4)_2SO_4$ / liter
6.0 g NaCl / liter
0.6 g $MgSO_4$ / liter
0.795 g $CaCl_2 \cdot 2H_2O$ / liter

DILUTION OF RUMEN CONTENTS

1. Add 180 ml of sterile reduced ADS to a previously steamed Waring Blender cup and pass a vigorous stream of CO_2 into the blender.
2. Weigh out 20 g of rumen ingesta into a previously steamed beaker and transfer ingesta to the blender cup. A pipette can be used to aid in the transfer.
3. Blend vigorously for two minutes, while directing a stream of CO_2 into the vortex of the mixing contents.

4. This 1:10 dilution of rumen contents is then serially diluted in 9.0 ml ADS tubes out to the 10^{-11} dilution (final tube thus contains 1×10^{-11} g rumen contents/ml). Each dilution tube should be shaken 30 times before sub-sampling.

MPN ASSAY

1. Three MPN broth tubes are inoculated with 1.0 ml from each dilution tube, beginning with the 10^{-6} dilution (18 total tubes). The MPN tubes thus contain 10^{-6}, 10^{-7}, 10^{-8}, 10^{-9}, 10^{-10}, 10^{-11} g per tube.
2. After two weeks, growth of the cellulolytic bacteria is estimated by visible loss of cellulose and total bacterial growth by a decrease in pH (measured on pH meter).
3. A typical set of readings might be as follows:

Dilution	Visible loss of cellulose	Decrease in pH*
10^{-6}	3	3
10^{-7}	3	3
10^{-8}	2	3
10^{-9}	0	3
10^{-10}	0	1
10^{-11}	0	0

*Tubes with a decrease in pH greater than 0.2 units are scored as positive.

Numbers are then estimated from a three tube MPN table (attached to the end of this Expt.). It is desirable that your sample has been diluted to extinction, i.e., no growth.

4. The MPN table is based on 10-fold dilutions, and the MPN value represents the number of organisms present in the next lower dilution. For example, using visible loss of cellulose as a criterion, reading the 10^{-7}, 10^{-8}, 10^{-9} tubes (3, 2, 0) from the table, gives an MPN of 93×10^6 cellulolytic bacteria per gram of rumen contents. For total bacterial concentration (decrease in pH), the 10^{-9}, 10^{-10}, 10^{-11} tubes (3, 1, 0) give an MPN number of 43×10^8 total bacteria per gram of rumen contents.
5. A more accurate estimate of bacterial numbers can be obtained by using a five tube MPN assay and reading from an appropriate MPN table; however, the increase in accuracy may be slight and considerably more time and media are required.

GENERAL REFERENCES

Bryant, M. P. and L. A. Burkey. 1953. Cultural methods and some characteristics of some of the more numerous groups of bacteria in the bovine rumen. *Journal of Dairy Science*, **36**, 205-217.

Dehority, B. A., P. A. Tirabasso and A. P. Grifo, Jr. 1989. Most-probable-number procedures for enumerating ruminal bacteria, including the simultaneous estimation of total and cellulolytic numbers in one medium. *Applied and Environmental Microbiology*, **55**, 2789-2792.

Grubb, J. A. and B. A. Dehority. 1976. Variation in colony counts of total viable anaerobic rumen bacteria as influenced by media and cultural methods. *Applied and Environmental Microbiology*, **31**, 262-267.

MPN Table for Three Tube Assay

Tubes positive				Tubes positive				Tubes positive			
10 ml	*1.0 ml*	*0.1 ml*	*MPN*	*10 ml*	*1.0 ml*	*0.1 ml*	*MPN*	*10 ml*	*1.0 ml*	*0.1 ml*	*MPN*
0	0	1	3	1	2	0	11	2	3	3	53
0	0	2	6	1	2	1	15	3	0	0	23
0	0	3	9	1	2	2	20	3	0	1	39
0	1	0	3	1	2	3	24	3	0	2	64
0	1	1	6	1	3	0	16	3	0	3	95
0	1	2	9	1	3	1	20	3	1	0	43
0	1	3	12	1	3	2	24	3	1	1	75
0	2	0	6	1	3	3	29	3	1	2	120
0	2	1	9	2	0	0	9	3	1	3	160
0	2	2	12	2	0	1	14	3	2	0	93
0	2	3	6	2	0	2	20	3	2	1	150
0	3	0	9	2	0	3	26	3	2	2	210
0	3	1	13	2	1	0	15	3	2	3	290
0	3	2	16	2	1	1	20	3	3	0	240
0	3	3	19	2	1	2	27	3	3	1	460
1	0	0	4	2	1	3	34	3	3	2	1100
1	0	1	7	2	2	0	21	3	3	3	1100+
1	0	2	11	2	2	1	28				
1	0	3	15	2	2	2	35				
1	1	0	7	2	2	3	42				
1	1	1	11	2	3	0	29				
1	1	2	15	2	3	1	26				
1	1	3	19	2	3	2	44				

From Jacobs & Gerstein's Handbook of Microbiology, Copyright 1960, D. Van Nostrand Company, Inc., Princeton, N. J.

Experiment No. 5. Effect of diet on total and cellulolytic rumen bacterial concentrations.

OBJECTIVES

1. Demonstrate procedures for reading MPN tubes and estimation of concentration from a three tube MPN table.
2. Determine total and cellulolytic rumen bacterial concentrations in rumen contents using ADS and MPN medium prepared in Expt. 4.

EXPERIMENTAL PROCEDURE

1. Obtain a sample of rumen contents from an available fistulated animal if possible, otherwise from a slaughter house. The sample of rumen contents can be taken at any time during the day; however, in most studies comparing the effect of various treatments or diets on rumen populations in animals fed once daily, rumen samples are taken just prior to feeding.
2. Dilute rumen contents in ADS as demonstrated in Expt. 4.
3. Set up a three tube MPN assay for dilutions 10^{-6}, 10^{-7}, 10^{-8}, 10^{-9}, 10^{-10}, 10^{-11} (Demonstrated in Expt. 4).

REFERENCES

Bryant, M. P. and I. M. Robinson. 1961. An improved nonselective culture medium for ruminal bacteria and its use in determining diurnal variation in numbers of bacteria in the rumen. *Journal of Dairy Science*, **44**, 1446-1456.

Caldwell, D. R. and M. P. Bryant. 1966. Medium without rumen fluid for nonselective enumeration and isolation of rumen bacteria. *Applied Microbiology*, **14**, 794-801.

Dehority, B. A. and J. A. Grubb. 1980. Effect of short-term chilling of rumen contents on viable bacterial numbers. *Applied and Environmental Microbiology*, **39**, 376-381.

Grubb, J. A. and B. A. Dehority. 1975. Effects of an abrupt change in ration from all roughage to high concentrate upon rumen microbial numbers in sheep. *Applied Microbiology*, **30**, 404-412.

Mackie, R. I., F.M.C. Gilchrist, A. M. Robberts, P. E. Hannah and H. M. Schwartz. 1978. Microbiological and chemical changes in the rumen during the stepwise adaptation of sheep to high concentrate diets. *Journal of Agricultural Science, Cambridge*, **90**, 241-254.

Maki, L. R. and E. M. Foster. 1957. Effect of roughage in the bovine ration on types of bacteria in the rumen. *Journal of Dairy Science*, **40**, 905-913.

358 Rumen microbiology

Experiment No. 6. Enumeration and isolation of rumen bacteria with solid media.

OBJECTIVES

1. To observe the laboratory procedures involved in the anaerobic preparation of slant and roll tube media.
2. To observe the procedures for inoculating and preparing roll tubes.
3. Demonstrate techniques used for the transfer of pure cultures, viewing of live mounts with phase microscopy and preparation of Gram-stained smears.
4. Preparation of rumen fluid-glucose-cellobiose-agar (RGCA) slants.

EXPERIMENTAL PROCEDURES

MEDIA

Directions for preparing rumen fluid-glucose-cellobiose-agar (RGCA) slants are as follows for a 300 ml batch:

- 45.0 ml Mineral Solution I*
- 45.0 ml Mineral Solution II*
- 0.3 ml of 0.1% Resazurin solution
- 0.45 g of Glucose
- 0.45 g of Cellobiose
- 4.5 g of Agar
- 75.0 ml of Distilled water
- 120.0 ml of Rumen fluid (Supernatant obtained from centrifugation at 1000 x g for 10 minutes).

*See Expt. 4 for composition.

NOTE: - for roll tube medium, agar concentration is increased to 2% (6.0 g) and 0.15 g of soluble starch is added (RGCSA roll tubes).

The medium is gassed with O_2 free CO_2 and brought almost to boiling with a Bunsen burner. It is then sealed anaerobically, the stopper wired in place and autoclaved for 5 min at 121°C. The flask is then placed in a water bath at about 45°C, opened anaerobically under CO_2 and the following added:

- 10.0 ml of 12% Na_2CO_3
- 5.0 ml of 3% cysteine - HCl

Continue gassing for about 10 min and check pH with meter. When pH of the medium falls below 7, it is tubed anaerobically under CO_2 into 16 x 150 mm culture tubes in approximately 7.0 ml aliquots. The tubes are then autoclaved in racks for 20 minutes at 15 lb pressure (121°C). Remove racks and tilt slants while the medium is still liquid and allow to solidify in that position.

NOTE: - for roll tubes, 18 x 150 mm culture tubes are used and 4.0 ml aliquots are added to each tube.

INOCULATION OF ROLL TUBES

1. Add 180 ml of reduced anaerobic dilution solution (ADS) to a previously steamed Waring blender container, under a strong stream of CO_2.
2. Weigh out 20 g of rumen ingesta into a previously steamed beaker, and then add to blender container.
3. Blend vigorously for two minutes, directing the stream of CO_2 into the vortex during that period.
4. With a wide-mouth pipette, transfer 1.0 ml to a tube containing 9.0 ml of reduced ADS. Continue dilutions using 9.0 ml ADS tubes. Each dilution tube should be shaken 30 times before subsampling.
5. Eight 18 x 150 mm tubes, each containing 4.0 ml RGCSA medium, will be inoculated with one ml of the 1×10^{-7}, 1×10^{-8} and 1×10^{-9} dilutions, for a total of 24 tubes. The agar medium in these tubes will be melted before starting, and held in a 45°C water bath until inoculated.
6. After inoculation, tubes are rolled in cold water so that a thin agar film is well-distributed over the entire inner surface.
7. After incubation at 38°C for 7 days, four tubes at each dilution will be used for isolating pure cultures and the remaining four roll tubes will be used to count baterial numbers.

TRANSFER OF PURE CULTURES AND MICROSCOPIC OBSERVATION

1. Procedures used for transferring pure cultures from laboratory stock culture collection will be demonstrated.
2. Phase microscopic observation of bacteria:
    a. With a sterile loop, transfer a loop-full of the water of syneresis from an 18-20 hour RGCA slant into a drop of distilled water on a microscope slide.
    b. Cover with a glass cover slip and examine under the phase microscope.
3. Gram Stain:
    a. With a sterile loop, transfer a loop-full of the water of syneresis from

an 18-20 hour RGCA slant to a slide and spread. Allow to air-dry, then briefly heat fix.
b. Stain for 1 min with crystal violet, wash in tap water.
c. Apply Lugol's iodine solution for 1 min, wash in tap water.
d. Decolorize in 95% ethyl alcohol for 30 seconds.
e. Counterstain with safranin for 15 seconds, wash and dry with heat.
f. Examine slide microscopically under oil-immersion objective.

REFERENCES

Bryant, M. P. and L. A. Burkey. 1953. Cultural methods and some characteristics of some of the more numerous groups of bacteria in the bovine rumen. *Journal of Dairy Science*, **36**, 205-217.

Dehority, B. A. 1966. Characterization of several bovine rumen bacteria isolated with a xylan medium. *Journal of Bacteriology*, **91**, 1724-1729.

Dehority, B. A. 1969. Pectin-fermenting bacteria isolated from the bovine rumen. *Journal of Bacteriology*, **99**, 189-196.

Hungate, R. E. 1950. The anaerobic mesophilic cellulolytic rumen bacteria. *Bacteriological Reviews*, **14**, 1-49.

Experiment No. 7. Counting roll tubes and isolation of pure cultures of rumen bacteria.

OBJECTIVES

1. Demonstrate counting colonies in roll tubes.
2. Isolation of bacteria from single colonies in a roll tube and inoculation into RGCA slants.
3. Provide each student with two or three inoculated slants.

EXPERIMENTAL PROCEDURE

1. Four to seven days after inoculation of the roll tubes, 2 or 3 colonies will be picked for each student. That is, the colony will be picked with a needle and stab-inoculated into an RGCA slant. Each student will incubate the slant tubes and after several daily transfers, observe them under the phase scope and do a Gram stain.
2. A demonstration of counting bacterial colonies in the roll tubes will be given, preferably after 7 days incubation or 14 days if cellulose is the only substrate.
3. Each student will be expected to describe their bacterial isolates, i.e., visual estimation of purity, motility, shape, Gram stain and cell measurements.

REFERENCES

Bryant, M. P. and L. A. Burkey. 1953. Cultural methods and some characteristics of some of the more numerous groups of bacteria in the bovine rumen. *Journal of Dairy Science*, **36,** 205-217.

Hungate, R. E. 1966. *The Rumen and Its Microbes.* Academic Press. New York, N.Y.

Stewart, C.S. and M. P. Bryant. 1988. The rumen bacteria. In: *The Rumen Microbial Ecosystem* (P. N. Hobson, ed.) pp 21-75. Elsevier Science Publishers Ltd. London, England.

Experiment No. 8. Enumeration of rumen fungi.

OBJECTIVES

1. Prepare MPN medium for counting rumen fungi.
2. Compare rumen fungal concentrations between sheep fed an all roughage and high concentrate diet.

EXPERIMENTAL PROCEDURES

1. Prepare the following fungal MPN medium:

   300 ml

   - 45.0 ml Mineral solution I*
   - 45.0 ml Mineral solution II*
   - 0.3 ml of 0.1% Resazurin solution
   - 0.3 ml of 0.1% Hemin solution
   - 0.3 g Glucose
   - 0.3 g Cellobiose
   - 0.3 g Maltose
   - 0.3 g Xylose
   - 0.6 g Trypticase
   - 0.15 g Yeast extract
   - 1.35 ml VFA mixture
   - 75.0 ml 3% cellulose suspension
   - 60.0 ml of Rumen Fluid (Supernatant from centrifugation at 1000 x g for 10 min)
   - 15.0 ml of distilled H_2O

   *See Expt. 4 for composition.

   Gas with CO_2 and heat carefully over burner. When medium is fairly well reduced, add:
   10.0 ml of 12% Na_2CO_3

   Continue gassing for about 20 min, then add:
   5.0 ml of 3% cysteine-HCl

   Gas for an additional 10-15 min and check pH. If pH is outside the range of 6.6 to 6.9, adjust as required with NaOH or H_3PO_4. Total volume is 257 ml. This is a reduction of 14.3% of total volume. Tube anaerobically in 6.0 ml aliquots into 16 x 150 mm tubes. Autoclave in tubes at 15# for 20 min.

Just prior to use, 1.0 ml of antibiotic solution is added to each tube. The 1.0 ml is $1.0/7.0 \times 100 = 14.3\%$.

Antibiotic solution:

The final concentrations of antibiotics in the medium should be:
   2000 U penicillin and 130 U streptomycin per ml. Thus the antibiotic solution must contain 14,000 U of penicillin and 910 U of streptomycin per ml.

Approximate concentrations of commercial antibiotics are:
   Penicillin = 1600 U per mg.
   Streptomycin = 763 U per mg.

Need to check label before making up your antibiotic solution.

2. Prior to the morning feeding, obtain samples of rumen contents from two animals, one fed all roughage and the other high concentrate.
3. Using the same procedure for dilution of rumen contents as described in Expt. 4, dilute out 10^{-7} and inoculate three MPN tubes with each dilution from 10^{-2} up to 10^{-7}.
4. After 14 days, determine growth by visible loss of cellulose and decrease in pH, and use MPN table given in Expt. 4 to estimate total and cellulolytic fungal concentrations.
5. Using a loop, place some of the cellulose remaining in a positive tube on a glass slide with a coverslip and observe the fungal rhizoid and sporangia under the microscope.

REFERENCE

Obispo, N. E. and B. A. Dehority. 1992. A most probable number method for enumeration of rumen fungi with studies on factors affecting their concentration in the rumen. *Journal of Microbiological Methods*, **16**, 259-270.

INDEX

Abomasum, 21
Abrupt ration change, 275, 277
Acetitomaculum ruminis, 257
Acetogenic bacteria, 256
    distribution, 257
Adenosine triphosphate (ATP), 325
Aerobic microorganisms, 34
Alpaca, 10
Aminoethylphosphonic acid (AEP), 325
Amylase
    in rumen bacteria, 248
Anaerobic glove box, 278
Anaerobic lactobacilli, 253
Anaeromyces
    A. elegans, 297
    A. mucronatus, 297
Anaerovibrio, lipolytica, 327
Anoplodinium, 47
Antimicrobials, 279
Arabans, 210
Artificial saliva, 169
Ass, 6

B vitamins, 329
Bacillus, 258
Bacteria
    antagonism between species, 333
    attached to rumen epithelium, 284
        composition, 284-286
        concentration, 285-287
    authentic species, 177
    species composition, 272
    epimural, 285
    exogenous in the rumen, 259
    distribution, 287
    history, 157
    in vitro cultivation
        pure cultures, 157-159.
        mixed cultures, 157
    in vivo-in vitro methods, 157, 158
        vivar technique, 158
        in situ or synthetic fiber bags, 158
    hemicellulose fermenting species, 210
    hemicellulolytic enzymes, 224

    isolation
        anaerobic glove box, 159
        habitat-simulating medium, 160
        roll tubes, 159
    pectin fermenting species, 29
    starch digesters, 243
    strain designation, 177
    vitamin requirements, 330-331
    washed suspensions, 157
Bacterial cells
    attached to feed, 26
    extracellular glycoprotein coat, 283
    free and attached, 279
    location in rumen (compartments), 168
Bacterial concentrations
    culture or viable counts, 269
        comparison to direct counts, 269
    differential counts
        amylolytic bacteria, 277
        carbohydrate utilizers, 278
        cellulolytic bacteria, 279
        lactate utilizers, 277
        starch, xylan and pectin utilizers, 276
        xylanolytic bacteria, 279

    direct counts, 266
    effect of antibiotics, 279
    incubation time, 270
    inhibition, 333
    factors affecting the concentration
        effect of diet, 274
        frequency of feeding, 273
        level of feeding, 274
        position sampled, 275
    hay particle size, long versus ground or
        pelleted, 276
    in fluid fraction, 265
    in particulate fraction, 265
    MPN procedure, 272
    plating techniques, 278
    sampling site, 272
Bacterial interactions, 332
Bacterial media
    factors effecting counts, 271
    habitat simulating (RGCA), 270
    medium 10, 270
    medium 98-5, 270

365

366 Rumen microbiology

medium RGCSA, 271
selective medium, 272
Bacterial subpopulations
   attached to feed particles, 280
      dislodging, 283
      effect of storage at zero degrees C, 281
      effect of surfactants, 282
      quantitation with ^{15}N, 282
   attached to rumen epithelium, 280
   free in fluid, 280-281
Bacteriocins, 200
Bacteroides amylophilis, 201, 245
Bacteroides ruminicola, 211
Bacteroides succinogenes, 178
Biohydrogenation, 327
   bacterial species involved, 328
Biological value of microbial protein, 321
Birds, 4
Bison, 78
Blepharoconus krugerensis, 52, 138, 140
Blepharocorythidae, 44, 48, 52
Blepharoprosthium parvum, 52
Borrelia, 250
Bos indicus, 130
Bos taurus, 130
Buetschlia
   B. parva, 51
   B triciliata, 52
   diurnal variation, 92
Buetschliidae, 44, 48, 51, 52
Butyrivibrio alactacidigens, 254
Butyrivibrio fibrosolvens, 178, 210, 229, 329
   cellulose digestion from forages, 197, 239
   description, 183
   gram stain, 184
   lipid hydrolysis and biohydrogenation, 327-328
   plasmids, 185
   proteolytic activity, 254
      free or cellular, 255
   serological analysis, 184
   strain relatedness, 184

Caecomyces
   C. communis, 296
   C. equi, 296
Caribou, 137
Caloscolex, 44, 62, 135
Camel, 10
   bactrian, 135
   dromedary, 135
Capybara, 6, 7, 138
Cecum fermentors, 6
Cecum-colon fermentors, 6
Cellodextrins, 332
Celloxylanase, 225
Cellulolytic species, 178
   adhesion to and detachment from cellulose, 192
   cocultures, 199, 201
   DNA hybridization, 201
   guanine plus cytosine (G+C) base content, 201
   in cecum of guinea pig, horse, rabbit, sheep 288
   in feces of human, rabbit and horse, 288
   mechanisms of adhesion, 195
   mineral requirements, 189
   minor rumen species, 186
   16S rRNA sequences, 201
   stomach of Langur monkey, 288
   sugar composition of extracellular polysaccharides (EPS), 201
   unknown nutrient requirements, 189
   vitamin requirements, 188
   volatile fatty acid requirements (VFA), 187, 188
Cellulose, 1
   solubility in cupriethylene diamine, 162
   relationship to hemicellulose, 209
Cellulose digestion
   cross feeding, 200
   effects of forage maturity, 197
   effects of soluble carbohydrates, 190
   from intact forages, 196-198
   inhibition between cellulolytic species, 199
   purified cellulose, 196, 197
   synergism, 199
Charonina
   C. equi, 52
   C, nuda, 52
   C. ventriculi, 52
   diurnal variation, 92
Chemical reactor, 1
Chemotaxis, 102
Chevrotain forestomach, 12
Chickens, 5
   cecal bacteria, 288
Chitin, 295, 324
Chitin synthase, 324
Chloramphenicol, 300
CLA (conjugated linoleic acids), 328
Clostridium, 178
   C. chartatabidum, 186
   cellulolytic species, 186
   spore-former, 186
Clostridium longisporum
   forage digestion, 198
Cockroach, 4
Coenzyme M, 253
Colon fermentors, 6
Conjugation, 43
Coprophagy, 8
Corynebacterium, 284

Cross feeding, 332
Cycohexamide, 308
Cycloposthidae, 62

D-Alanine, 325
Dall sheep, 137, 140
Dasytricha
    cultivation, 112
    fermentation products, 102
    morphology, 49,51
Dasytricha hukuokaensis, 51
Dasytricha kabanii, 51
Dasytricha ruminantium, 51
    requirement for bacteria, 110
    separating from rumen contents, 102
    substrates fermented, 102, 104
Deer
    Ezo, 135
    Fallow, 137
    Red, 137
    white-tailed, 134
Defaunation
    by isolation, 143
    with DSS, 142
Detrition, 25
Diaminopimelic acid, 168
    as internal marker, 325
    in *S. bovis*, 244
Digestion
    rumen, 25
Dinosaurs, 141
Dioctyl sodium sulfosuccinate (DSS), 142
Diplodiniinae
    ciliary zones, 54, 56
    classification, 44-47
    genera, 45,46 57-59
    metabolism, 106
    morphology, 58
    skeletal plates, 57
Diplodinium, 57
Diploplastron, 47
Ducks, 5

Elephant, 6, 140
Elk, 137
Elytroplastron, 47, 59, 130
Emu gastrointestinal tract, 4
Endopolygalacuronate lyase, 235
Enoploplastron, 47, 58
Entodiniinae, 44, 47,54
Entodiniomorphs
    cultivation, 113
Entodinium
    caudal spination, 55
    E. longinucleatum, 55
    metabolism, 105
    morphology, 54, 55

Entodinium alces, 133, 140
Entodinium anteronucleatum, 133
Entodinium bursa, 113
Entodinium caudatum, 105, 112, 113, 116, 120
Entodinium dalli, 140
Entodinium dubardi, 143
Entodinium exiguum, 106, 112, 120
Entodinium ovibos, 134
Entodinium quadricuspis, 133
Entodinium spinonucleatum, 134
Eodinium, 47
Epidinium, 44, 59, 61,130
Epidinium caudatum, 108, 115, 120
Epidinium ecaudatum, 107
Epiplastron, 44, 59, 138
Eremoplastron, 47
Escherichia coli, 258
Esophageal groove, 11, 20
Eubacterium cellulosolvens
    description, 185
    formerly *Cillobacterium cellulosolvens*, 185
    pectin digestion, 231
Eubacterium ruminantium, 211
    description, *213, 250*
Eubacterium limosum, 233
Eubacterium uniforme, 212, 213
Eubacterium xylanophilum, 212, 213
Eudiplodinium, 47, 58
Eudiplodinium bubalus, 134
Eudiplodinium maggii, 107
Eudiplodinium medium, 107
Eukaryote, 326

Factors controlling rumen passage
    feed intake, 26
    physical form, 26
    particle specific gravity, 26
Facultative anaerobes, 257
Fibrobacter intestinalis, 178
Fibrobacter succinogenes, 166, 178,192, 229
    adhesion to particulate matter, 283
    carbohydrates fermented and end
        products, 180
    cellulase enzymes, 181, 194
    cellulose digestion, 190
    forage cellulose digestion, 197, 239
    physiological characteristics, 179
Fish, 4
Fistula, 22
Fistulation procedure, 22
Flagellate protozoa
    occurrence, 3, 43, 73
    morphology, 66, 67
    mistaken identification, 295
    rumen species, 66
Fluid turnover time, 115

Forages
    structural carbohydrate composition, 209
Forage evaluation, 164
Foregut fermentation, 8
Forestomach
    sacciform, 10
    tubiform, 10
Functional specific gravity, 26, 27
Fungal fermentation
    catabolite repression, 302
    forages, 304, 308
    grains, 305
    purified structural carbohydrates, 302
    soluble carbohydrates, 302
Fungal inhibition
    by rumen bacteria, 309
    by normal end products, 307
    by pure cultures of cellulolytic bacteria, 306-307
Fungal synergism
    effect on cellulose and xylan digestion, 306
    with methanogens, 305
Fungal zoospores, 43, 295
    chemotaxis, 296, 298
    encystment, 298
    germination, 298
Fungi
    characteristics, 298
    classification, 297
    concentrations, 300, 310
        in different sections of GI tract, 311
    effect of concentrates, 300
    effect of frequency of feeding, 300
    enumeration
        MPN procedures, 300
        roll tubes, 300
    enzymes
        polysaccharide degrading, 303
        proteolytic, 303
    genera and species, 296
    haem-containing compounds, 298
    in saliva, 311
    interactions, 334
    isolation methods, 300
    isolated from various herbivores, 296
    life cycle, 298, 312
    nutritional requirements, 301
    occurrence in various animal species, 311
    optimum growth conditions, 301
    physical disruption of plant cells, 309
    rhizoids, 297
        anucleate, 297
        nucleated, 297
    sporangia, 297
    thallus, 298
    thallus types, 297
        endogenous, 297
        exogenous, 297
        monocentric, 297
        polycentric, 297
    vitamin requirements, 330
Fusobacterium, 284
Fusobacterium polysaccharolyticum, 186

Galactans, 210
Geese, 4,5
Giraffe, 137
Glutamate dehydrogenase, 248
Glutamine synthetase, 248
Grouse, 5
Guanaco, 10
Guinea pig, 6,7,182

Hamster rat, 8
Hemicellulose, 1, 163
    comparison between digestion of isolated and intact, 222
    composition, 209, 211
    degradation, 215, 226
    differences between forages, 222
    digestion from intact forages, 219
    digestion of isolated hemicellulose
        by cellulolytic species, 214-218
        by hemicellulolytic species, 217-219
        rate and extent, 216
        sequential addition of cultures, 223
    determination in plants, 209
    ethanol soluble and insoluble, 215
    relationship to cellulose, 209
    solubilization, 226
    synergism, 220-221, 223
    utilization, 215, 226
Hemicellulolytic enzymes, 224
Herbivore, 1
Hindgut fermentation, 1
    bacteria, 4,5, 7,9
    protozoa, 3,7,9
Hippopotamus forestomach, 8, 9
Hoatzin, 4
Holotrich protozoa
    chemotaxis, 87-92
    effects of feed restriction, 93
    effect of osmolality, 93
    establishment in rumen, 93
    growth cycles, 86
    sequestration and migration, 87-92
Horse hindgut, 6
Hungate technique, 258
Hydrogenosomes, 103

Ingestion and rumination of feed, 22
Inhibition
    among bacteria, 333
Insect digestive tract, 3

in vitro fermentation, 160
  accumulation of end products, 166
  cellulose digestion from forages, 161
  closed system, 158, 166
  continuous culture system, 158, 168
  effect of maturity and lignification, 161, 163
  effect of particle size, 161
  fermentation capacity, 167, 168
  hemicellulose and pectin digestion from forages, 163
  inoculum, 161, 166, 282
  limitations, 171
  rumen simulation technique (Rusitec), 168
  validity, 165
in vivo fermentation, 239
  interactions, 239
Isobutyric acid, 187
Isovaleric acid, 187
Isotrichidae, 44, 48, 49
Isotricha
  fermentation products, 101
  morphology, 49, 50
  I. jalaludinii, 50
  I. intestinalis, 50
  I. prostoma, 50
  separating from rumen contents, 103
  substrates fermented, 101, 104

Kangaroo, 10, 138

Lachnospira multiparus, 222-223, 229, 239
  description, 233
  pectinolytic enzymes, 234
Lactobacillus, 258, 284
Lactobacillus lactis, 254
Lactobacillus ruminis, 254
Lactobacillus vitulinus, 254
Langur monkey, 288
Lignin, 210
Linoleic acid, 328
Linolenic acid, 328
Lipid metabolism, 327
  biohydrogenation, 327
  hydrolysis, 327
Llama, 10
  stomach anatomy, 11

Mammals, 6
Marsupials, 10
Mastication, 25
Maturity of forage
  effect on cellulose digestion, 197
  effect on hemicellulose digestion, 220
Megasphaera elsdenii, 329
  description, 252
  occurrence in humans and pigs, 252, 288

Metadinium, 47, 58
Methanobacterium ruminantium, 252
Methanobacterium formicicum, 253
Methanobrevibacter ruminantium
  description, 253
  in human feces, 288
  in Langur monkey, 288
  methane production, 252
Methanogenic bacteria, 252
Methanomicrobium mobile, 253
Methanosarcina barkeri, 253
2-Methylbutyric acid, 187
Methylcellulose, 194
Microaerophile, 35
Microbial interactions, 330, 333, 335
Microbial lipids, 329
Microbial markers
  external, 324
  ideal criteria, 322
  internal, 324
  purines, 324
Microbial protein
  bacteria, 321
    amino acid composition of pure cultures, 322
  effect of diet, 322
  fungi, 321
  nitrogen content, 323
  passage to hindgut, 322, 323
  protozoa, 321
  true digestibility, 321
Microcetus lappus, 92
Micrococcus, 284
Minimum pH
  cellulolytic bacteria, 30
  protozoa, 121
Monensin, 279
Mongolian gazelle, 135
Monkeys
  family Cercopithecidae, 7
  family Colobinae, 7, 8
Moose, 133, 137, 140
Most probable number assay, 272
Mouse deer, 12
Multi-chambered stomachs, 8
Mutualism, 147

^{15}N, 326
1,4-naphthoquinone, 250
Neocallimastix
  N. frontalis, 296
  N. hurleyensis, 296
  N. patriciarum, 296
  N. variablis, 296
Net protein utilization, 321
Nucleic acids, 325

370 Rumen microbiology

Obligate anaerobe, 34
Oligonucleotide probes, 326
Oligoisotricha bubali, 49, 51, 130
Omasum, 20, 142
Opisthotrichum, 44, 60, 61, 138
Ophryoscolecidae
    orientation, 53
    subfamilies, 54
Ophryoscolecinae
    ciliary zones, 54
    classification, 45-47
    genera, 59
    skeletal plates, 60
Ophryoscolex, 44, 60, 61, 108
    geographic distribution, 129
Ophryoscolex purkynjei, 108, 120
Orpinomyces
    O. bovis, 296
    O. intercalaris, 297
    O. joyonii, 296
Ostracodinium, 47, 58
Ostracodinium tiete, 134
Ostrich gastrointestinal tract, 4
Oxygen toxicity, 34
Oxytetracycline, 300

^{32}P, 326
PABA (*p*-Aminobenzoic acid), 188
Pangaea, 141
Parabundleia ruminantium, 52
Paraisotricha, 52
Paraisotrichidae, 44, 52
Parentodinium africanum, 62, 63, 138, 140
Passage of feed from the rumen, 23
PCR (polymerase chain reaction), 326
Pectin, 1,163, 209
    bonds in grass and legume, 238
    composition, 229
    concentration in forages, 229
    degradation, 235
    digestion by rumen bacteria, 231
        coculture with cellulolytic or
            hemicellulolytic, 238
    enzymes involved in digestion
        depolymerases, 234
        pectinesterases, 234
    fermentation of isolated pectin, 235
    method of determination, 229
    synergism in digestion, 237
    utilization, 235
Peccary forestomach, 8,9
Pectinophilic bacteria, 232
Penicillin, 308
Peptostreptococcus elsdenii, 252
Peptostreptococcus sp., 232, 239
    description, 234
Phospholipids, 329

Pig stomach, 9
Pingus minutus, 52
Piromonas, 296
Piromyces
    P. citronii, 296
    P. communis, 296
    P. dumbonica, 296
    P. mae, 296
    P. minutus, 296
    P. rhizinflata, 296
    P. spiralis, 296
Polymorphella bovis, 52
Polyplastron, 47, 59
Polyplastron multivesiculatum, 106, 107, 114
    geographic distribution, 129
Preruminants, 12
Prevotella ruminicola, 193, 229
    description, 212
    in hemicellulose digestion, 211, 239
    genotypes, 213
    hemin requirement, 212
    nitrogen sources, 213
    pectinolytic enzymes, 234
    proteolytic activity, 254
    subspecies *brevis*, 212
    subspecies, *ruminicola*, 212
    VFA requirement, 213
Prokaryote, 326
Propionibacterium, 258, 284
Proteolytic bacteria, 254
    in New Zealand cows, 256
Protozoa, ciliate
    antagonism between species, 93
    cannibalism, 94
    cellulolytic activity, 108
    ciliary zones, 44, 47
    classification, 43
    cytoalimentary system, 64
    defaunation, 142
    dividing cells, 78
    effects of absence, 143-146
    effect of pH on growth, 120
    essentialness, 143
    establishment in rumen, 74
    fauna composition
        effect of diet, 131
        rangifer-type, 137
    faunation, 73
    generation time, 115
    geographic distribution, 129
        similarity among locations, 130, 134
    growth cycles, 86
    in omasum, 142
    lysis, 141
    origination of species, 140
    oxygen tolerance, 103
    phylogeny, 63

passage, 141
population types, 93, 94
predation, 94, 334
  bacteria and fungi, 334
requirement for bacteria, 110
role, 141, 145
specificity
  host, 136, 137
  protozoan, 136, 139
total numbers in rumen, 75, 76, 85
turnover in rumen, 75, 141
ultrastructure, 62
vitamin requirements, 330
Protozoal concentrations
  after starvation, 82
  distribution among animal species, 132, 136
  diurnal variation, 83
  effect of diet, 75, 133
  effect of energy level, 77
  effect of feed level, 82
  frequency of feeding, 81
  in different geographical locations, 131, 132
  minimum pH, 121
  pH effects, 78
  physical form of feed, 82
  effect of volume, 76
  in rumen contents, 74, 75
  influence of other factors, 80
Pseudoruminants, 10
Purines, 325
Pyloric sphincter, 21

Quokka, 10

Rabbit hindgut, 6
Reindeer, 137, 183
Reptile, 4
Resistant sporangium, 311
Rhamnose, 210
Rhea gastrointestinal tract, 4
Rhinoceros, 6
Rifampin, 251
rRNA (ribosomal ribonucleic acid), 326
  analysis pitfalls, 326
Rumen environment
  buffering capacity, 30
  dry matter, 32, 36
  osmotic pressure, 31, 36
  oxidation-reduction potential, 33, 36
  pH, 28, 36
  rumen gases, 33
  surface tension, 33
  temperature, 27, 36
Rumen-reticulum anatomy, 19
Rumen volume
  Effect of diet and volume, 24
Rumination, 25

Ruminobacter amylophilis, 201
  description, 245
  proteolytic activity, 254
Ruminococcus
  biotypes, 183
  genus description, 181, 182,
  in cecal contents of guinea pig, 182
  in rumen of reindeer and musk-oxen, 183
Ruminococcus albus, 178
  forage cellulose digestion, 197, 239
  forage hemicellulose digestion, 212
  forage pectin digestion, 230
  phenylacetic acid (PAA) requirement, 189
  phenylpropanoic acid (PPA) requirement, 189
  species description, 182
Ruminococcus flavefaciens, 166, 178, 192
  adhesion to plant material, 283
  chain formation, 182
  forage cellulose digestion, 197, 239
  forage hemicellulose digestion, 212
  forage pectin digestion, 230
  type species, 181
Ruminococcus schinkii, 257
Ruminomyces, 296

^{35}S, 326
Sable antelope, 137
Salinomycin, 279
Saliva
  composition, 23, 30
  volume per day, 23
Salmonella, 258
Sampling procedures
  through a fistula, 266
  at slaughter, 266
  stomach tube, 266
Selective media, 272
Selenomonas ruminantium, 193
  description, 246
  proteolytic activity, 254
  selective medium for isolation, 247
  ureolytic activity, 247
  variety *bryanti*, 247
  variety *lactilyticas*, 247, 327
  VFA requirement, 247
Sequential addition of cultures, 223
Sheep hindgut, 6
Sphaeromonas, 296
Spirochetes, 235, 250-251
Sporangium, 298
Springbok, 137
Staphylcoccus, 284
Starch digestion
  relative activity of different species, 248
Stearic acid, 328
Streptococcus, 258, 284

Streptococcu bovis, 232, 243
    description, 244
    intracellular pH, 245
    pectinolytic enzymes, 234
    strain differences, 244
    vitamin requirements, 244
Streptomycin, 308
Strict anaerobe, 35
Stomach tube, 266
Succinimonas amylolytica
    description, 246
Succinivibrio dextrinosolvens, 229
    description, 249
    ureolytic activity, 249
    requirement for vitamin K-like compound, 250
Superoxide anion, 35
Symbiosis, 27
Synergism
    in hemicellulose digestion, 220-221
    among bacteria, 332

Tapir, 6
Teff hay, 219
Termite digestive tract, 3
Transmission electron microscopy, 236
Tree sloths, 8
Treponema, 250, 288

Treponema saccharophilum, 233
Treponemes, 232-233
    pectinolytic enzymes, 235
Turkey, 5
Turnover times
    liquid, 23,25
    solids, 23-25

Vaccenic acid, 328
Valeric acid, 187
Veillonella alcalescens, 288
    description, 251
Vitamin B_{12}, 188, 329
Vitamin K, 329
Vitamin synthesis, 329
    concentration in rumen, 330
Vicuña, 10

Wallaby, 10
Warthog, 6
Wild ruminants, sampling, 266

Xylanase, 212
Xylobiase, 212

Zebra, 6